Fractures of the Distal Radius

Springer

New York
Berlin
Heidelberg
Barcelona
Budapest
Hong Kong
London
Milan
Paris
Santa Clara
Singapore
Tokyo

Diego L. Fernandez, M.D.

Orthopaedische Chirurgie FMH

Jesse B. Jupiter, M.D.

Associate Professor, Orthopaedic Surgery
Harvard Medical School, and
Director, Orthopaedic Hand Service
Massachusetts General Hospital

Fractures of the Distal Radius

A Practical Approach to Management

With 371 illustrations in 698 parts

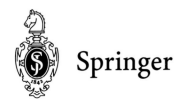
Springer

Diego L. Fernandez
Orthopaedische Chirurgie FMH
Mittelstr. 54
3012 Bern, Switzerland

Jesse B. Jupiter
Director, Orthopaedic Hand Service
Massachusetts General Hospital
ACC 527, 15 Parkman Street
Boston, MD 02114 USA

Library of Congress Cataloging-in-Publication Data
Jupiter, Jesse B.
    Fractures of the distal radius / Jesse B. Jupiter, Diego L. Fernandez.
      p. cm.
    Includes bibliographical references and index.
    ISBN 0-387-94239-4. – ISBN 3-540-94239-4
    1. Radius – Fractures. I. Fernandez, Diego L. II. Title.
    [DNLM: WE 820 J95f 1995]
    RD557.J68 1995
    617.1'57 – dc20
    DNLM/DLC
    for Library of Congress   94-45533

Printed on acid-free paper

Production managed by Karen Phillips; manufacturing supervised by Rhea Talbert.
Typeset by Best-set Typesetter Ltd., Hong Kong.
Printed and bound by Maple-Vail Book Manufacturing Group, York, PA.
Printed in the United States of America.

9 8 7 6 5 4 3 2 1

ISBN 0-387-94239-4 Springer-Verlag New York Berlin Heidelberg
ISBN 3-540-94239-4 Springer-Verlag Berlin Heidelberg New York

Dedicated to our Fathers

Leoncio Diego Fernandez, M.D.
Samuel Jacob Jupiter

"There is a dead medical literature and there is a live one. The dead is not all ancient and the live is not all modern."

Oliver Wendell Holmes

Foreword

by Henry J. Mankin

At first glance at this volume, it is easy to ask "why so much about so little?" After all the distal radius is only a small part of the body and its fractures, although common, are really not exactly a life- or limb-threatening issue. Admittedly it is a fracture that we often do not deal with well, but is that really worth an entire volume? How wrong one would be with that attitude! How truly inappropriate is such a view of this truly spectacular and well-written compendium of important technology and information!

Fractures of the Distal Radius is truly a remarkable effort and one that by all standards offers the reader a practical guide to the diagnosis and management of distal radius fractures and their sequellae. Each of the management chapters provide the reader with methods of identifying the injury, techniques of anesthesia, reduction, fixation, immobilization, aftercare, potential complications and their management and expected and achieved outcomes. All types of injuries are detailed, and all methods of treatment including closed techniques are described. This it would seem would be sufficient for a book about an injury, especially one as frequently encountered and as seemingly prosaic as fractures of the radius. As important as that goal is, however, it is not alone the purpose, nor in this essayist's opinion, the principal achievement of this remarkable volume.

The book has been written by two outstanding surgeons who not only describe the lesions and the best treatment on the basis of their own experience, but in addition provide the readers with a broad panoply of methodology for the management of the injuries based not just on what is successful in their own hands, but on a careful assessement of an extraordinarily voluminous body of literature. No stone lies unturned by Drs. Fernandez and Jupiter in providing the reader with every recorded classification system and their strengths, weaknesses and difficulties of application. At the same time they offer as their choice the new Fernandez approach which to this reader seems to make sense out of potential chaos and confusion. This alone is perhaps worth the price of the volume and is a truly valuable contribution.

Of perhaps greater interest to some of us is the evident fact that the authors display for this day and age, a rather astounding reverence for history. The first chapter clearly demonstrates this point and despite its lack of direct application to management of the injured patient (which after all is what the book is about) is for some of us, the most edifying and entertaining section. It describes in remarkably clear fashion the extraordinary, centuries-old struggle since the time of ancient Greece to define and describe this very common injury. Faced with the complex anatomy of the wrist, lack of anatomical specimens of the fractures (very few autopsies were done then or even now for injuries about the wrist), and of course the absence of imaging studies, the ancients were appropriately puzzled by the injury and the ensuing deformities. Fractures and dislocations were confused with one another and the putative site of injury (as in the eponymically immortalized Abraham Colles' case) was often far from the place which we now know is the actual location of the fracture. It is amazingly evident that Smith, Barton, Colles, Dupuytren, Malgaigne, Goyrand, Petit, Cotton and the rest (including Velpeau... presumbably of shoulder immobilization fame, who gave the deformity the name of "talon de fourchette" or the "silver fork deformity") all described features of these often eponymously immortalized injuries prior to the first X-ray picture taken by Wilhelm Conrad Roentgen just about 100 years ago (and appropriately for this volume of his wife's hand and wrist!). The struggle for definition of the fact of these injuries is eloquently described by the authors, in many cases by direct quotes from thsee ancient sources and in fact, really paraphrases the development of modern medicine throughout the centuries. Seminal observations by ancient scholars using the tools of their day add a bit to knowledge. Others in the next generation, or even next century, build on these data with new observations until with modern technology and systems of study we come upon what passes for current-day "truth." This is true until another generation extends these observations and establishes yet another plateau of knowledge. This then is the way of learning about disease, and no more careful assessment of the role of such a process can be encountered than is found in the exposition of the diagnosis, classification, and management of fractures of the distal radius in this very book. We are indebted to the authors for this remarkable and stunning exposition of the history of what has been mistaken by many modern clinicians to be a straight-forward problem, but has been clearly shown by them to be a tangled and sometimes confusing web of fact and fancy surrounding a series of complex anatomical and functional problems.

Henry J. Mankin, M.D.
Chief of the Orthopedic Service
Massachusetts General Hospital;
Edith M. Ashley Professor of Orthopaedics
Harvard Medical School

Foreword

by Maurice E. Müller

This outstanding book on the fractures of the distal radius has been written by two surgeons famous for their expertise in this area. Diego Fernandez began to contribute to our knowledge in this area in the late 1970s in Berne where he was responsible for the surgical care of all wrist and hand injuries at the University Orthopaedic Department. It was during this time that he began to formulate the guidelines for the classification and treatment of fractures of the distal radius. During the years that followed, fractures of the distal radius were almost always among the subjects of his lectures given on the occasion of AO courses and Meetings of Hand Surgery Societies, in both North and South America. The many discussions held on these occasions with world authorities gave him the opportunity to broaden and mature his concepts. Publications on the classification and treatment of these injuries as well as on the treatment of complications of hand fracture followed. This brought him international acceptance and greatly accelerated his academic career in Switzerland. On this occasion he has collaborated with his close friend Jesse Jupiter who is equally world famous for his many contributions to the pathomechanics and treatment of fractures of the distal radius. Jesse Jupiter is the chief of the Upper Extremity Service at the Massachusett's General Hospital in Boston. In this position he is involved not only in clinical care of extremely difficult upper extremity problems, but also in related clinical and basic research. The close collaboration of the two experts has resulted in a book which is destined to become a milestone in the literary contributions of this subject.

The two authors discuss not only their own experience but make frequent references to English, European, and particularly to French literature. Unquestionably one of the main features of this book is the authors' extensive discussion of over 20 published classification systems of injuries to the distal radius and of the correlation between the diagnosis, the surgical treatment, and the prognosis. The authors point out that in metaphyseal fractures an appreciation of the mechanism of injury is usually enough to effect a successful closed treatment. The open treatment of fractures, on the other hand, places much greater demands on the surgeon. Here the authors have chosen the methodology of the Comprehensive Classification of Fractures (CCF)* in which the classified fractures are organized in a hierarchical system of triads, in an ascending order of severity of the prognosis, be it for the type (or family), group or subgroup. In order to give the injury full expression, they had in many instances to utilize as well the qualifications giving information on the associated lesion of the ulna and radio-ulnar joint. The authors evaluated the classification as being easily reproducible and reliable. The detailed morphological categorization of the fractures made it possible to establish an exact

*Müller M.E., Nazarian S., Koch P., Schatzker J.: *The Comprehensive Classification of Fractures of Long Bones*, Springer-Verlag Heidelberg-New York, 1990.

diagnosis and clear guidelines to treatment correlated with the prognosis of the outcome. In evaluating the CCF, the authors found that although the system of classification was designed for all fractures of the long bones, it gave them the best practical guide to the selection of either closed or open treatment of fractures of the distal radius.

I recommend this book very strongly to all those concerned with the care of fractures of the distal radius. The text contains well over 400 illustrations which clearly describe the authors' concepts and make it easy for the reader to master most of the recommended procedures. The book appeals to the expert in this area because the authors describe many very specialized procedures including the arthroscopically aided reduction and fixation of the difficult C2 and C3 fractures. It will also serve well as a reference book because of its scope and superb bibliography.

Maurice E. Müller, M.D.
Berne, 1st of July 1995

Preface

by Jesse B. Jupiter

In 1980, while traveling in Switzerland as an AO Fellow, I first met Diego Fernandez. I was quite struck by his knowledge and experience but probably most impressed by the fact that he was developing sufficient experience to contemplate a text on the management of fractures of the distal radius. Up to that point I was under the impression that this was a relatively solved problem.

Influenced by his insight and experience, I began on my own to critically assess this problem and develop my own experience and understanding of the complexities inherent in this particular injury pattern.

Spurned on by our mutual interest and keen friendship, Diego posed the possibility of this collaborative effort which I immediately adopted with great enthusiasm.

The search through the literature was enlightening, not only in providing a great understanding of this particular injury but also in revealing much of the evolution of our specialty. As with all such efforts, one must pay tribute to the investigators in the distant and immediate past. In my own case, I was greatly influenced by people such as Martin Allgöwer, Thomas Rüedi, Richard Smith, and Harold Kleinert in their encouragement in my own development to pursue subjects of interest and to provide me with the role models of physician-surgeon-scholar to emulate.

Contemporary colleagues and friends such as Hill Hastings, Uli Büchler, Jurg Brennwald, and Charles Melone have provided continuous stimulation and insight into the various aspects of this subject. The cross fertilization of their ideas and management tactics is amply reflected throughout this text.

A text such as this reflects an inordinate amount of support in its inception and completion. Much credit must be given to my transcriptionist, Michel Tresfort, who continued to keep things in place despite the numerous changes, editions and deletions.

While the amount of effort put forth to complete such a text must place certain demands on one's personal life, my wife, Beryl, and children, Stacy and Ben, were less impacted by this effort than many of my previous publications by virtue of the fact that I managed to write much of this early in the morning and late at night, as it truly was a "labor of love" that maintained my interest and enthusiasm despite the time of day or night.

But it is back to Diego Fernandez to whom I give the greatest acknowledgements, as the collaborative effort here, more than the production of a scholarly work, has cemented a long-lasting friendship.

Jesse B. Jupiter, M.D.
Boston Massachusetts
June 1995

Preface

by Diego L. Fernandez

Since the beginning of my orthopaedic career, having been exposed to hand surgery by Eduardo Zancolli in Buenos Aires and later as a staff member in Orthopaedic Surgery of the University of Berne, I became increasingly interested in the management of wrist trauma. The fracture of the distal radius, being one of the most frequent injuries of the human skeleton, attracted my attention early on due to its rich variety of anatomical forms, the complexity of intraarticular disruption, as well as associated injuries to adjacent soft tissues, carpal structures, and radioulnar ligaments. Further exposure to the management of early and late complications of distal radius fractures stimulated even more the search for an algorithm of treatment in order to optimize functional recovery. In 1977 Maurice Müller assigned to me the task of analyzing fractures of the distal radius and ulna for the preparation of his comprehensive *Fracture Classification of Long Bones*. This, daily clinical experience, together with the material gathered through the years, influenced the decision to write a book on the management of these common but not always easy fractures. However, this was not going to be an easy task since at that time I was running the trauma service at the Kantonspital in Aarau.

At this point in time, two very dear friends joined in to help me in the preparation of the manuscript. One of them, Richard Ghillani, revised and corrected the original chapters I had written during his stay in Switzerland, and finally he co-authored the chapter on radiocarpal fracture-dislocations. And then came Jesse Jupiter, who, with his overwhelming energy, interest, and dedication, gave the final thrust to the editing process along with the hard working staff of secretaries in Boston. The fact that Jesse had also accumulated clinical material and a rich experience on this subject made it even more challenging, since, during our discussions criticism and re-assessment of what was being written was updated constantly. In spite of the continual search for new techniques and modern methods of fixation, we decided on writing about the current, worldwide accepted procedures based on the analysis of our own results and those of other experts in this particular field. Newer techniques under current evaluation, such as special plate design, dynamic external fixation, and bone substitutes will in the near future provide the answer to whether or not better functional results with improved technology are still achievable.

I would first like to thank Jesse's magnificent effort and for his devoted friendship, then Richard Ghillani for his encouragement and kindness, and finally my secretary, Silvia Wüthrich, for her kind cooperation during the preparation of the manuscript. Lastly, a word of thanks to my teachers in orthopaedic surgery, my father, Eduardo Zancolli, and Maurice Müller who played a definitive role in my life, and without whose stimulation and guidance orthopaedic surgery would not be so much fun.

Diego L. Fernandez, M.D.
Berne, Switzerland

Contents

Chapter One

The Fracture of the Distal End of the Radius: An Historical Perspective

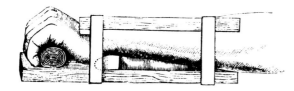

Many and excellent are the treatises which have appeared from time to time on the subjects of dislocation of the wrist, and fractures of the inferior surface of the radius... the abundance of theorizing has been productive of confusion worse confounded, but in many of the most valuable monographs, discrepancies are more apparent than real, and some sort of order is attainable from the seeming chaos.

T.K. Cruse, 1874

The history of the distal radius fracture is a fascinating one, for it intertwines historical precedent, the nobility of surgical tradition, and the inevitable conflict attendant to strong surgical personalities. Although it is inconceivable that this common injury was thought to be not a fracture but rather a carpal dislocation until the end of the eighteenth century, descriptions of what surely were fractures abound in the literature from the time of Hippocrates onward.[20] Yet, as pointed out by Cruse in 1874, failure to differentiate the two on clinical grounds was not so surprising as

The very peculiar and anomalous signs of Colles' fracture, the absence of crepitus and mobility, and the many points of difference on its symptomatology and morbid anatomy from what is usual in fractures are abundant reasons for a mistake so frequently made.[10]

The history of the distal radius fracture can best be viewed in three specific epochs, the first being that of recognition, the second that of definition, and the third that of therapeutic. As will become evident, much of the energy and enthusiasm of early investigators was directed as much at demonstrating the inadequacies of their contemporaries' viewpoints as to providing new insight into the understanding or, for that matter, treatment of this injury.

Yet, the story must begin with Hippocrates, who described traumatic injuries about the wrist in the following terms:

The joint of the hand is dislocated either inward or outward, most frequently inward.

Hippocrates further went onto describe four distinct directions of dislocations, and this influence extended for nearly two thousand years through the writings of Galen, Palladius, Celsus, Duvernay, and Fabricius.[10] Much of these investigators' work was directed at describing the positions of dislocations and their effect on digital motion. Even a casual overview of their writings would certainly reflect the fact that the injuries they so described could well have been, and more likely were, fractures of the distal end of the radius. By the same token, it is remarkable that even in the first quarter of the nineteenth century,[37] the positions of carpal dislocation were described very much in the same manner as they were described by Hippocrates over two thousand years before.

Recognition

Although most would be willing to offer Abraham Colles as the single individual who should be given the most credit for directing the attention of his contemporaries to the underlying truths of these injuries,[7,32] there are two men who in fact must be given their rightful place in the historic adventure associated with this fracture. Notwithstanding the fact that many today call these fractures Colles' fractures, it was probably J.L. Petit who early in the eighteenth century may have suggested the carpal dislocations to be in some instances fractures of the end of the radius.[33] Although Petit suggested the application of anterior and posterior "compresses" to the region of the deformity, in contrast to the traditional use of tight bandaging, his writings reflect what could best be described as a lack of commitment to suggest to his contemporaries that these lesions were other than carpal dislocations.

Whereas Petit's writings raise at best only a hint that he was becoming suspicious that these injuries might in fact be fractures, it was Claude Pouteau in the latter part of the eighteenth century who, without question, recognized the lesion of the fracture of the distal end of the radius with dorsal displacement of the distal fragment.[35] In a work published posthumously in 1783, Pouteau pointed out the almost universal error in diagnosing these fractures as carpal dislocations. He stated:

These fractures are most often taken for contusions, luxations incomplete, or for separation of the radius from the ulnar at their junction near the wrist.

Pouteau attributed the distal radius fracture to a sudden and energetic contraction of the pronator quadratus and described clinical symptoms which he felt to be consistent with these injuries, as well as various forms of treatment.

Unfortunately, during the succeeding three decades following Pouteau's publications, there remained only occasional mention in the literature of the possibility that the traumatic dislocation of the carpal area could be anything but a joint dislocation. Desault alluded to the combination of a fracture and dislocation but did little to shed any light on distinguishing between the two and any alteration in treatment.[11,12]

In 1814 appeared the now famous article by Abraham Colles. Although he never had the opportunity to dissect a specimen (which might well explain why he suggested that the fracture took place 1½ inches proximal to the radiocarpal joint), Colles must be permitted to share the limelight for credit in discovering the true nature of this injury.[7] Colles in his article made certain to assuage his contemporaries with regard to the likely reasons for confusion by stating:

The injury to which I wish to direct the attention of surgeons has not, as far as I know, been described by any author: indeed, the form of the carpal extremity of the radius would rather incline us to question its being liable to fracture. The absence of crepitus and of other common symptoms of fracture together with the swelling, which instantly arises in this, as in other injuries of the wrist, render the difficulty of ascertaining the real nature of the case very considerable.

He goes on to further state:

While the absence of crepitus and of the other usual symptoms of fracture rendered the diagnosis extremely difficult; a recollection of the superior strength and thickness of this part of the radius, joined to the mobility of its articulation with the carpus and ulnar, rather incline me to question the possibility of a fracture taking place at this part of the bone.

Yet, in contrast to many of those who preceded him, Abraham Colles was quite confident in his observations and was able to make a very firm commitment to this lesion as he stated:

I cannot conclude these observations without remarking, that were my opinion to be drawn from those cases only which have occurred to me, I should consider this as by far the most common injury to which the wrist or carpal extremity of the radius and ulnar are exposed. During the last three years I have not met with a single instance of Desault's dislocation of the inferior end of the radius, while I have had opportunities of seeing a vast number of the fractures of the lower end of this bone.

Colles not only offered treatment, which will be discussed later on, but even outcome when he suggested:

One consolation only remains, that the limb will at some remote period again enjoy perfect freedom in all of its motions and be completely exempt from pain: the deformity, however, will remain undiminished through life.

Although Colles' impact has permeated through the years following his seminal article, it likely had nowhere nearly as much influence over contemporary medical and surgical care as did Dupuytren and his contemporaries. A great change took place in medical science in the early nineteenth century under the influence of French physicians. Dupuytren based his observations, to a large extent, on post-mortem examinations that not only demonstrated convincingly, to both him and his colleagues, that of these injuries were fractures, but also revealed the morphology of the fracture patterns.[14] His role as chief of the Hôtel Dieu in Paris provided him with ample clinical opportunity for study of these injuries. He stated in no uncertain terms that he believed these to be common injuries:

I have for a long time publicly taught that fractures of the carpal end of the radius are extremely common; that I had always found these supposed dislocations of the wrist turn out to be fractures; and that, in spite of all which has been said upon the subject, I have never met or heard of one single well authenticated and convincing case of the dislocation in question. I have also stated that, in all the wrists I had dissected with this view, I had never met with a dislocation as the consequence of a fall on the palm of the hand.

He further went on to suggest:

As to the frequency of fractures of the radius at its lower part, I apprehend that there are no longer two opinions, whatever may be thought of the impossibility, or at least extreme rarity of dislocations.

Two contemporaries of Duputyren played a preeminent role in further advancing the understanding that the injury to the terminal end of the forearm was a fracture rather than carpal dislocation. The first is Malgaigne, who published work on the distal radius at nearly the same time as Dupuytren was espousing his own concepts.[26] He noted that falls on the hand may produce a variety of fracture patterns and associated deformities. He identified a variety of injuries and noted that there were no age limits to such lesions. The frequencies of fractures hospitalized at the Hôtel Dieu were identified at this time by Malgaigne (Table 1.1).

In addition, Malgaigne provided a list of fracture types as a result of a fall on the palm. His understanding of the nature of the injury was quite extraordinary, as he suggested that a fall landing on the entire palm as opposed to the thenar or hypothenar eminence might result in a different injury pattern. He identified the various injuries in terms of his own experience (Table 1.2).

Table 1.1. Fractures seen at the Hôtel Dieu.[26]

year	Number of fractures	Number of distal radius fractures
1818	81	4
1827	109	10
1828	110	5
1830	101	6

A second French surgeon contemporary to Dupuytren was Goyrand. Goyrand's essay appeared in 1832.[18] Although he confirmed that these injuries were indeed fractures, and that the majority of fractures of the distal fragment were dorsally displaced, in some instances he noted that displacement could be in a volar or palmar direction.

Table 1.2. Types of fractures or dislocations resulting from a fall on the palm in Malgaigne's experience.[26]

Type	Frequency
Fracture of radius, inferiorly	Common
Fracture of radius, inferiorly with incomplete luxation ulna	Common
Fractures of both bones, inferiorly	Rare
Fracture of radius, inferiorly, with complete luxation ulna	Rare
Fracture in general with opening and soft parts	Rare
Fracture of radius, inferiorly with compound luxation ulna	Rare
Luxation forward of forearm on wrist, or luxation backwards of carpus on forearm	Two doubtful cases
Luxation of radius with fracture of radius	1 case
Luxation of radius alone	No case
Backward luxation of forearm on wrist, or forward luxation of carpus on forearm	No case
Fracture of ulnar inferiorly	No case

Definition

From the time of Dupuytren onwards, most came to accept the fact that the vast majority of injuries to the wrist, particularly those associated with falls on the palm, were indeed fractures rather than dislocations. The subsequent literature reflects an enthusiasm for identifying specific characteristics of the fractures as well as the mechanisms of injury. It is of interest to also note how often authors would point out the inaccuracies of their contemporaries! The vast majority of observations were based upon post-mortem or post-amputation specimens, the latter attesting to some of the inherent risks of having medical attention for these injuries.

Dupuytren made a number of observations based on post-mortem specimens. He noted:

Usually fractures of the lower end of the radius are simple but sometimes they are comminuted. I have seen some specimens in which the lower fragment was split vertically into two portions. M. Flaubert, surgeon-in-chief at l'Hôtel Dieu at Rouen, showed me in 1832 the radius of a mechanic who, after a fall on the wrist and foot, died of a diseased liver. This bone was broken about six lines above the joint: the styloid process was detached and drawn up; and from the center of the articulation a radiating fracture extended in various directions.[14]

In 1839, Voillemier, also a French contemporary of Dupuytren, brought forth to the medical community several interesting and provocative observations as to the patterns of the distal radius fracture.[23,41] He suggested that with higher energy of trauma, there was a direct transmission of the force of injury into the carpal end of the radius, with impaction of the distal fragment onto the proximal fragment:

The upper or broken margin of the lower fragment and also the ulnar margin, undergo very little displacement; while the lower or articular surface, and the radial margin are carried backwards, upwards, and outward.

He suggested that comminution would occur if the proximal radius continued its action almost as a wedge splitting the distal fragment. Although Voillemier did not have access to post-mortem specimens of acute injuries, but rather to longstanding healed fractures which he cut with a saw, he did raise some interest with his observation that instead of being oblique, as had been

Figure 1.1. Cross section of specimen with healed distal radius fracture. From Frank H. Hamilton, *A Practical Treatise on Fractures and Dislocations*. Reprint of 1860 edition. (san Francisco: Norman Publishing, 1991). Courtesy of Norman Publishing.

Figure 1.2. Specimen from Bigelow's collection demonstrating evidence of impaction and comminution of the articular surface. From Frank H. Hamilton, *A Practical Treatise on Fractures and Dislocations*. Reprint of 1860 edition. (san Francisco: Norman Publishing, 1991). Courtesy of Norman Publishing.

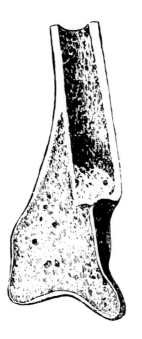
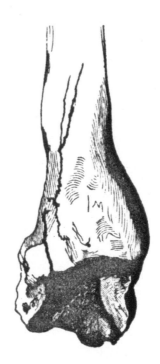

generally supposed, the fractures in his specimens appeared almost universally transverse from the palmar to the dorsal surface, and only on occasion did he suggest that the fracture line had been slightly oblique in a radial to ulnar direction. One should bear in mind, however, that these observations were made on specimens that had remote fractures with healing and evidence of callus (Fig. 1.1). Voillemier's concepts of impaction as the mechanism of injury and of the morphology of the fractures influenced a number of subsequent investigators, including Callender[5] and Bigelow[3] (Fig. 1.2).

In 1837, Diday suggested that the obliquity of the fracture permitted the distal fragment to be displaced upwards and proximally, with a variable amount of overriding of the distal fragment, which he felt represented a common feature of this injury.[13] Diday went on to suggest that the overriding and subsequent shortening affected the normal relationships of the radioulnar joint.

Alternative definitions of fracture patterns were offered by a number of investigators during the early part of the nineteenth century. The definition of a shearing-type fracture continues to be attributed to Dr. John Rhea Barton, who published his important paper in 1838.[1] Barton described the fracture line as oblique from the articular margin upwards and backwards, separating and displacing the distal portion with only a portion of the posterior margin of the articular surface being injured. He noted that this could be similarly found on the palmar surface, though considerably less commonly. Although Barton was not able to document his work with fresh post-mortem specimens of injury, his descriptions were highly suggestive of the shearing-type injury that bears his name:

The only important change, which takes place in consequence of this fracture is, that the concave surface of the extremity of the radius, which receives and articulates with the three first carpal bones is converted as it were into an oblique surface by the loss of a portion of its marginal ridge; commonly by the separation of an entire piece, sometimes by the crushing of its substance. . . .

It sometimes happens, though rarely, that the fracture of a similar character to the one just described, occurs on the palmar side of the radius, from the application of a force against the back of the hand whilst it is bent forward to its ultimate degree. Whenever the fracture takes place in front, the end of the radius projects over the wrist on the dorsal side and the carpal bones and fragment rise out of their proper situation and form the tumor on the palmar side thus reversing the deformity of the arm.

The fact that Barton did not have autopsy specimens suggested to a number of subsequent investigators that he was more likely than not describing extra-articular bending-type fractures, which have subsequently been known as Colles' or Smith's fractures. In fact, Malgaigne alluded to a case seen by M. Lenoir, who treated a patient who was thought to have had a dislocation of his hand in a backwards direction. The patient died, and Lenoir was able to observe at autopsy that a considerable fragment had been broken from the dorsal lip of the articular surface. This fragment had become displaced dorsally and proximally, carrying with it the carpal bones.[26]

Stimson suggested three good reasons why this fracture should not be known as a Barton's fracture:[39]

1. it was likely a Colles' fracture;
2. the lesion that he was supposed to be describing was actually observed by M. Lenoir and mentioned by Voillemier[41] and Malgaigne;[26] and
3. it may well have been more a complication than a standard fracture.

Furthermore, in 1839 Letenneur presented a case of a volar dislocation of the wrist accompanied by a fracture of the anterior ridge of the radius seen in autopsy specimens.[24]

Fractures featuring anterior or palmar displacement of the distal fragment were described by R.W. Smith of Dublin, who published a monograph in 1847 in which he firmly not only identified this lesion but also established Colles' fracture as the rightful eponym for the entity of a fracture of the distal end of the radius.[31,38] The fact that he, too, was from Dublin led many, from that time on, to call fracture of the distal radius the "Irish" fracture. Yet undoubtedly this fracture pattern was described by Goyrand[18] in 1832 and a by number of his other French contemporaries. Smith suggested that the lesion was the result of a fall on the back of the hand:

The situation of the fracture is from half an inch to an inch above the articulation: It is accompanied by great deformity, the principal features of which are a dorsal and palmar tumor and a striking projection of the head of the ulnar at the posterior and inner part of the forearm; the dorsal tumor occupies the entire breadth of the forearm but is most conspicuous internally, where it is constituted by the lower extremity of the ulnar displaced backward; from this point the inferior outline of the tumor passes obliquely upwards and outwards corresponding in the lateral direction to the lower end of the superior fragment of the radius. Immediately below the dorsal swelling there is a well-marked sulcus deepest internally below the head of the ulna, directed nearly transversely, but ascending a little as it approaches the radial border of the forearm.

He goes on to say:

The palmar is less remarkable than the dorsal tumor; formed principally by the lower fragment of the radius, it is obscured by the thick mass of flexor tendons which cross in front of the carpus, but towards the ulnar border of the limb there is a considerable projection, which marks the situation of the pisiform bone, passing down to its attachment into which can be seen the tendon of the flexor carpi ulnaris thrown forward in strong relief. The transverse diameter of

Figure 1.3. The classic drawing of Smith depicting the clinical appearance of the hand with an anterior displaced fracture.

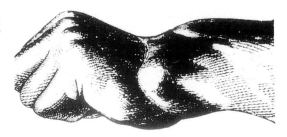

the forearm is not much altered, but the anteroposterior is considerably increased and the radial border of the limb becomes concave at its lowest part. (Fig. 1.3)

Because Smith did not do anatomic dissections of acute injuries but rather of healed bones, he needed to defend his observations:

I cannot speak with accuracy as to the anatomical characteristics of the injury, having never had an opportunity of examining after death the skeleton of the forearm in those who had during life met with this accident . . . but still I feel satisfied that the injury is a fracture of the lower end of the radius with displacement of the lower fragment along with the carpus forwards, and of the head of the ulnar backwards, and that it has not infrequently been mistaken for dislocation of the carpus forwards and of the bones of the forearm backwards.

Several years later, in 1865, G.W. Callender reviewed his observations of 36 specimens in the museums associated with the various schools of medicine in London.[5] He supported Voillemier's concept of impaction of the distal fragment into the proximal fragment (this is understandable, as these investigators studied skeletons with healed fractures and therefore mature callus):

They show clearly enough that the cause of each deformity is the impaction of the proximal into the distal portion of the bone.

He noted that in falls on the hand:

Weak cancellous tissue is broken across and the wedge-like end of the compact wall is driven into the distal portion of the bone not always in the same direction and is there firmly impacted.

Callender did attempt to explain the deformity associated with these fractures:

The carpal extremity may, however, be driven by the original incident to one side or the other, as may be seen in many of the specimens a displacement explaining the manner in which the impaction is established.

Callender, in reviewing the various specimens, also identified the lesions attributed to Goyrand and Smith, as well as fractures involving disruption of the articular surface, which may well have been initially described by Voillemier (Fig. 1.4). In describing the anterior displaced fractures, he related two instances when these were observed. The first is a clinical case in which the hand struck the ground in a flexed position at the wrist:

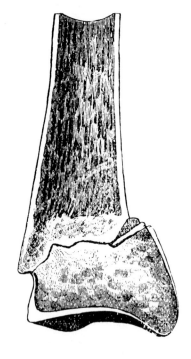

Figure 1.4. An anatomical specimen of a Smith's fracture. From Frank H. Hamilton, *A Practical Treatise on Fractures and Dislocations.* Reprint of 1860 edition. (San Francisco: Norman Publishing, 1991). Courtesy of Norman Publishing.

There was a well marked prominence of the forearm about three-quarters of an inch above the wrist joint and opposite it on the palmar surface was a considerable depression. The lower fragment of the radius was inclined at an oblique angle to the palmar surface. Reduction could not be effected. Ten months later, the deformity persisted with good rotation, exaggerated flexion, and an inability to extend the hand beyond a straight line with the forearm.

Callender also observed a specimen of an anterior displaced fracture pattern:

This kind of impaction is seen in a specimen in the Museum of the Westminster Hospital. The carpal extremity of a radius has been fractured and the ulnar is broken at its styloid process. The distal end of the radius is displaced forwards and outwards chiefly in the last-named direction, but there is no rotation of the shaft on its long axis.

Callender described a case of an intraarticular impacted fracture which more likely than not was among those described by Voillemier:

In a case previously referred to there was a comminuted fracture of the radius extending into the wrist-joint, but, there was no displacement and no deformity existed during life.

A discussion of the development of definitions of fracture patterns of the end of the radius would not be complete without mentioning that Velpeau must be given the credit for the term "silver fork deformity" or "talon de fourchette."[30]

A number of authors tried to produce a more accurate anatomic definition of the ulnar side of the distal radius fracture. Nélaton noted that "either the internal lateral ligament ruptures or the styloid apophysis of the ulnar to which it is attached breaks off."[29]

Later in the nineteenth century, Cameron noted:

It is usually affirmed that the prominence of the lower end of the ulnar is due to dislocation of that bone; the internal lateral ligaments being ruptured and the radioulnar ligament and the triangular fibrocartilage being more or less stretched and torn; and I have no doubt that this very generally happens. But another injury is certainly common viz, fracture and complete separation of the tip of the ulnar styloid process.[6]

Mechanism

Consistent with early investigators' descriptions of the morphology of the fractures was their interest in putting forth their own interpretation of the fracture mechanism. Although many of the theories had their own individual insights, it is reasonable to look at the concepts of the early investigators in three main perspectives.[34]

The first was shared by only a few investigators. The foremost of these was Pouteau, who suggested that some, but not all, fractures of the distal radius occurred as a result of muscular action.

The second theory was that the impact was directly transmitted into the radius itself as a result of the fall. This theory was favored by Malgaigne, Dupuytren, and Goyrand, among others. These investigators felt that the radius fractured at its weakest point as a consequence of the impact between the ground below and the weight of the body above.

The third group of theories related to the position of the hand and forearm at the time of impact. LeComte[22] and others suggested that the anterior volar carpal ligaments sustained the forces of both tension and compression and were fundamental in the development of these fractures. More information regarding the early theories can be found in the discussion of the fracture mechanism in Chapter 2.

Treatment

The evolution of treatment for the distal radius fracture in the nineteenth century was very much representative of the problems attendant on the inherent tendency to keep within surgical tradition which became contrasted with the need for new developments as greater understanding of the problem evolved. Ultimately it became commonplace to see each surgeon attempt to imprint his own individuality onto both reduction maneuvers and immobilization techniques. The literature reflects a wide range of concepts and techniques, to the point that the fracture appeared to be treated in innumerable ways depending upon the individual surgeon's preference and ingenuity. Hamilton reflected upon this when he stated:

I must also enter my protest against many or all of those carved splints which are manufactured, hawked about the country, and sold by mechanics, who are no surgeons; with the fossa for each styloid process, a ridge to press between the bones, and various other curious provisions for supposed necessities, but which never find in any arm their exact counterparts, and only deceive the inexperienced surgeon into neglect of the proper means for making a suitable adaption. They are the fruitful source of excoriations, ulcerations, inflammations, and deformities.[19]

Among the more common forms of treatment for what were thought from antiquity to be carpal dislocations was bandaging the hand and forearm with linen wraps or other means of attempting tight control over the deformity once it was reduced. This carried over along with the addition of supports when it became recognized that these injuries were more often than not fractures of the distal radius. Malgaigne notes that Cline of London recommended the addition of straight splints for the forearm to be placed above the rolled bandages.[26] These splints were not permitted to extend lower than the wrist so that when the forearm was suspended in a sling in a state of semipronation, the hand would fall on its own weight to the ulnar side.

Colles early on quite clearly described his approach to both fracture reduction and immobilization:

Let the surgeon apply the fingers of one hand to the seat of the suspected fracture and, locking the other hand in that of the patient, make a moderate extension, until the observed limb is restored to its natural form.

On splintage, Colles stated:

It is obvious that, in the treatment of this fracture, our attention should be principally to guard against the carpal end of the radius being drawn backwards. For this purpose, while assistants hold the limb in a middle state between pronation and supination, let a thick and firm compress be applied transversely on the anterior surface of the limb, at the seat of the fracture, taking care that it should not press on the ulna; let this be bound on firmly with a roller and then let a tin splint, formed to the shape of the arm, be applied to both its anterior and posterior surfaces. In cases where the end of the ulnar has appeared much displaced, I have laid a very narrow wooden splint along the naked side of this bone. This latter splint I now think should be used in every instance, as, by pressing the extremity of the ulnar against the side of the radius, it will tend to improve the displacement of the fractured end of this bone. It is scarcely necessary to observe that the two principal splints should be much more narrow at the wrist than those in general use, and should also extend to the roots of the fingers spreading out as to give a support to the hand.

Dupuytren described his method of reduction:

For the purpose of accomplishing the proper adjustment of this form of fracture, the limb should be separated from the trunk, and the back of the hand turned upwards, the forearm being semi-flexed on the upper arm.

The assistant whose business it is to make counter-extension grasps the inferior part of the upper arm, whilst another assistant makes gradual exten-

sion on the hand directing it at the same time toward the ulnar side of the forearm. The surgeon places himself on the outer side of the limb, presses with both hands the fleshy part of the forearm, both before and behind into the interosseous space; and then by suitable manipulation brings the fractured ends into apposition. Reduction is effected without difficulty but it is not always so easy to keep the ends of the bone in proper relation.

Dupuytren goes on to describe his method of immobilization:

When the first part of the operation is achieved, I apply the usual apparatus for fractures of the forearm—that is to say a bandage for the hand, two graduated compresses on the anterior surface of the forearm and two on the posterior and over these two broad splints: the whole is to be made fast by several turns of the same bandage in which the hand has been rolled.

Dupuytren noted the tendency of the hand to deviate radially and attempted to control this:

Recently, however, I have devised the addition of a cubital splint to the ordinary apparatus. It consists of a steel plate about 15 inches long, an inch and one quarter wide, and one line in thickness. It is divided into two parts, one straight and the other semi-circular and corresponding at the commencement of its curve to the wrist: the concavity of the latter division has five studs, placed at equal distances from each other. The ordinary apparatus for fractures of the forearm being applied, the straight part of this splint is to be fastened against the inner margin of the ulnar with a roller: a pad is then placed between the inner side of the wrist and the lower end of the splint, so as to separate them: the hand is afterwards drawn toward the convexity of the curved portion of the splint and the tapes by which they are kept in contact are passed around the second metacarpal bone and made fast to the studs in its concavity. It is not difficult to understand the modus operandi of this apparatus: the pad serves at once to correct the projection and (apparent) curvature of the ulnar and to act more efficiently on the fracture; whilst the abduction of the hand, through the agency of the external lateral ligaments of the wrist, tends to preserve the accurate adjustment of the fragments. I have, by the above method, succeeded to my entire satisfaction in curing these troublesome fractures, without any deformity or sacrifice of the rotatory motions of the forearm.

Nélaton[29] and Goyrand, as well as others, used a similar type of device. Blandon and also Welch used wood instead of steel for this type of *attelle cubitale* of Dupuytren[19] (Fig. 1.5).

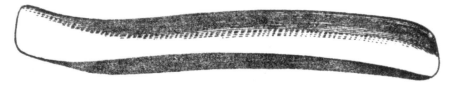

Welch's palmar splint

Figure 1.5. The splint developed by Welch. From Frank H. Hamilton, *A Practical Treatise on Fractures and Dislocations*. Reprint of 1860 edition. (san Francisco: Norman Publishing, 1991). Courtesy of Norman Publishing.

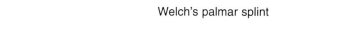

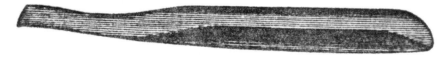

Welch's dorsal splint

Goyrand described his approach:

The forearm is to be flexed slightly on the arm; then extension with inclination of the hand to the ulnar is to be made, and counter-extension being done by assistants, the surgeon presses the fragment into place. Anterior and posterior graduated compresses, the pieces of stout cloth folded several times are then placed over the palmar and dorsal surface of the radius below the compresses—compresses are to force the muscle into the interosseous space for the purpose of correcting the tendency of the broken radius to the ulna . . . the pads are secured by a bandage, two splints, the lower borders of which extend to the termination of the pads are carefully adjusted. In cases of great deformity, Dupuytren's attelle cubitale *is to be added.*

Nélaton stated:

Dupuytren and Goyrand, imitated in this by other surgeons, sought by inclining and slightly flexing the hand towards its ulnar edge, to produce a permanent extension upon the lower fragment of the radius and to exercise pressure upon the dorsal surface of this fragment by means of the extension tendency of the fingers that pass at this pad. But this extension, supposing it be possible, appears to me useless.

Rather, Nélaton used graduated compresses upon the dorsal surfaces of the carpus and upon the lower fragment of the radius, and then splints were applied on the dorsal and volar surface secured with a roller (Fig. 1.6). Only when the fragment displacement was pronounced did he appear to add the ulnar splint of Dupuytren. An additional splint has been attributed to Nélaton, the so-called pistol splint (Fig. 1.7), but this too appears to be somewhat controversial, as Nélaton's writings do not describe such a device nor did others who investigated the development of the pistol splint.[36]

The pistol splint was a preformed splint constructed with a bend or pistol shape that would hold the hand and wrist in some palmar flexion and ulnar deviation, avoiding the need for the ulnar splint. It would appear from some of the early investigators that the combination of tight bandaging in conjunction with the confining nature of this *attelle cubitale* led to a number of associated problems with stiffness of the hand and wrist, as will be discussed later in this chapter. This type of device was amended by Bond, who placed the pistol-shaped splint on the palmar surface[15] (Fig. 1.8).

In 1842, Huguier presented a new device which used two splints anteriorly and posteriorly which extended beyond the fingers. A sort of collar arose from around the carpus from which anteriorly and posteriorly four tapes extended to the elements of the splints beyond the fingers. These tapes were drawn tightly so as to make an extension on the hand and tied to the splints. Huguier suggested that Goyrand's approach for correction of the initial fracture displacement by manipulation did not serve a purpose and felt that his device could accomplish as well as maintain the position. The lack of subsequent enthusiastic support for this approach no doubt was based upon the problems that must have occurred in association with this form of bandaging.[19]

Fenger in Copenhagen in 1847 also pointed out the deficiencies of the splint technique of Dupuytren and colleagues.[15]

The hand is first to be brought into a position of strong flexion and the forearm is then placed on an oblique plane, with the carpus highest, the hand being permitted to hang freely down the perpendicular end of the plane. The tendons of the extensor muscles are thus brought into a position which enables them to assist in keeping the reduced fragments of the bone in proper relation . . . The patient is to be kept in bed but the hand is not confined, the seat of the fracture covered only by an evaporating lotion.

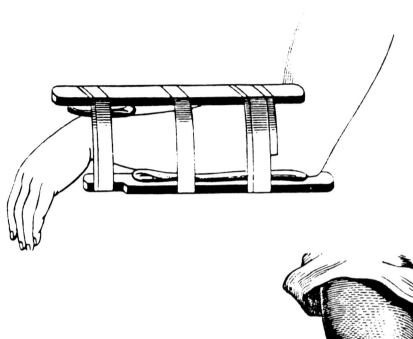

Figure 1.6. The splint described by Nélaton. Reprinted with permission. Richardson BW: *Dublin Q J Med Sci*, 1871.

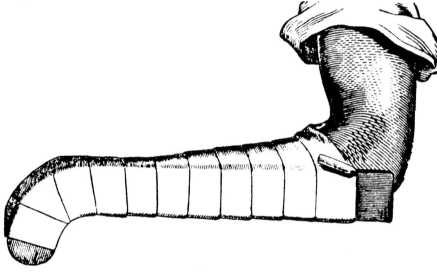

Figure 1.7. The pistol splint attributed to Nélaton. From Frank H. Hamilton, *A Practical Treatise on Fractures and Dislocations.* Reprint of 1860 edition. (san Francisco: Norman Publishing, 1991). Courtesy of Norman Publishing.

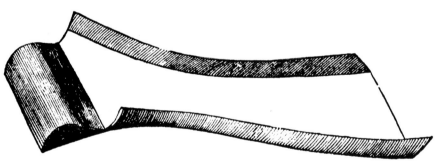

Figure 1.8. An early American splint for distal radius fractures was that devised by Bond. From Frank H. Hamilton, *A Practical Treatise on Fractures and Dislocations.* Reprint of 1860 edition. (san Francisco: Norman Publishing, 1991). Courtesy of Norman Publishing.

When Fenger's work was presented by Dr. Hodgkin to the Royal Medical and Surgical Society in 1847, an interesting and enlightening discussion followed. One individual, Mr. Arnott, stated:

The nature of this accident was described thirty years ago by Colles of Dublin, whose description had been reproduced by Smith of Dublin, in his recently published work. Dr. Smith described the fracture from an examination of twenty specimens, and has given nine or ten illustrations of the appearances. He was fully aware of the difficulty attending the diagnosis and treatment of this, having himself suffered, many years since, having had his arm broken not far above the articulation, and could bear witness to the pain and extremely disagreeable sensations attending the application of Dupuytren's bandage. He was inclined to think favorably of Professor Fenger's method, by which the extension was produced by the weight of the hand acting through the medium of the capsular ligament, and was glad that Dr. Hodgkin had made it known to them.[15]

This approach described by Fenger was reported by other authors, including Velpeau, who noted in 1846 that he had tried Fenger's plan, although he found the results not very satisfactory. Velpeau ended up by recommending incorporation of the splint and compresses, keeping the fingers immobile.[40]

Malgaigne criticized the approach recommended by a number of his contemporaries, especially Huguier and Velpeau:

Without discussing here the comparative value of the two appareils, I believe that this could scarcely be endured by the patients and M. Diday tells us that in the trials which he has made, the pain produced by the extension was so great that he was compelled to renounce it.[26]

Malgaigne felt that there were three indications for reduction of the fracture: reestablishment of the interosseous space, correction of the deformity of the radiocarpal articulation, and prevention of an abduction deformity of the hand. Malgaigne described a method of manipulative reduction in which extension and counterextension performed by an assistant were followed by the surgeon's pressing the distal fragment into position. He maintained his reduction using anterior and posterior splints and compresses which terminated at the wrist. These were applied in such a manner to put the most pressure on the distal radial fragment with a minimum of interference with the mobility of the hand and wrist. Malgaigne also recommended lateral splints that would act on the inner border of the ulnar and other splints on the outer border applying pressure on the radial styloid. The pressure was distributed by pads, and he urged that the hand be left free, somewhat similar to the method described by Cline. Parenthetically, this form of splintage continues to the present in many areas of the world, including the traditional treatments in Asia (see Chapter 5).

A splint that sought to control the fracture somewhat akin to that of Dupuytren and the strategically applied splints recommended by Malgaigne was devised by Professor Gordon of Belfast, Ireland.[17] Instead of using iron, as did Dupuytren's splint, this splint used a piece of wood attached to the standard anterior splint which overlapped the radius and had a bevel within the wood which would be located immediately under the fracture (Fig. 1.9). Gordon's splint proved popular in Ireland and Great Britain but did not appear to influence those on the continent of Europe or in North America.

A thorough description of the development and application of splintage

Figure 1.9. Gordon's splint controlling the hand and wrist in ulna deviation and palmar flexion but leaving the hand free for mobility. From Frank H. Hamilton, *A Practical Treatise on Fractures and Dislocations.* Reprint of 1860 edition. (san Francisco: Norman Publishing, 1991). Courtesy of Norman Publishing.

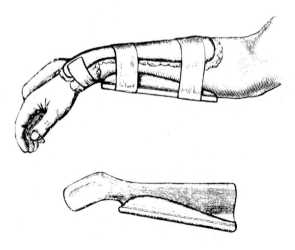

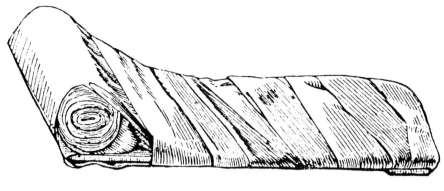

Figure 1.10. The splint constructed by Hays. From Frank H. Hamilton, *A Practical Treatise on Fractures and Dislocations.* Reprint of 1860 edition. (san Francisco: Norman Publishing, 1991). Courtesy of Norman Publishing.

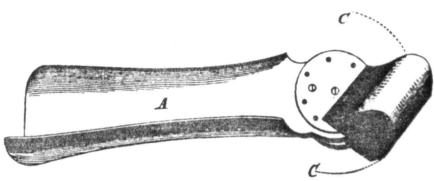

Figure 1.11. The splint devised by E.P. Smith attempted to hold the hand in a fixed position. From Frank H. Hamilton, *A Practical Treatise on Fractures and Dislocations.* Reprint of 1860 edition. (san Francisco: Norman Publishing, 1991). Courtesy of Norman Publishing.

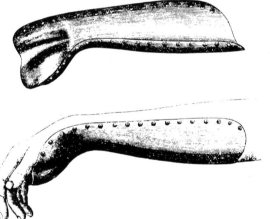

Figure 1.12. The metallic splint devised by Levi. Note the American interest in supporting the hand out to the metacarpophalangeal joints with a palmar support. From Frank H. Hamilton, *A Practical Treatise on Fractures and Dislocations.* Reprint of 1860 edition. (san Francisco: Norman Publishing, 1991). Courtesy of Norman Publishing.

for distal radius fractures in North America can be found in the work of Hamilton.[19] He noted that there appeared to be a general tendency in North America to have the contoured curved splint placed on the palmar surface with the straight splint on the dorsal surface of the forearm, in contrast to the method used on the European continent. In North America the palmar splint terminated at the metacarpophalangeal joints, whereas in the European approach the palmar splint ended at the distal radius.[27] This enabled the hand to be maintained in a contained position, over either a hard block or a pad of appropriate size. Hamilton noted the evolution in North America of ready-made splints; among the earliest were those constructed by Hays in Philadelphia (Fig. 1.10) and soon after by E.P. Smith and Levi (Figs. 1.11 and 1.12).

Hamilton developed his own approach:

Having restored the fragments to place, in case of Colles' fracture, by pressing forcibly upon the back of the lower fragment, the force being applied near the

Figure 1.13. The splints applied by Hamilton. Note the rolled bandages on the hand. From Frank H. Hamilton, *A Practical Treatise on Fractures and Dislocations.* Reprint of 1860 edition. (San Francisco: Norman Publishing, 1991). Courtesy of Norman Publishing.

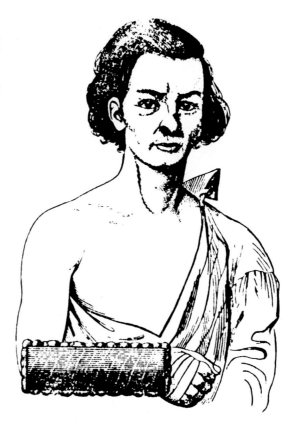

styloid apophysis of the radius, the arm is to be flexed upon the body and placed in a position of semi-pronation; when the splints are to be applied and secured with a sufficient number of turns of the roller, taking special care not to include the thumb, the forcible confinement of which is always painful and never useful. (Fig. 1.13)

Hamilton appeared quite concerned about the difficulties that the various splints appeared to present with regard to swelling of the hand and associated stiffness and loss of function. He noted:

The first application of the bandages to be only moderately tight and as the inflammation and swelling developed in these situations with rapidity, they should be attentively watched and loosened as soon as they become painful. It must be borne in mind that to prevent and control inflammation in this fracture, it is the most difficult and by far the most important object to be accomplished, while to retain the fragment once reduced is comparatively easy and unimportant . . .

Any moderate, or even considerable malposition of the lower fragment, after a fracture of the radius, is not sufficient in itself to occasion anchylosis. It is true that in the fracture now under consideration, the direction of the articular surface of the radius is changed. But of what consequence is this so long as the carpal bones with which alone this bone is articulated preserve their relation to the radius unchanged? . . .

During the first seven to ten days, therefore, these cases demand the most assiduous attention; and we had much better dispense with the splint entirely than to retain them at the risk of increasing the inflammatory action. Indeed, I have no doubt that very many cases would come to a successful determination without splints if only the hand and arm were kept perfectly still in a suitable position until bony union was affected.

The difficulties and morbidity attendant to the use of tight roller banding with or without a variety of supportive splints are pervasive in the early literature related to the management of the distal radius fracture in the nineteenth century. Dupuytren quite clearly pointed this out:

The two succeeding cases are not only interesting as fractures of the radius, but they are further deserving of attentive consideration on account of the serious complications which accompany them, and which were the consequence of forgetting an important precept. More than once, indeed, it has occurred that the surgeons have been so intent on preserving fractures in their proper position, that the extreme constriction employed has actually caused destruction of the parts. A piece of advice which I have frequently given, and which I cannot too often repeat is, to avoid tightening too much the apparatus for fractures during the first few days of its being worn; for the swelling which supervenes is always accompanied by considerable pain and may be followed by gangrene. It cannot, therefore, be too urgently impressed upon young practitioners, to pay attention to the complaints which the patients make; and to visit them twice daily, and relax the bandages and straps as need may be, in order to obviate the frightful consequences which may spring from not heeding this necessary precaution; by carefully attending to this point I have been saved the painful alternative of ever having to sacrifice a limb for complications which its neglect may entail.

Dupuytren presents as an example a case:

Antoine Rilard, age 44, fractured his right radius whilst going down into a cellar in February 1828 and went at once to the hospital of la Charité. When the fracture was reduced (it was near the base of the bone) an apparatus was applied, but fastened too tightly; and, not withstanding the great swelling, and the acute pain which the patient endured, it was not removed until the fourth day when the hand was cold and edematous, and the forearm red, painful, and covered with vesications. Leeches, poultices, and fomentations were applied, and followed by some alleviation of the local symptoms, though there was much constitutional disturbance. At the close of a fortnight from the accident, the palmar surface of the forearm presented a point where fluctuation was supposed to exist; but one bistoury was plunged into it, no matter followed. Portions of the flexor muscles subsequently sloughed, and the skin subsequently mortified. The only recource was amputation, which was performed above the elbow, six weeks after his admission; and he afterwards recovered without the occurrence of any further untoward symptoms.

Dupuytren presents another dramatic example:

In nearly every instance the swelling of the limb requires that careful attention should be paid to the bandage or straps, by which the apparatus is confined. Similar accidents are likely to result from the employment of an immovable apparatus, of which an example occurred in the practice of M. Thiery, one of my pupils. He was summoned to visit a young girl, on whom such an apparatus had been applied for a supposed fracture of the radius. After suffering excruciating torment, the forearm mortified, and amputation was the only recource; on examining the limb no trace of fracture could be discovered. Had a simple apparatus been here employed, and properly watched, this patient's limb would not have been sacrificed.

The physicians in the nineteenth century were not immune to medical-legal problems associated with difficulties in the management of fractures of the distal radius. An illustrative but certainly not the only reported instance of medical-legal proceedings was described by Hamilton:

November 21, 1851, a boy ten years old living in the town of Andover, Mass., had his left hand drawn into the picker of a woolen mill, producing several severe wounds of the hand and a fracture of the radius near its middle. One of the wounds was situated directly over the point of fracture, but whether it communicated with the bone or not was not ascertained. A surgeon was called, who closed the wounds, covered the forearm with a bandage from the hand to above the elbow, and applied compresses and splints. This lad made no complaint, his appetite remained good, and his sleep continuing undisturbed, until the third day when he began to speak of a pain in his shoulder; on the same day it was noticed that his hand was rather insensible to the prick of a pin. Early on the morning of the fourth day his surgeon being summoned, found him suffering more pain and quite restless; and on removing the dressings, the arm was discovered to be insensible and actually mortified from the shoulder downwards. Opiates and cordials were immediately given to sustain the patient, and fomentations ordered.

On the sixth day a line of demarcation commenced across the shoulder, and on the 21st day, the father himself removed the arm from the body by merely separating the dead tissues with a feather. Subsequently a surgeon found the head of the humerus remaining in the socket and removed it, the epiphysis having become separated from the diaphysis. The boy now rapidly got well.

In the year 1853, this case became the subject of a legal investigation, in the course of which Dr. Pilsbury, of Lowell, Mass. declared that in his opinion this unfortunate result had been caused by too tight bandaging, and by neglecting to examine the arm during four days.

On the other hand, Drs. Hayward, Bigelow, Townsend, and Ainsworth, of Boston with Kimbell of Lowell, Drs. Loring and Pierce of Salem believe that the death of the limb was due to some injury done to the artery near the shoulder joint; and in no other way could they explain the total absence of pain during the first two days; nor could they regard this condition as consistent with the supposition that the bandage occasioned the death of the limb.

Conner in 1881 in the Cincinnati *Lancet* pointed out to his colleagues the difficulty in changing their approach to these fractures.[8] As the standard at that time continued to be tight bandaging and confining splints, Conner had visited Gordon in Belfast and became impressed with alternative techniques. By the same token, he recognized the problems attendant to changing the standards of medical care at the time and stated to his colleagues:

I would advise you in your practice to use splints and usually approved dressings. If under such circumstances, having exercised due care and ordinary skill, an unfortunate result follows, you will be protected, not against trouble but against adverse legal judgement. While on the other hand, you would have hard work today to escape pecuniary liability if a bad result should occur in a case treated by a simple wrist band and forearm sling. I have no doubt that many a man and woman in the next twenty years will be positively and severely damaged by the employment of authorized and standard methods of treating fractures of the lower end of the radius but the community at large has no right to complain if it suffers because experiments are not made, and new methods of treatment not adopted. As the laws are now, if you employ a hitherto untried method, you do it at your own risk. This malpractice suit business is much more than generally supposed a two-edged sword.

With these descriptions in mind, one can appreciate the evolution of the work of Lucas de Championnière.[16,25] This surgeon published two books and some 35 papers on the treatment of injuries to bone and joints incorporating manipulative techniques. When he began his work, the approach was very

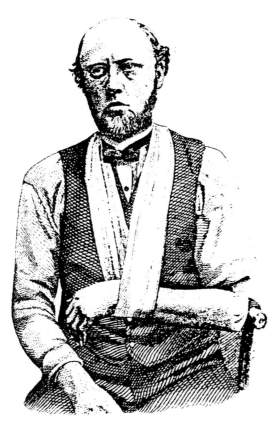

Figure 1.14. As suggested by Lucas-Championnière, a stable fracture could well be treated in a sling, permitting the hand and wrist to lie in ulna deviation and some palmar flexion. Reprinted with permission. Moore EM: A new treatment for Colles' fractures of the radius. *Trans NY State Med Soc* 233–244, 1870.

much as it had been for centuries: to reduce a fracture and apply a supportive dressing which was not to be removed until union was complete; if it had to be changed, no motion was allowed, since motion was thought to interfere with the formation of callus. Lucas-Championnière rather suggested that both massage and mobilization should be combined with support of the limb in such a manner that the surgeon would take continuous heed to avoid the associated morbidity of these commonplace approaches to fractures in general and those of the distal radius in particular. Lucas-Championnière recommended with distal radius fractures to begin mobilization and massage of the digits and wrists quite quickly after reduction and application of immobilization. Massage would avoid the site of fracture but extend more proximally up the forearm and encourage mobilization of the elbow. Furthermore, on those fractures which appeared to be stable and without undue deformity, either before or after reduction, he recommended a sling that allowed the hand and wrist to fall into ulnar deviation (Fig. 1.14).

The end of the nineteenth century saw the impact of roentgenology perhaps as much in the understanding of the distal radius fracture as anywhere else.[2,9] It quite clearly defined the fracture patterns and the results of treatment. Thus the discussions in the literature became much more standardized, as did the management approaches. As Morton stated in a study published in 1907 regarding the radiology of distal radius fractures:

The state of the lower fragment was a fertile source of discussion in the pre-roentgen ray days.[28]

The enormous impact of imposing figures such as Böhler[4] and Robert Jones[21] influenced succeeding surgeons—both in continental Europe and in the Anglo-Saxon world—bringing the understanding and management of most distal radius fractures very much to that which is understood today (Fig. 1.15).

Figure 1.15. The splints used by Robert Jones for uncomplicated Colles' fractures.

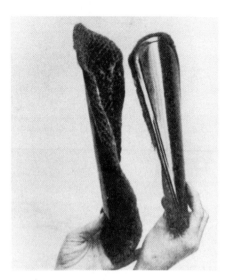
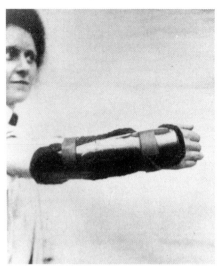

References

1. Barton JR: Views and treatment of an important injury of the wrist. *Medi Examiner* 1: 365–368, 1838.
2. Beck C: Colles' fracture and the roentgen rays. *Medi News* February: 230–232, 1898.
3. Bigelow HJ: Reports of medical societies. *Boston Med Surg J* 99, 1858.
4. Böhler L: Die funktionelle Bewegungsbehandlung der "typischen Radiusbrüche." *Munch Medizin Wochensch* 20: 33, 1923.
5. Callender GW: Fractures injuring joints—Fractures interfering with the movements at the wrist and with those of pronation and supination. *Saint Bartholomews Hosp Rep* 281–298, 1865.
6. Cameron HC: Fracture of the lower extremity of the radius (Colles'). *Glasgow Med J* X: 97–103, 1878.
7. Colles A: On the fracture of the carpal extremity of the radius. *Edinburgh Med Surg J* 10: 182–186, 1814.
8. Conner C: Fractures of the lower end of the radius. *Cincinnati Lancet* April 23: 371, 1881.
9. Cotton FJ: The pathology of fractures of the lower end of the radius. *Ann Surg* 32: 194–218, 1900.
10. Cruse TK: Essay on wrist joint injuries. *Trans NY State Medi Soc* III: 56–118, 1874.
11. Desault PJ: *Oeuvres chirurgicales ou exposés de la doctrine et la pratique de P.J. Desault par Xavier Bichat.* Paris: Méguignon, 1801.
12. Desault PJ: *A Treatise on Fractures and Luxations.* Philadelphia: 1817.
13. Diday M: Mémoire sur les fractures de l'extremité inférieure du radius. *Arch Gen Med* XIII: 141, 1837.
14. Dupuytren G: *On the Injuries and Diseases of Bone.* Translated by F.G. Clark. London: Sydenham Society, 1847.
15. Fenger: On fracture of the lower extremity of the radius—Royal Medical and Chirurgical Society. *L Lancet* May 8: 487–488, 1847.
16. Gibbon JH: Lucas-Championnière and mobilization in the treatment of fractures. *Surg Gynecol Obstet* XLIII: 271–278, 1926.
17. Gordon A: *Fractures of the Lower End of the Radius.* London VIII: 1875.
18. Goyrand G: Memoire sur les fractures de l'extrémité inférieure du radius qui simulent les luxations du poignet. *Gaz Med* 3: 664–667, 1832.
19. Hamilton FH: *A Practical Treatise on Fractures and Dislocations.* Philadelphia: Blanchard & Lea, 1860.
20. Hippocrates: *Genuine Works.* Translated by F. Adams. London: Sydenham Society, 1849.
21. Jones R: *Injuries of the Joints.* London: Henry Frowde and Hodder & Stoughton—Oxford University Press, 1915.
22. LeComte O: Recherches nouvelles sur les fractures de l'extremité inférieure du radius. *Arch Gen Med* 52–81, 1860.
23. LeGoffres M: *Précis iconographiques de bandages, pansements et appareils.* Paris: 1858.

24. Letenneur M: *Bull Soc Anat*. Converted No Journal, 1838.
25. Lucas-Championnière J: Traitement des fractures du radius et du péroné par le massage. Traitement des fractures pararticulaires simples compliquées de plaie sans immobilisation, mobilisation et massage. *Bull Mem Soc Chir Paris* 12: 560, 1886.
26. Malgaigne J: *A Treatise on Fractures* Translated by John Packard. Philadelphia: JB Lippincott, 1859.
27. Moore EM: A new treatment for Colles' fractures of the radius. *Trans NY State Med Soc* 27, 1870.
28. Morton R: A radiographic survey of 170 cases clinically diagnosed as "Colles' fracture." *Lancet* March: 731–732, 1907.
29. Nélaton A: *Eléments de pathologie chirurgicale*. Germer Bailliere, 1844.
30. Packard JH: Velpeau quoted in Malgaigne JF: *A Treatise on Fractures*. Philadelphia: JB Lippincott, 16, 1859.
31. Peltier LF: Eponymic fractures: Robert William Smith and Smith's fracture. *Surgery* 1035–1042, 1959.
32. Peltier LF: Fractures of the distal end of the radius. An historical account. *Clin Orthop Rel Res* 187: 18–22, 1984.
33. Petit JL: *L'Art de guérir les maladies de l'os*. Paris: L. d'Houry, 1705.
34. Pilcher LS: Reason versus tradition in the treatment of certain injuries of the wrist joint. *Proc Med Soc County Kings* 1–19, 1878.
35. Pouteau C: *Oeuvres posthumes de M. Pouteau. Mémoire, contenant quelques réflexions sur quelques fractures de l'avant-bras sur les luxations incomplettes du poignet et sur le diastasis*. Paris: Ph-D Pierres, 1783.
36. Richardson BW: Lessons from surgical practice. *Dublin Q J Med Sci* LII 104: 295–299, 1871.
37. Sanson M: *Dictionnaire de médecine et de chirurgie pratique*. Paris: 1832.
38. Smith RW: *A Treatise on Fracture in the Vicinity of Joints and on Certain Forms of Accidental and Congenital Dislocations*. Dublin: Hodges and Smith, 1847.
39. Stimson LA: *Treatise on Fractures*. Philadelphia: Henry Lea's Son & Co., 1883.
40. Velpeau C: *Boston Med J* XXXV: 213, 1846.
41. Voillemier M: Histoire d'une luxation complète et récente du poignet en arrière suivit de réflexions sur le mécanisme de cette luxation. *Arch Gen Med* 6: 401–417, 1839.

Chapter Two
Epidemiology, Mechanism, Classification

My own feeling is that whatever their fallibility, eponyms illustrate the lineage of surgery and bring to it the color of old times, distinguished features, ancient sieges and pestilences, and continually remind us of the international nature of science . . . [50]

M. Ravitch, M.D.

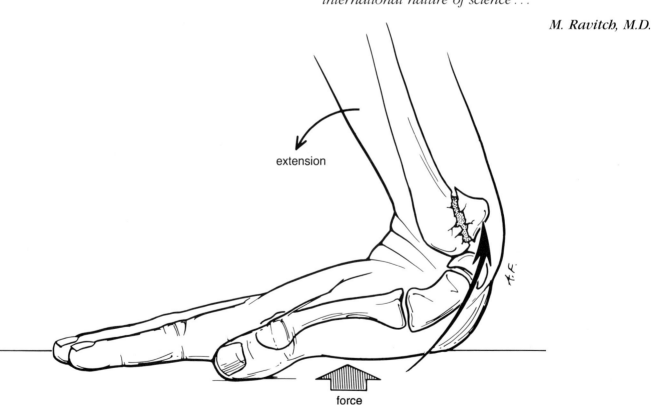

extension

force

Epidemiology

Incidence

Fracture of the distal end of the radius has been estimated to account for upwards of one-sixth of all fractures seen and treated in emergency rooms.[19,20,47] Given its frequency, it is somewhat surprising that little has been written outside of the Scandinavian literature regarding its epidemiologic features.[1,4,5,14,24,33,40,47,60] By the same token, the Scandinavian studies have provided us a relatively clear understanding of a number of features of the distal radius fracture, including incidence, age and sex prevalence, mechanisms, and in some cases, associated risk factors. From a compilation of data generated by epidemiologic studies, it is evident that distal radius fractures are more common in women, increase in incidence in both sexes with advancing years, and resnet more frequently from falls from level ground than from higher-energy trauma.

The commonplace nature of the distal radius fracture was evident even in the early literature which began to define these injuries as fractures. Dupuytren noted in 1829 that of 109 fractures treated in the Hôtel Dieu, 23 had their "seat" in the forearm. In 1830, of 97 fractures, 22 belonged to the forearm, with 16 involving the radius alone.[12]

At the Massachusetts General Hospital in the third decade of the twentieth century, fractures of the distal end of the radius accounted for 11 percent of all fractures cared for at the hospital.[65]

In one of the earlier Scandinavian studies, Alffram and Bauer reviewed all the forearm fractures treated in Malmö, Sweden, over a 5-year period from 1953 to 1957.[1] The urban population of Malmö at that time was slightly more than 200,000 people. In this study, nearly 2000 fractures of the distal radius were recorded, which represented 74.5 percent of all the forearm fractures reported over that period. Most distal radius fractures occurred in two distinct age groups—between 6 and 10 years and between 60 and 69 years. Among the patients 60 years of age and older, women outnumbered men sevenfold!

Of interest, 25 years later Bengner and Johnell looked again at the incidence of forearm fractures in Malmö over a 2-year period encompassing 1980 and 1981.[4] The population at this time was 234,000. These authors recorded 1990 cases of distal radius fractures, of which 1914 were fractures within 3 cm of the radiocarpal joint, 35 were radial styloid process fractures, and 41 were displaced epiphyseal fractures. Only 104 cases of diaphyseal fractures of the radius, ulna, or both were documented.

In the follow-up Malmö study, women showed a peak age-specific incidence in childhood as well as a dramatic increase after the age of 50 years. In men, there was also a peak in childhood and a moderate increase after the age of 70 years. The biggest variation from the preceding study of Alffram and Bauer 25 years before occurred in men after the age of 70, with an increase of almost six times that seen in the years 1953 to 1957 (Table 2.1).

It is also noteworthy that in the study of Bengner and Johnell, 45 percent of patients with distal radius fractures had additional skeletal injuries. These included fractures of the proximal humerus in 22 women (12 ipsilateral) and 1 man, and trochanteric hip fractures in 17 women (4 ipsilateral) and 2 men (both ipsilateral).

Schmalholz in 1981 through 1982 looked at the incidence of distal radius fractures in a different location in Sweden, within the catchment area of Södersjukshuset, Stockholm, which served a population of 210,400 persons over the age of 15 years.[56] In total, 1536 fractures were recorded in 1528

Table 2.1. Fractures of the distal forearm during 1980 and 1981 in relationship to age and sex. Total number and age-specific annual incidence per 10,000 inhabitants in Malmö, Sweden.

Age (yrs)	Women		Men	
	No.	Incidence	No.	Incidence
0–9	47	22	78	34
10–19	86	32	132	47
20–29	33	10	32	9
30–39	62	20	47	15
40–49	53	19	38	15
50–59	258	77	39	13
60–69	401	120	34	12
70–79	322	124	50	30
>80	181	161	21	45

Reprinted with permission. Begner U, Johnell O: Increasing incidence of forearm fractures. *Acta Orthop Scand* 56: 158–160 1985.

patients. These comprised 1495 Colles' fractures (8 bilateral) and 41 Smith's fractures. Eighty-four percent of the cases involved women, with a mean age of 66 years (range, 16 to 96). Among the men, the mean age was 49 years (range, 16 to 95).

Schmalholz observed the age-specific incidence among women to increase rapidly above the age of 45 years, reaching a maximum at 65 years.

A study was undertaken by Solgaard and Petersen in Denmark in 1981 with a regional population of 224,705 individuals over the age of 20 years. Distal radius fractures were recorded in 394 women and 99 men.[60] The mechanism of fracture was a fall on level ground in 87 percent of women and 64 percent of men, with the remainder mostly the result of traffic accidents and falls from a height. Eight Smith's fractures and two Barton's fracture-dislocations were identified.

The final Scandinavian study of note is that of Falch in Norway in 1983.[14] Here, too, the vast majority of fractures were observed to occur in women, with the incidence rising sharply in the years surrounding menopause. Although the incidence of fracture was seen also to increase in men with advancing age, this increase was far less than that in women.

Sennwald reviewed the distal radius fractures treated at the St. Gallen Orthopaedic Clinic from 1980 to 1982.[58] Over these 3 years, 653 fractures were seen. Of these, 200 were in patients aged 30 or under, 102 in patients between 31 and 51, and the remaining 351 in patients 51 or over. In patients below the age of 30, the fracture was seen more often in males (69 percent); between 30 and 51 years men and women were equally affected; and after 51 years, women were greatly affected (86.6 percent).

An epidemiologic study was also performed in the United States by Owen and colleagues.[47] These investigators looked at the incidence of distal radius fractures among the adult residents 35 years and older of Rochester, Minnesota over a 30-year period (1945 to 1974). They recorded 125 distal radius fractures in 1137 residents. Women were affected six times as often as men, and the age-specific incidence in women increased steadily until the age of 60 to 64, when it appeared to level off. Among the men, the incidence rates increased early but stopped rising around ages 50 to 54. In this study as well, the vast majority of fractures occurred from low-energy falls, as only 8 percent were associated with more severe trauma such as motor vehicle accidents.

Risk Factors

As the incidence of distal fractures is highest in aging women, the development of postmenopausal osteoporosis has been implicated by most as a critical risk factor. Yet this has been challenged by several investigators who have suggested that women with distal radius fractures had nearly the same mineral content of bone when compared to age-matched controls without fracture.[21,25,26]

Another explanation, rather than osteoporosis, has been offered which suggests that the pattern of distal radius fracture is consistent with the pattern of falling in the aging population.[10,23] Falls in late middle-aged women are more common than in men, whereas both sexes will be equally affected in extreme old age. Secondly, the change in manner of falling associated with aging may also play a pivotal role in fracture patterns. Middle-aged individuals are more likely than not to attempt to stop their fall, landing on an outstretched hand, whereas the more elderly are less likely to react in such a way and more likely to land directly on their hip.[7]

To support these contentions, two studies have implicated postural instability or "sway" as an important risk factor in developing a fracture of the distal radius.[10,23] These studies suggested that perimenopausal and postmenopausal women with fractures of the distal radius represent a subset of individuals who are prone to recurrent falls when compared to control patients matched for age, sex, and associated medical illnesses. The tendency toward postural instability was not seen to nearly this degree in middle-aged men, implying that they have fewer fractures than women not because they have osteoporosis but because they tend to fall less often.

Classification

There are few areas of skeletal injury where eponymic descriptions have enjoyed such longevity as in fractures of the distal end of the radius.[48] Although their use may provide a comfortable frame of reference for communication among clinicians, they have no longer proven effective in delineating the individual characteristics of specific fractures.

To be effective, a classification system must accurately depict the type and severity of the fracture to serve as a basis both for treatment and for evaluation of the outcome of the treatment.[43] As fractures of the distal radius are commonplace and are readily visualized on routine radiographs, it should come as no surprise that a number of investigators have attempted to create more objective classification systems.[8,16,18,30,38,39,45,46,54,55] While the various classifications have attempted to provide a more accurate representation of the variety and extent of fracture patterns, some have proven more helpful than others in predicting outcome.

Although we believe many prior classifications to be of historic interest, it is relevant to review these, as each in its own way has advanced our understanding of the distal radius fracture.

Historic

As discussed by Lidström in his exhaustive monograph on the distal radius fracture, early classifications were based upon:[30]

1. The fracture line
2. The direction of displacement of the distal fragment

3. The degree of displacement of the fracture
4. The extent of articular involvement
5. Any involvement of the distal radioulnar joint

Destot in 1923 classified the fractures as either anteriorly or posteriorly directed.[11] Within these two major groups, differentiation was made with respect to the direction of the line of the fracture.

Taylor and Parsons in 1938 also divided the fractures into two major groups, but in their classification injuries to the triangular fibrocartilage were considered an important distinguishing feature.[62]

Nissen-Lie in 1939[45] (Fig. 2.1) and Gartland and Werley in 1951[18] (Fig. 2.2A) developed classification systems based on the presence of extraarticular or intraarticular involvement, the presence or absence of comminution, and the presence or absence of angular deformity. Unfortunately, in neither system was a grading established to quantitate the extent of fracture displacement.

Lidström in 1959 extended these criteria into six groupings with descriptive identification of the direction of displacement[30] (Fig. 2.2B). In addition, this classification further expanded on the nature of the articular involvement.

In 1965, Older et al. published a classification system that not only graded dorsal angulation, the presence and extent of comminution, and the direction and extent of displacement, but also identified the presence of shortening of the distal radial fragment in relation to the distal ulna[46] (Fig. 2.2C). This feature has subsequently been considered by some investigators to offer a greater prognostic value of outcome.[22]

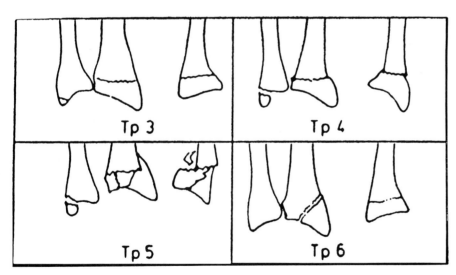

Figure 2.1. *Nissen-Lie classification*

Type 1: A fracture at the junction of the shaft and distal extremity of the radius, i.e., somewhat more proximal than the most common fractures. This type occurs only in children aged 1–15 years and is often the green-stick type (not illustrated).

Type 2: Slipping of the epiphysis with dorsal displacement, often with a dorsally avulsed triangular fragment of the radius. Occurs in the age range 10–20 years (not illustrated).

Type 3: Minimal displacement.

Type 4: Dorsal angulation, extraarticular, no comminution.

Type 5: Intraarticular comminuted.

Type 6: Fractures of the radial styloid.

Type 7: Fracture with dorsal displacement (not illustrated). Reprinted with permission. Solgård S: Classification of distal radius fractures. *Acta Orthop Scand* 56: 249–252, 1984.

Figure 2.2A. *Gartland and Werley classification*

Group 1: Simple Colles' fracture with no involvement of the radial articular surface.
Group 2: Comminuted Colles' fracture with involvement of the radial articular surface.
Group 3: Comminuted Colles' fracture with involvement of the radial articular surface with displacement of the fragments.
Group 4: Extraarticular, undisplaced (added for completeness by Solgård, 1985).

Figure 2.2B. Lidström classification (1959):

Group I: Minimal displacement.
Group II: Fractures with posterior displacement.
Group IIA: Extraarticular, dorsal angulation.
Group IIB: Fracture with merely dorsal angulation involving the joint but without comminution of the articular surface.
Group IIC: Fracture with complete displacement not involving the joint surface.
Group IID: Fracture with complete displacement but without comminution of the articular surface.
Group IIE: Fracture with complete displacement and comminution at the joint surface .
Group III: Fracture with volar displacement (not illustrated).

Figure 2.2C. *Older et al. classification (1965)*

Type I: Nondisplaced.

1. Loss of some volar angulation and up to 5 degree of dorsal angulation.
2. No significant shortening—2 mm or more above the distal radius.

Type II: Displaced with minimal comminution

1. Loss of volar angulation or dorsal displacement of distal fragment.
2. Shortening—usually not below the distal ulna but occasionally up to 3 mm below it.
3. Minimal comminution of dorsal radius.

Type III: Displaced with comminution of the dorsal radius.

1. Comminution of distal radius
2. Shortening—usually below the distal ulna.
3. Comminution of the distal radius fragment—usually not marked and often characterized by large pieces

Type IV: Displaced with severe comminution of the radial head

1. Comminution of dorsal radius marked.
2. Comminution of the distal radial fragment—shattered
3. Shortening—usually 2–8 mm below the distal ulna
4. Poor volar cortex in some cases.

Figure 2.2D. *Frykman classification (1967):*

Type 1: Extraarticular.
Type 2: A Type 1 with fracture of distal ulna.
Type 3: A Radiocarpal joint involved.
Type 4: A Type 3 with fracture of distal ulna.
Type 5: Distal radioulnar joint involved.
Type 6: Type 5 with fracture of distal ulna.
Type 7: Radiocarpal and radioulnar joints both involved.
Type 8: Type 7 with fracture of distal ulna.
Reprinted with permission. Jenkins NH: The unstable Colles' fracture. *J Hand Surg* 14B: 149–154, 1989 Edinburgh, UK: Churchill Livingstone.

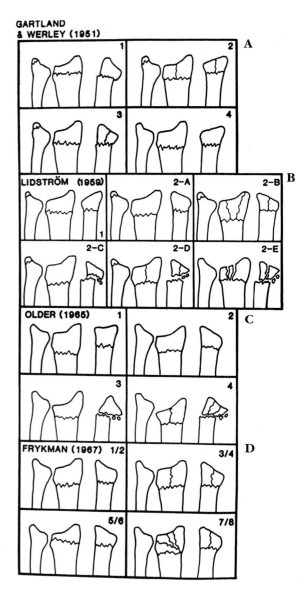

In 1967 Frykman established a system of classification that identified individual involvement of the radiocarpal and radioulnar joints as well as the presence or absence of a fracture of the ulnar styloid process.[17] While this system has had widespread use in subsequent literature, it unfortunately does not allow quantification of the extent or direction of the initial fracture displacement, the degree of comminution, or shortening of the distal fragment (Fig. 2.2D). As such, it suffers in its ability to offer a prognostic value in evaluating the outcome of the proposed treatment for the individual fracture.

Of interest, Colles-type fractures formed the predominant lesion classified by these early investigators. In fact, little specific attention was paid to radiocarpal articular fracture-dislocations since Barton's[2] and Letenneur's[28] early writings. Ehalt in 1935 depicted a number of fracture patterns similar to those described by Barton.[13] Thomas in 1957 included the volar fracture-dislocation as his Type II classification of distal radius fractures with volar displacement[63] (Fig. 2.3).

Contemporary Classifications

More contemporary classifications have been developed for extraarticular as well as intraarticular fractures, emphasizing both fracture patterns and treatment issues. Jenkins in 1989 in a study reviewing prior classifications added his own based upon the presence and distribution of comminution[22] (Fig. 2.4). Jenkins continued the emphasis on the relationship of comminution to the intrinsic stability of the fracture following manipulative reduction.[46,59]

An additional classification was developed by Rayhack, which further emphasizes prognostic aspects of the different fracture groupings.[51] His classification differentiates extra- and intraarticular fractures, displaced and non-displaced fractures, and the reducibility and stability of the individual patterns (Fig. 2.5).

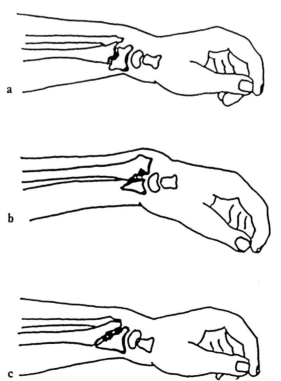

Figure 2.3. *Thomas classification of volar displaced fractures*

A. Type I: An extraarticular fracture with palmar angulation.
B. Type II: An intraarticular fracture with volar and proximal displacement of the distal fragment along with the carpus.
C. Type III: An extraarticular fracture with volar displacement of the distal fragment and carpus.

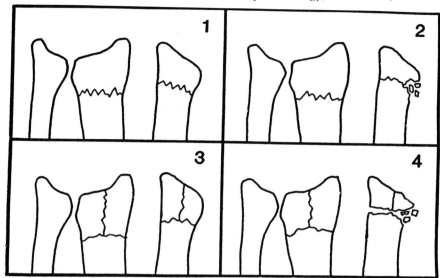

Figure 2.4. *Jenkins classification based entirely upon comminution*

Group 1: No radiographically visible comminution.
Group 2: Comminution of the dorsal radial cortex without comminution of the distal fragment.
Group 3: Comminution of the fracture fragment without significant involvement of the dorsal cortex.
Group 4: Comminution of both the distal fragment and the dorsal cortex. As the fracture line involves the distal fracture fragments in groups 3 and 4, intraarticular involvement is very common within these groups Such involvement is not, however, inevitable and nor does it affect the fracture's placement within the classification.

Reprinted with permission. Jenkins NH: The unstable Colles' fracture. *J Hand Surg* 14B: 149–154, 1989 Edinburgh UK: Churchill Livingstone.

Fifure 2.5. *Rayhack classification of distal radius fractures*:
Type 1: Nonarticular, nondisplaced.
        Nonarticular, displaced.
        1. Reducible,* stable.
        2. Reducible,* unstable.
        3. Irreducible.*
Type 3: Articular, nondisplaced.
Type 4: Articular, displaced. A.Reducible,* stable. B.Reducible,* unstable. C.Irreducible.*

Reprinted with permission. Rayhack J: Symposium Distal Radius Fractures. In Cooney W ed. *Contemporary Orthopaedics*. Vol. 21: July 1990. Bobit Publishing Co.

PROPOSED RAYHACK CLASSIFICATION
OF DISTAL RADIAL FRACTURES

I.   Non-articular   Non-displaced

II. Non-articular   Displaced

     A. Reducible*   Stable
     B. Reducible*   Unstable
     C. Irreducible*

III. Articular   Non-Displaced

IV. Articular   Displaced

     A. Reducible*   Stable
     B. Reducible*   Unstable
     C. Irreducible*

*(By ligamentotaxis only)

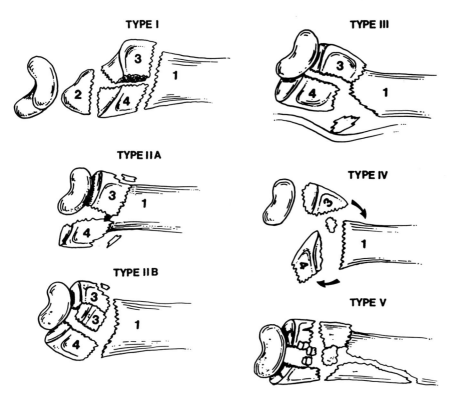

Figure 2.6. *Melone classification of intraarticular fracture*
Type I: Stable fracture. Non-displaced or variable displacement of the medial complex
     as a unit. No comminution. Stable after closed reduction
Type II: Unstable "Die-punch." Moderate or severe displacement of the medial com-
     plex as a unit with comminution of both anterior and posterior cortices.
     Separation of the medial complex from the styloid fragment. Radial shortening
     > 5–10 mm. Considerable angulation usually exceeding 20 degrees.
     IIA: Reducible.
     IIB: Irreducible.
Type III: "Spike" fracture. Unstable. Displacement of the medial complex as a unit as
     well as displacement of an additional spike fragment from the comminuted
     radial shaft.
Type IV: Split fracture. Unstable. Medial complex severely comminuted with wide
     separation and/or rotation of the distal and palmar fragments. Type V: Explosion
     injuries.

Reprinted with permission. Melone CP Jr: Distal radius fractures. Patterns of articular
fragmentation. *Orthop Clin No Am* 24: 239–253, 1993. Philadelphia: WB Saunders Co.

In 1984 Melone observed that the components of the radiocarpal articular
fractures appeared to fall into four basic parts[39] (Fig. 2.6):

1. The radial shaft
2. The radial styloid
3. The dorsal medial fragment
4. The palmar medial fragment

The medial fragments and their strong ligamentous attachments with the
proximal carpal bones and the ulnar styloid have been termed the "medial
complex" by Melone. The extent and direction of these fragments form the
basis of this classification as well as a prognostic view of the fracture type's
reducibility and intrinsic stability.

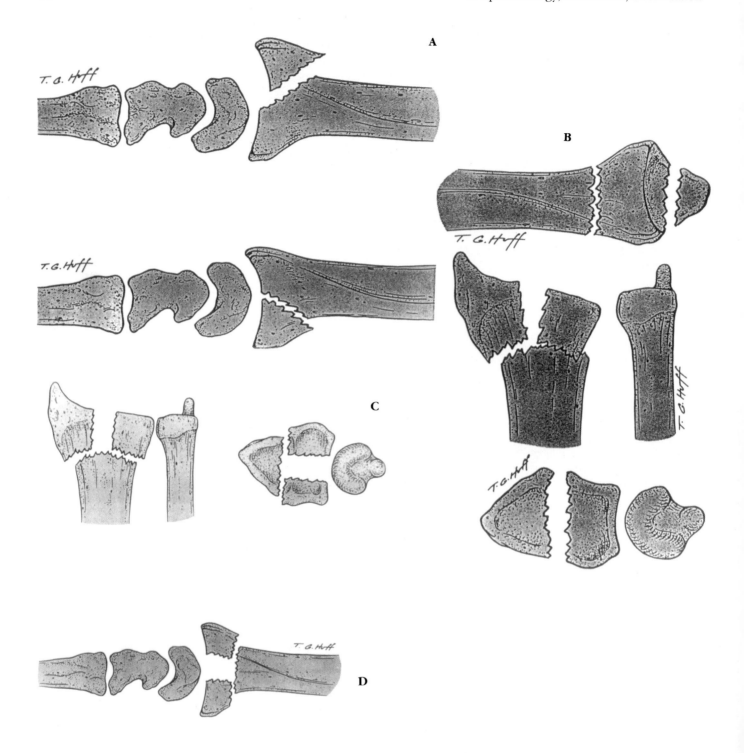

Figure 2.7. *McMurtry classification of intraarticular fractures.*
A. Two-part: the opposite portion of the radiocarpal joint remains intact.
B. Three-part the lunate and scaphoid facets of the distal radius separate from each other and the proximal portion of the radius.
C. Four-part, similar to the three-part except that the lunate facet is further divided into volar and dorsal fragments.
D. Five-part: includes a wide variety of comminuted fragments (not illustrated).

McMurtry in 1990 defined an intraarticular fracture to include any fracture that extends into the radiocarpal or radioulnar joint and is displaced more than 1 to 2 mm.[38] These fractures can further be subdivided into (1) two-part, (2) three-part, (3) four-part, and (4) five-part fractures. A "part" was defined as a fragment of bone of sufficient size to be functionally significant and capable of being manipulated and/or internally stabilized (Fig. 2.7).

An additional classification specific to intraarticular fractures was developed by the Mayo Clinic, emphasizing the role of the specific articular contact areas.[42] The classification was formulated to include the specific articular surfaces of the distal radius and highlight fracture components involving these articulations (Fig. 2.8).

A "universal classification" was proposed by Cooney et al. in a published symposium on fractures of the distal end of the radius[8] in 1990. The classification was based on the basic divisions of intra- versus extraarticular and stable versus unstable fractures. The extraarticular fractures were identified as Type I (undisplaced, stable) and Type II (displaced, unstable). Intraarticular fractures were also separated into intraarticular, undisplaced, stable (Type III) and intraarticular, displaced, unstable (Type IV). The Type IV fracture was further subdivided into Type IVA for intraarticular, stable fractures after reduc-

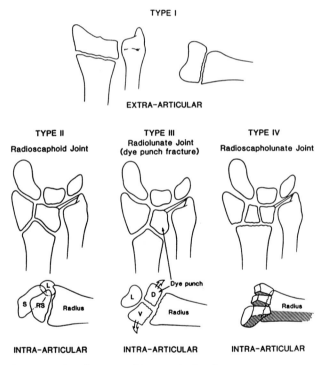

Figure 2.8. *The Mayo classification of intraarticular fractures*
Type I: An intraarticular undisplaced fracture of the radiocarpal joint.
Type II: A displaced intraarticular fracture of the radioscaphoid joint involving a significant portion of the articular surface of the distal radius (more than a radial styloid fracture.
Type III: A displaced intraarticular fracture of the radiolunate joint that often presents as a "die-punch" fracture of the lunate fossa. A displaced fracture component into the distal radioulnar joint is common.
Type IV: A displaced intraarticular fracture involving both radioscaphoid joint surfaces and usually involving the sigmoid fossa of the distal radioulnar joint. This fracture is usually comminuted.

Reprinted with permission. Missakian M, Cooney WP, Amadio PC et al: Open reduction and internal fixation for distal radius fractures. J Hand Surg 17: 745–755, 1992.

Figure 2.9. Universal classification of distal radius fractures as proposed by Cooney et al.

Type I: Nonarticular, undisplaced
Type II: Nonarticular, displaced.
Type III: Intraarticular, displaced
Type IVA: Intraarticular, reducible, stable
Type IVB: Intraarticular, displaced, reducible, unstable.
Type IVC: Intraarticular, irreducible. Type IVD Complex (not illustrated).

Reprinted with permission. Cooney WP, Agee JM, Hastings H et al. Symposium: Management of intraarticular fractures of the distal radius. *Contemp Orthop* 21: 71–104, 1990. Bobit Publishing Co.

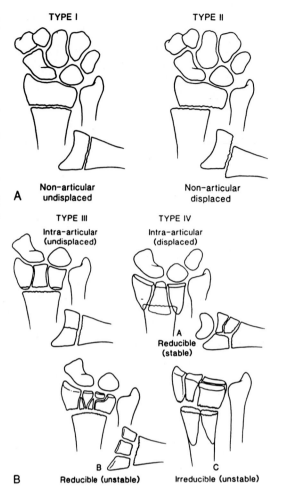

tion; Type IVB for unstable fractures after reduction; Type IVC for unstable and irreducible fractures; and Type IVD for complex fractures (Fig. 2.9).

Another treatment-oriented classification is that of Sennwald and Segmüller who in 1984 established a classification based, in their view, on "anatomical, physiological, and mechanical foundations" to help formulate treatment considerations[58] (Table 2.2). They categorized the quality of bone as either normally mineralized immature, normally mineralized adult, or bone under-

Table 2.2. Sennwald and Segmüller classification.

Quality of bone	Site	Typology
Normally mineralized, immature	Metaphyseal, epiphyseal	Epiphysis—single fragment (mono block) Epiphysis—marginal fracture (split block)
Normally mineralized Adult bone	Metaphyseal, epiphyseal	Epiphysis—split fracture
Men < 60 Women < 40		Epiphysis—single fragment *Simple*—Barton or split *Comminuted*—
Bone undergoing demineralization Men ≥ 60 Women ≥ 40	Metaphyseal	Epiphysis—single fragment (impacted)

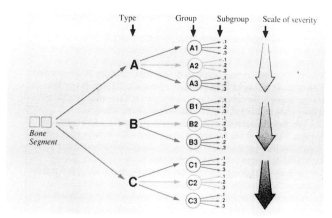

Figure 2.10. *The comprehensive classification of fractures of long bones*[43]
Types: A,B,C.
Groups: $A_1,A_2,A_3,B_1,B_2,B_3,C_1,C_2,C_3$
Subgroups: .1, .2, .3. The arrows show the increasing gravity, difficulty of management, and less favorable prognosis as they progress from A_1 to C_3.

going demineralization. They further identified the site of fracture (metaphyseal or diaphyseal) and extent of fracture fragments ("monoblock" or single-fragment split fracture such as Barton's, or comminuted fractures).

Perhaps the most inclusive classification of both intra- and extraarticular fractures has been developed by Maurice Muller and collaborators.[15,43] This system is adaptable for computerized documentation of all fractures of the long bones. Each bone and segment of the individual bone is given a number, with the forearm coded 2 and its distal segment 3. Three basic types (A, B, C), nine main groups (A_1, A_2, A_3; B_1, B_2, B_3; C_1, C_2, C_3), and 27 subgroups (.1, .2, .3) can be identified. Documentation of additional ulnar lesions will produce 144 possible combinations of distal radius fractures (Fig. 2.10).

The three basic types include extraarticular fractures (Type A), partial articular fractures (Type B), and complete articular fractures (Type C) (Fig. 2.11).

The main groups and subdivisions further define each possible fracture pattern.

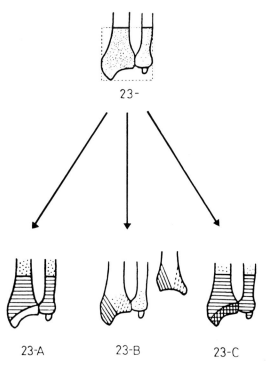

Figure 2.11. *Distal radius*
A: Extraarticular fracture.
B: Partial articular fracture.
C: Complete articular fracture.

A   **EXTRA-ARTICULAR:** Fractures neither affect the articular surface of the radiocarpal nor the radioulnar joints.

A1 Extra-articular fracture, of the ulna, radius intact

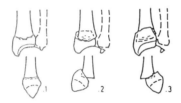

   1 styloid process
   2 metaphyseal simple
   3 metaphyseal multifragmentary

A2 Extra-articular fracture, of the radius, simple and impacted

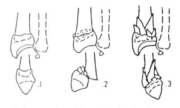

   1 without any tilt
   2 with dorsal tilt (Pouteau-Colles)
   3 with volar tilt (Goyran-Smith)

A3 Extra-articular fracture, of the radius, multifragmentary

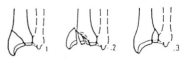

   1 impacted with axial shortening
   2 with a wedge
   3 complex

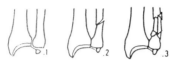 **B**   **SIMPLE ARTICULAR:** Fracture affects a portion of the articular surface, but the continuity of the metaphysis and epiphysis is intact

B1 Partial articular fracture, of the radius, sagittal

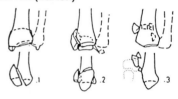

   1 lateral simple
   2 lateral multifragmentary
   3 medial

B2 Partial articular fracture, of the radius, dorsal rim (Barton)

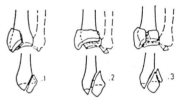

   1 simple
   2 with lateral sagittal fracture
   3 with dorsal dislocation of the carpus

B3 Partial articular fracture, of the radius, volar rim (reverse Barton, Goyrand-Smith II)

   1 simple, with a small fragment
   2 simple, with a large fragment
   3 multifragmentary

Type A: Extraarticular fractures: The fracture involves neither the radiocarpal nor the radioulnar joint (Fig. 2.12).

Type B: Partial articular fractures: The fracture involve only part of the articular surface, while the rest of that surface remains attached to the diaphysis.

Type C: Complete articular fractures: The articular suface is disrupted and completely separated from the diaphysis. The severity of these fractures depends on whether its articular and metaphyseal components are simple or multifragmentary.

Classification of Ulnar Lesions

In most cases, it is the fracture of the distal radius that will be primarily responsible for the final outcome. Therefore, the different types of associated injuries involving the distal ulna and radioulnar articulation have not generally been included in classifications (Fig. 2.15). These include:

C   COMPLEX ARTICULAR: Fracture affects the joint surfaces (radio-ulnar and/or radio-carpal) and the metaphyseal area

c

C1 Complete articular fracture, of the radius, articular simple, metaphyseal simple

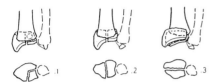

1 postero-medial articular fragment
2 sagittal articular fracture line
3 frontal articular fracture line

C2 Complete articular fracture, of the radius, articular simple, metaphyseal multifragmentary

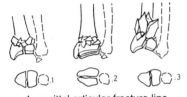

1 sagittal articular fracture line
2 frontal articular fracture line
3 extending into the diaphysis

C3 Complete articular fracture, of the radius, multifragmentary

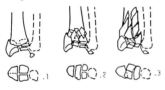

1 metaphyseal simple
2 metaphyseal multifragmentary
3 extending into the diaphysis

Figure 2.12. (*far left*) the distal radius is shown in the anatomic position. The reader is looking at the *palmar surface* in the anteroposterior views and at the radial border of the forearm in the lateral views so that dorsal is to the left and palmar is to the right. Type A—See figure text.

Figure 2.13. (*center*) Type B—See figure text.

Figure 2.14. (*right*) Type C—See figure text.

1. Tear of the triangular fibrocartilage and/or distal radioulnar ligaments
2. Fracture of the ulnar styloid and/or distal radioulnar ligaments
3. Fracture of the neck of the ulna
4. Metaphyseal multifragmented fracture of the ulna
5. Fracture through the ulnar head
6. Multifragmented articular fracture of the distal ulna

Many fractures of the distal radius are associated with either a tear of the triangular fibrocartilage and/or an avulsion fracture of the ulnar styloid. An ulnar styloid fracture will be seen in many distal radius fractures, whereas a fracture of the neck of the distal ulna occurs in only 3 to 5 percent of cases. In addition, if initial angulation or displacement of the distal radial fragment is greater than 25 to 30 degrees in the sagittal plane, a complete disruption of the volar and dorsal radioulnar ligament is almost always the case, provided there is no associated fracture of the ulnar neck.

Figure 2.15. Classification of ulnar lesions—
See text.

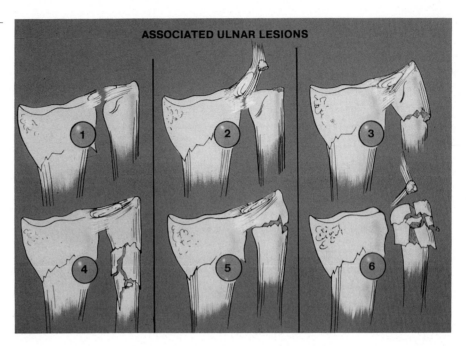

As a greater understanding of distal radius fracture develops, it is clear that the ulnar lesions should be recorded, because they may require specific treatment at the time of the accident or because they may be responsible for painful posttraumatic sequelae after the fracture has healed. With the exception of the A_1 group, which contains the isolated extraarticular fracture of the distal ulna, the specific ulnar lesion should be added to the distal radius fracture classification.

Authors' Preference

Two classification systems have evolved which identify the fracture types to a large degree on the basis of the mechanism of the fracture. Castaing introduced this approach in 1964, identifying extra- and intraarticular patterns, direction of deformity, and various patterns of distal ulna and radioulnar joint injury[6] (Fig. 2.16).

Castaing's approach has been expanded by Fernandez and forms the basis of the authors' approach to fractures of the distal radius.[15]

Fernandez Classification

Despite the exhaustive capabilities of computerized documentation of the Comprehensive Classification of Fractures (CCF),[43] in its present form it does not provide treatment recommendations. For this reason, a more simplified approach has been developed and will form the basis for the discussion of distal radius fracture treatment in this book.

It is our feeling that the understanding of the mechanism of the distal radius fracture has enormous importance in the overall management of the problem. It is for this reason, more than any other, that we have chosen to base our classification groups in a way that emphasizes the mechanism of injury rather than the more traditional radiologic characteristics. As a greater understanding of distal radius fractures develops, it is apparent that associated ligamentous injury, carpal bone subluxation or fracture, and concomitant soft tissue lesions tend to occur in direct relationship to the force and direction of the injury.

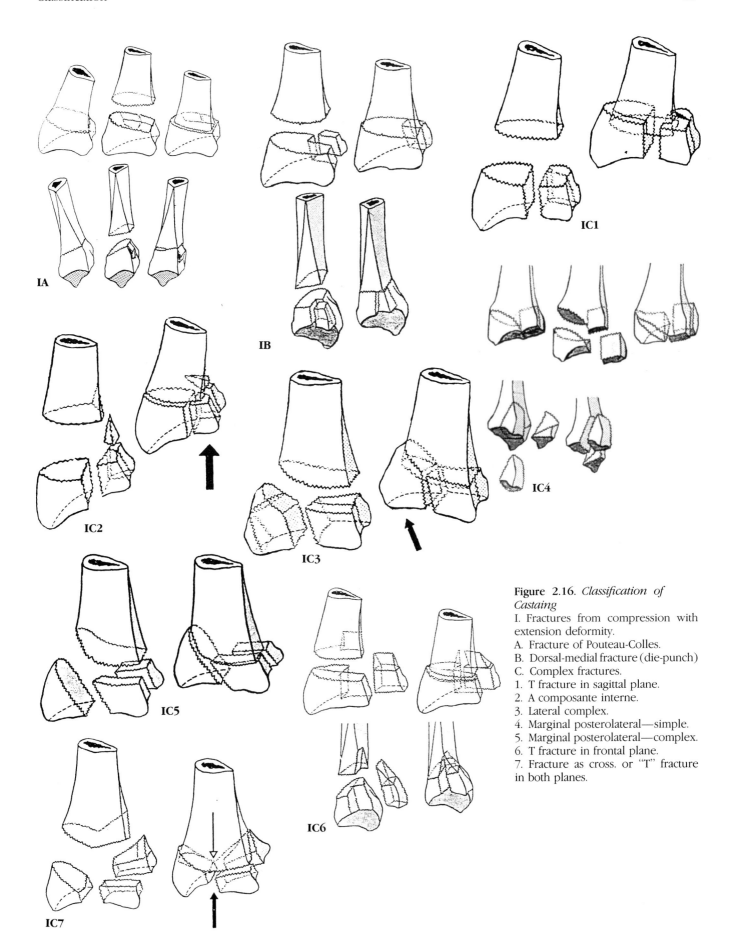

Figure 2.16. *Classification of Castaing*

I. Fractures from compression with extension deformity.

A. Fracture of Pouteau-Colles.

B. Dorsal-medial fracture (die-punch)

C. Complex fractures.

1. T fracture in sagittal plane.

2. A composante interne.

3. Lateral complex.

4. Marginal posterolateral—simple.

5. Marginal posterolateral—complex.

6. T fracture in frontal plane.

7. Fracture as cross. or "T" fracture in both planes.

II. Fractures from compression with flexion deformity.
A. Fractures of Goyrand-Smith.
B. Anterior marginal—simple.
C. Anterior marginal—antero-externe (simple) D.Anterior marginal—complex

Reprinted with permission. Castaing J: Les fractures récente de l'extrémíte inferieure du radius chez l'adulte:. *Rev Chir Orthop* 5. 581–696, 1964.

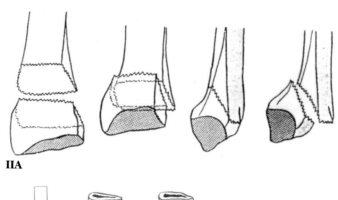

IIA

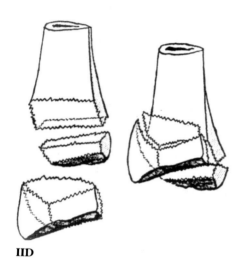

IID

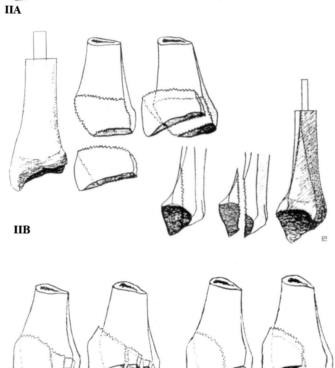

IIB

IIC

Assessment of the mechanism of injury has in fact been a matter of interest since it became apparent that these injuries were fractures and not dislocations.[9,31,44,49,52,53,61]

Observers have long since recognized that "luxations" and/or fractures of the distal end of the radius are often associated with a direct impact on the extended hand and wrist. It is curious to read early observations of situations that resulted in a distal radius fracture. Take, for example, MacLeod's description in 1879:[34]

A young man contended with an older and stronger man in a test of strength by placing elbows on a table, interlocking fingers and then pressing back upon each other, palm to palm. The hand of the young man became violently extended until finally something gave way, with development of sharp pain in the radius and with the well-marked deformity characteristic of fracture of the inferior extremity of that bone.

Some time later, in 1917, Pilcher wrote:[49]

The writer [Pilcher] had his own interest in it [radius fracture] as a boy when one of his playmates fell upon his outstretched hand and was picked up with a "broken and crooked wrist".

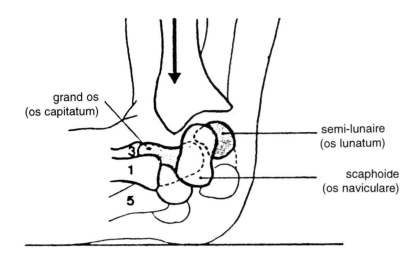

grand os
(os capitatum)

semi-lunaire
(os lunatum)

scaphoide
(os naviculare)

Figure 2.17. The theory of Destot is that the force of the body weight is transmitted through the carpus directly to the distal metaphysis of the radius where the cortex is thinnest. Reprinted with permission. Castaing J: Les fractures récente de l'extrémité inferieure du radius chez l'adulte. *Rev Chir Orthop* 5. 581–696, 1964.

When immediately after graduating he spent some months in a country district looking for practice, he found it when one of his neighbors fell out of an apple tree and sustained a wrist fracture.

Again, some years later, he essayed his fortune in a city, he was helped mightily by a friend who had the misfortune to fall down a flight of icy steps one wintry day and fractured the base of his radius.

Early investigators attempted to understand the fracture mechanism by reproducing distal radius fractures in cadavers, for the most part in static loading experiments. As detailed in the monographs of Lidström (1959)[30] and later Frykman (1967),[17] several basic theories developed from the early experiments.

1. Blow and Counter-Blow Theory

This concept was initially put forth by Dupuytren (1834)[12] and supported by several succeeding investigators.[2,11,35,44,57,64] This theory suggested that it is the force of the body weight which is transmitted through the carpus directly to the distal radius specifically at the distal metaphysis where the cortex is thinnest. With the advent of x-ray, Destot and Gallois observed that when the wrist was extended, the carpal bones came up against the distal radius at the moment of fracture at the same time as the radial head impacted the distal humerus, with transmission of the force of impact directly to the lower part of the radius[11] (Fig. 2.17).

2. Ligament Avulsion Theory

This concept was first suggested early on by several investigators, including LeComte (1861).[27] The basis of this theory centered on the fact that the close anatomic relationship between the olecranon and distal humerus resulted in the ulna rather than the radius absorbing more of the impact of the fall. LeComte suggested that the force of injury was transmitted to the radius and volar radiocarpal ligaments, which then produced a traction force sufficient to create a fracture of the distal radius. This theory was not without its early critics.[2,32,41]

3. Bending Fracture Theory

Meyer in 1925 suggested that the characteristics of the distal radius fracture were influenced by three factors: the position of the hand, the surface upon which the impact occurred, and the velocity of the force.[41] Of interest is that he also observed the influence of the loss of integrity of the distal radioulnar joint on fracture displacement.

Lewis in 1950 expanded this approach by suggesting that at the moment of impact, the hand remains in place while the kinetic energy of the fall manifests itself as continued forward movement of the body.[29] The hyperextended position of the hand and wrist places an increased load on the volar radiocarpal ligaments while the proximal carpal row is pressed against the end of the distal radius. Using the analogy of a cantilever beam loaded beyond its limit of elasticity, Lewis considered failure of the beam (or distal radius) to have occurred as a result of a bending moment (Fig. 2.18).

The influence of the position of the hand and wrist at the moment of impact was also emphasized by Lilienfeldt (1885).[31] He noted that the type of fracture could be altered by changing one of two aspects, i.e., the position of the hand and the angle between the forearm and the surface of impact. He was able to reproduce fractures of the distal radius in cadavers when the angle of impact between the forearm and the surface on which the hand rested was between 60 and 90 degrees. If the hand rested in ulnar deviation, the fracture extended through the radial styloid, whereas ulnar styloid fractures appeared when the hand was in radial deviation at the time of loading.

Lilienfeldt also noted that he could produce a scaphoid fracture if the angle between the forearm and the surface of the impact was at least 90 degrees and the hand and wrist were both extended and radially deviated.

Frykman studied the mechanism of the distal radius fracture in both static and dynamic experiments in cadaveric models. He confirmed the observation of Lilienfeldt regarding the effect of the position of the hand and wrist and the development of a distal radius fracture versus a carpal bone fracture.

Castaing suggested that there was a certain amount of validity to each of the early theories of fracture mechanism. He additionally emphasized the possible

Figure 2.18. The concept of Lewis regarding the mechanism of distal radius fracture was based upon an analogy that the forearm in the position of impact was similar to a cantilever beam similarly loaded.

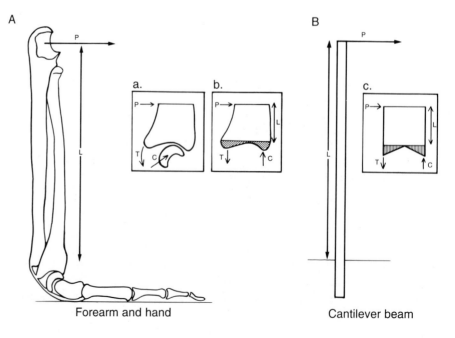

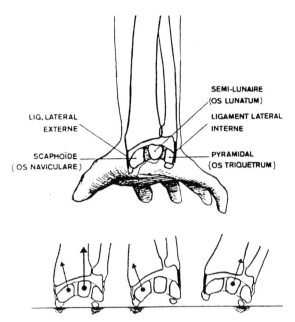

LIG. LATERAL
EXTERNE

SCAPHOÏDE
(OS NAVICULARE)

SEMI-LUNAIRE
(OS LUNATUM)

LIGAMENT LATERAL
INTERNE

PYRAMIDAL
(OS TRIQUETRUM)

Figure 2.19. Castaing suggested that the position of the hand at impact may be a major factor in the type of articular injury produced.

Reprinted with permission. Castaing J: Les fractures récentes de l'extrémité inferieure du radius chez l'adulte. *Rev Chir Orthope* No. 5: 581–696, 1964.

effect of the loading force passing asymmetrically through either the thenar or hypothenar eminence or producing somewhat different fracture patterns[6] (Fig. 2.19).

Castaing also supported the observations of others[18,36,49] who emphasized the rotational force associated with the production of dorsally displaced fractures, in most instances the distal fragment supinating with the pivot point being the distal radioulnar joint.

Based upon the specific mechanism of injury, the authors have divided the types of distal radius fractures into five major groups:

Type I: Bending fractures: The thin metaphyseal cortex fails due to tensile stresses with the opposite cortex, undergoing a certain degree of comminution (extraarticular Colles-Pouteau or Smith-Goyrand fractures) (Fig. 2.20).

Type II: Shearing Fractures of the Joint Surface: (Barton's and reverse Barton's fractures, radial styloid) (Fig. 2.21).

Figure 2.20. A: Schematic of a bending fracture of the metaphysis.

b. Bending fracture with dorsal displacement of the distal fragment in a 70-year-old female

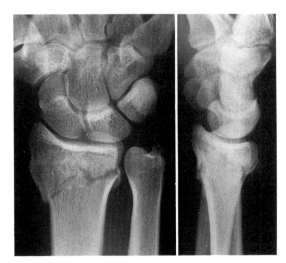

B

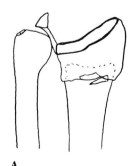

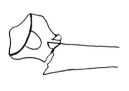

A

Figure 2.21. A. Schematic of a shearing fracture of the joint surface.
B. shearing fracture of the articular surface in a 28–year-old male from a motor-cycle accident

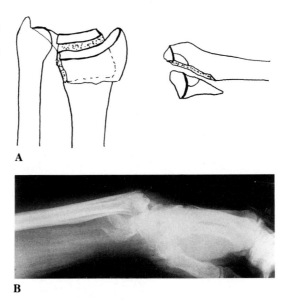

Figure 2.22. A. Schematic of a compression fracture.
B: compression fracture of the articular surface with a sagittal and coronal split of the articular surface in a 52–year-old female

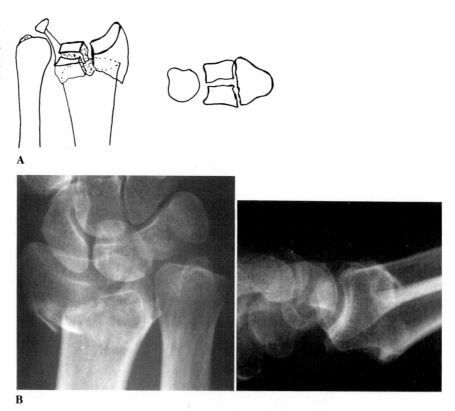

Type III: Compression Fractures of the Joint Surface: The articular surfaces are disrupted, with impaction of the subchondral and metaphyseal cancellous bone (intraarticular comminuted fractures of the distal radius) (Fig. 2.22).

Type IV: Avulsion Fractures: Fractures associated with ligamentous attachments (ulnar, radial, styloid) (Fig. 2.23).

Type V: Combined Fractures: Combinations of bending, compression, shearing, or avulsion mechanisms; usually high-velocity injuries (Fig. 2.24).

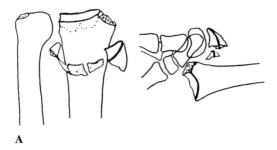

A

Figure 2.23. A: Schematic of avulsion fractures.
B: Complex fracture-dislocation of the radiocarpal joint with avulsion fracture and ligamentous injury associated with a fall from a roof by a laborer.

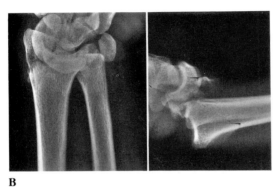

B

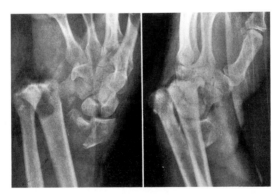

A *FR '90*

Figure 2.24. A: Schematic of a combined fracture.
B₁ & B₂: Two examples of complex fracture

B1

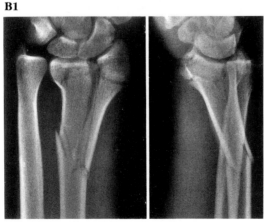

B2

Bending Fractures of the Metaphysis

With a fall on the extended hand and wrist, two forces will concentrate at the level of the wrist. These are the body thrust transmitted along the long axis of the radius, and an opposite reaction force occurring from the impact of the hand against the ground and acting in a proximal direction across the carpal bones. The impact of the scapholunate carpal complex transmits the forces of impact to the dorsal aspect of the radial articular facets, including a bending stress at the level of the metaphysis. The volar radial cortex fails due to tensile stresses, followed by compression on the dorsal aspect of the metaphysis, producing a variable amount of comminution of the dorsal cortex just proximal to the bony ridges of the extensor compartments. As a result, a certain amount of impaction of the cancellous bone in the dorsal aspect of the distal fragment is inevitable. This impaction or collapse of the cancellous bone of the distal fragment, particularly in the osteopenic patient, will result in a bony defect which becomes responsible for the commonly observed secondary displacement of the fracture following the initial reduction (Fig. 2.25).

We support the observations of Mayer,[36] Gartland and Werley,[18] and Castaing,[6] among others, that associated disruption of the distal radioulnar joint, when present, will add to the intrinsic instability of the distal metaphyseal fracture fragment along with playing an integral role in the postreduction stability of the fracture.

A fall on the outstretched hand with the forearm supinated and the elbow in

Figure 2.25. The mechanism of the bending fracture is that of the force of the body transmitted along the long axis of the radius against an opposite reaction force resulting from the impact of the hand against the ground (Colles' fracture).

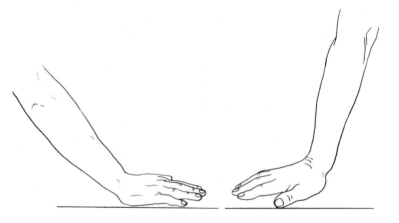

Figure 2.26. A fall on the outstretched hand with the forearm supinated and elbow in extension or a backwards fall onto the flexed wrist will produce a bending fracture with anterior displacement (Smith-Goyrand fracture).

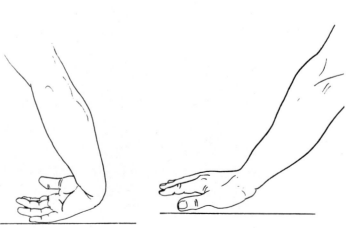

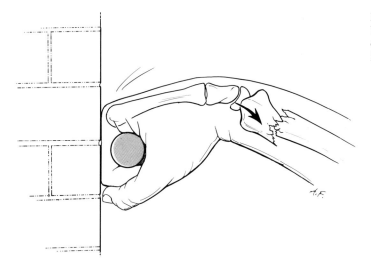

Figure 2.27. The extraarticular palmar bending fracture (Smith-Goyrand) can also occur from a direct blow to the clenched fist with the wrist in some palmar flexion.

extension will transmit the tension forces to the dorsal aspect of the metaphysis, with the compression forces now found on the volar or anterior surfaces (Fig. 2.26). This may also be seen to occur with a direct blow to the clenched fist, with the wrist held in a slightly palmar-flexed position (Fig. 2.27). This extra-articular bending fracture, long known as the Smith-Goyrand fracture, may have the metaphyseal line either transverse or slightly oblique, with comminution of the volar cortex to be expected in the osteopenic patient. In the frontal plane, either radial or ulnar deviation of the distal fragment may be seen, as well as pronation of the fragment with respect to the radial shaft.

Shearing Fractures of the Joint Surface

In younger patients, the mechanism described for volar bending fractures can shear off the volar lip of the radial articular surface, producing an articular fragment in conjunction with a volar subluxation of the carpus. This is due as well to the fact that the strong volar radiocarpal ligaments remain intact. This was described early on by Barton and also by Letenneur and is also known as the *fracture marginale antérieure*. These are extremely unstable because of the obliquity of the fracture line and are suitable for internal fixation.

Compression Fractures of the Joint Surface

Axial compression forces of a magnitude greater than those responsible for bending fractures are responsible for the more complex intraarticular fractures of the articular surface. These forces will ordinarily be associated with falls from a greater height, and comminution may be seen to extend into the distal third of the radius. Although the morphology of the intraarticular, disruption may vary, distinct patterns of articular injury have been identified by several investigators, including Castaing and Melone.

In some cases, disimpaction of the cartilage-bearing fragments may require limited open reduction and cancellous bone grafting to fill the resultant defect.

Avulsion Fractures of the Ligament Attachments

These fractures are a constant component of radiocarpal dislocations caused by a wrist torsional injury.[37] Radial or ulnar styloid fractures will be found in conjunction with radiocarpal fracture-dislocations. These injuries will generally require open reduction and stable fixation of the avulsed radial fragments. The high-energy nature of the fractures will often lead to soft tissue problems and the need for associated external fixation.

Combined Fractures

These injuries are the sequelae of high-energy impact and may present with one or more of the above-mentioned features; likely a combination of methods of fixation should be selected for treatment. Additional skeletal or soft tissue injury is commonplace.

Distal Radioulnar Joint Injuries

The authors have also applied a treatment-oriented approach to the classification of associated distal radioulnar joint (DRUJ) lesions. Since the final outcome following fracture union depends primarily on residual joint stability and posttraumatic arthritis, the classification parameters center upon the presence or absence of either distal radioulnar joint subluxation or dislocation of the ulnar head due to concomitant rupture of the triangular fibrocartilage complex and capsular ligaments and the degree of joint surface involvement (intraarticular fracture of the sigmoid notch and/or ulnar head).

Three basic types of distal radioulnar joint lesions have been established, depending upon the residual stability of the distal radioulnar joint after the fracture of the distal radius has been adequately reduced and stabilized. This implies that the anatomic relationships of the sigmoid notch to the ulnar head have been reestablished through an adequate restoration of the radial length and the sagittal and frontal tilt of the distal radial fragment. In certain high velocity injuries, these lesions may combine.

Type I: **Stable Lesions:** The distal radioulnar joint is clinically stable and the radiograph shows the radioulnar joint to be congruous. The primary stabilizers of the joint, including the triangular fibrocartilage complex and capsular ligaments, are intact. These include: (a) avulsion of the tip of the ulnar styloid and (b) a stable fracture of the neck of the ulna.

Type II: **Unstable Lesions:** The distal radioulnar joint is subluxated or dislocated. There is either (a) a massive substance tear of the triangular fibrocartilage complex or (b) an avulsion fracture of the base of the ulnar styloid.

Type III: **Potentially Unstable Lesions:** These reflect skeletal disruption of the distal radioulnar articular surfaces at either (a) the sigmoid notch (four-part fracture of the distal radius) or (b) the ulnar head.

The authors believe that these classifications further provide insight into the character of the individual fracture based upon displacement patterns, stability versus instability, associated lesions, including the distal radioulnar joint lesions, and even the children's fracture equivalent. This can be put into the form of a useful table to identify the specific aspects of the various subtypes (Tables 2.3 and 2.4).

Table 2.3. A Practical, Treatment Oriented Classification of Fractures of the Distal Radius and Associated Distal Radioulnar Joint Lesions. By Diego L. FERNANDEZ, M.D. PD

FRACTURE TYPES (ADULTS) BASED ON THE MECHANISM OF INJURY		CHILDREN FRACTURE EQUIVALENT	STABILITY/ INSTABILITY: high risk of secondary displacement after initial adequate reduction	DISPLACEMENT PATTERN	NUMBER OF FRAGMENTS	ASSOCIATED LESIONS: carpal ligament, fractures, median, ulnar nerve, tendons, ipsilat. fx upper extremity, compartment syndrome	RECOMMENDED TREATMENT
TYPE I BENDING FRACTURE OF THE METAPHYSIS		DISTAL FOREARM FRACTURE SALTER II	STABLE UNSTABLE	NON-DISPLACED DORSALLY (Colles-Pouteau) VOLARLY (Smith) PROXIMAL COMBINED	ALWAYS 2 MAIN FRAGMENTS + VARYING DEGREE OF METAPHYSEAL COMMINUTION (instability)	UNCOMMON	CONSERVATIVE (stable fxs) PERCUTANEOUS PINNING (extra- or intrafocal) EXTERNAL FIXATION (exceptionally BONE GRAFT)
TYPE II SHEARING FRACTURE OF THE JOINT SURFACE		SALTER IV	UNSTABLE	DORSAL RADIAL VOLAR PROXIMAL COMBINED	TWO-PART THREE-PART COMMINUTED	LESS UNCOMMON	OPEN REDUCTION SCREW-/PLATE FIXATION
TYPE III COMPRESSION FRACTURE OF THE JOINT SURFACE		SALTER III, IV, V	STABLE UNSTABLE	NON-DISPLACED DORSAL RADIAL VOLAR PROXIMAL COMBINED	TWO-PART THREE-PART FOUR-PART COMMINUTED	COMMON	CONSERVATIVE CLOSED, LIMITED, ARTHROSCOPIC ASSISTED, OR EXTENSILE OPEN REDUCTION PERCUTANEOUS PINS COMBINED EXTERNAL AND INTERNAL FIXATION BONE GRAFT
TYPE IV AVULSION FRACTURES, RADIO CARPAL FRACTURE DISLOCATION		VERY RARE	UNSTABLE	DORSAL RADIAL VOLAR PROXIMAL COMBINED	TWO-PART (radial styloid ulnar styloid) THREE-PART (volar, dorsal margin) COMMINUTED	FREQUENT	CLOSED OR OPEN REDUCTION PIN OR SCREW FIXATION TENSION WIRING
TYPE V COMBINED FRACTURES (I - II - III - IV) HIGH-VELOCITY INJURY		VERY RARE	UNSTABLE	DORSAL RADIAL VOLAR PROXIMAL COMBINED	COMMINUTED and/or BONE LOSS (frequently intraarticular, open, seldom extraarticular)	ALWAYS PRESENT	COMBINED METHOD

Table 2.4. Fracture of the Distal Radius: Associated Distal Radioulnar Joint (DRUJ) Lesions.

	Patho-anatomy of the lesion	Degree of joint surface involvement	Prognosis	Recommended treatment
Type 1 **Stable** (following reduction of the radius the DRUJ is congruous and stable)	A Avulsion fracture tip ulnar styloid B Stable fracture ulnar neck	None	Good	A+B Functional aftertreatment Encourage early pronation-supination exercises Note: Extraarticular unstable fractures of the ulna at the metaphyseal level or distal shaft require stable plate fixation
Type II **Unstable** (subluxation or dislocation of the ulnar head present)	A Substance tear of TFCC and/or palmar and dorsal capsular ligaments B Avulsion fracture base of the ulnar styloid	None	• Chronic instability • Painful limitation of supination if left unreduced • Possible late arthritic changes	A Closed treatment Reduce subluxation, sugar tong splint in 45° of supination four to six weeks A+B Operative treatment Repair TFCC or fix ulnar styloid with tension band wiring Immobilize wrist and elbow in supination (cast) or transfix ulna/radius with k-wire and forearm cast
Type III **Potentially unstable** (subluxation possible)	A Intraarticular fracture of the sigmoid notch B Intraarticular fracture of the ulnar head	Present	• Dorsal subluxation possible together with dorsally displaced die punch or dorso-ulnar fragment • Risk of early degenerative changes and severe limitation of forearm rotation if left unreduced	A Anatomic reduction of palmar and dorsal sigmoid notch fragments. If residual subluxation tendency present immobilize as in type II injury B Functional aftertreatment to enhance remodelling of ulnar head If DRUJ remains painful: partial ulnar resection, darrach or sauvé-kapandji procedure at a later date

References

1. Alffram PA, Bauer GCH: Epidemiology of fractures of the forearm. A biomechanical investigation of bone strength. *J Bone Joint Surg [Am]* 44A: 105–114, 1962.
2. Barton JR: Views and treatment of an important injury of the wrist. *Med Examiner* 1: 365–368, 1838.
3. Bähr F: Die typische Radiusfraktur und ihre Entstehung. *Z Chirur* 21: 841, 1894.
4. Bengner U, Johnell O: Increasing incidence of forearm fractures. A comparison of epidemiologic patterns 25 years apart. *Acta Orthop Scand* 56: 158–160, 1985.
5. Buhr AJ, Cooke AM: Fracture patterns. *Lancet* 1: 531–536, 1959.
6. Castaing J: Les fractures récentes de l'extremité inférieure du radius chez l'adulte. *Rev Chir Orthop* 50: 581–696, 1964.
7. Cook PJ, Exton-Smith AN: Fractured femurs, falls, and bone disorder. *J R Coll Physicians* 16: 45–49, 1982.
8. Cooney WP III, Agee JM, Hastings H II: Symposium: Management of intraarticular fractures of the distal radius. *Contemp Orthop* 21: 71–104, 1990.
9. Cotton FJ: The pathology of fractures of the lower end of the radius. *Ann Surg* 32: 194–218, 1900.
10. Crilly RG, Delaguerriere-Richardson, LD, Roth JH: Postural instability and Colles' fracture. *Age Aging* 16: 133–138, 1987.
11. Destot E, Gallois E: Recherches physiologiques et expérimentales sur les fractures de l'extremité inférieure du radius. *Rev Chir (Paris)* 18: 886–915, 1898.
12. Dupuytren G: Des fractures de l'extremité inférieure du radius simulant les luxations du poignet. *Orales Clini Chirurg* 1: 140, 1839.
13. Ehalt W: Die Bruchformen am unteren Ende der Speiche und Elle. *Arch Orthop Unfall Chir* 35: 397–442, 1935.
14. Falch JA: Epidemiology of fractures of the distal forearm in Oslo, Norway. *Acta Orthop Scand* 54: 291–295, 1983.
15. Fernandez DL: Avant-bras segment distal. In: *Classification AO des Fractures des Os Longs* edited by Müller ME, Nazarian S, Koch P. Berlin, Heidelberg, New York: Springer-Verlag, 1987, pp. 106–115.
16. Fernandez DL: Fractures of the distal radius. Operative treatment. AAOS Instructional Course Lectures 42: 73–88, 1993.
17. Frykman GK: Fracture of the distal radius including sequelae—Shoulder hand finger syndrome. Disturbance in the distal radioulnar joint and impairment of nerve function. A clinical and experimental study. *Acta Orthop Scand Suppl* 108: 1–155, 1967.
18. Gartland JJ, Werley CW: Evaluation of healed Colles' fractures. *J Bone Joint Surg [Am]* 33A: 895–907, 1951.
19. Golden GN: Treatment and prognosis of Colles' fracture. *Lancet* 1: 511–514, 1963.
20. Hollingsworth R, Morris J: The importance of the ulnar side of the wrist in fractures of the distal end of the radius. *Injury* 7: 263–266, 1976.
21. Horsman A, Norden BEC, Aaron J, Marshall DH: Cortical and trabecular osteoporosis and their relation to fractures in the elderly. In: *Osteoporosis: Recent Advances in Pathogenesis and Treatment* edited by Deluca HF, Frost HM, Jess WSS, Johnston CC, Parfitt AM. Baltimore: University Press, 1981, pp. 175–184.
22. Jenkins NH: The unstable Colles' fracture. *J Hand Surg* 14B: 149–154, 1989.
23. Kirschen AJ, Cape RDJ, Hayes KC, Spencer JD: Postural sway and cardiovascular parameters associated with falls in the elderly. *J Clin Exp Res Gerontol* 6: 291–307, 1984.
24. Knowelden J, Buhr AJ, Dunbar O: Incidence of fractures in persons over 35 years of age. *Br J Prev Soc Med* 18: 130–141, 1964.
25. Krolner B, Tondervold E, Toft B: Bone mass of the axial and the appendicular skeleton in women with Colles' fracture: Its relation to physical activity. *Clin Physiol* 2: 147–57, 1982.
26. Lamke B, Sjöberg HE, Sylven M: Bone mineral content in women with Colles' fracture: Effect of calcium supplementation. *Acta Orthop Scand* 49: 143–146, 1978.
27. LeComte O: Recherches nouvelles sur les fractures de l'extremité inferieure du radius. *Arch Gen Med* 5: 641, 1861.
28. Letenneur: *Soc Anat Bull* XIV, 1838, p. 162.
29. Lewis RM: Colles' fracture: Causative mechanism. *Surgery* 27: 427–436, 1950.
30. Lidström A: Fractures of the distal end of the radius. A clinical and statistical study of end results. *Acta Orthop Scand* 30 (*Suppl* 41): 1–118, 1959.
31. Lilienfeldt A: Ueber den klassischen Radiusbruch. *Arch Klin Chir* 27: 475, 1885.
32. Löbker K: Sitzung des medizinischer Vereins zu Greifswald. *Dtsch Med Wochenschr* 27: 475, 1885.

33. Lucht U: A prospective study of accidental falls and resulting injuries in the home among elderly people. *Acta Orthop Scand* 2: 105–120, 1971.
34. MacLoed J: Wrist fractures. *Br Med J* July: 39, 1879.
35. Malgaigne J: A Trcatise on Fractlcs, late by John Packand. Philadelyshia JB Cippinalt, 1859.
36. Mayer JH: Colles' fractures. *Br J Surg* 27: 629–642, 1940.
37. Mayfield JK, Johnson RP, Kilcoyne RF: Carpal dislocations: Pathomechanics and progressive perilunar instability. *J Hand Surg* 5: 226–241, 1980.
38. McMurtry RY, Jupiter JB: Fractures of the distal radius. In: *Skeletal Trauma*, edited by Browner BD, Jupiter JB, Levine AM, Trafton PG. Philadelphia: WB Saunders, 1992, pp. 1063–1094.
39. Melone CP r: Articular fractures of the distal radius. *Orthop Clin No Am* 15: 217–236, 1984.
40. Melton LJ, Riggs BL: Epidemiology of age-related fractures. In: *The Osteoporotic Syndrome. Detection, Prevention and Treatment*, edited by Avioli LV. New York: Grune and Stratton, 1983, pp. 45–72.
41. Meyer H: Der klassische Speichenbruch. *Klin Wochensch* 4: 554, 1925.
42. Missakian ML, Cooney WP III, Amadio PC, Glidewell HL: Open reduction and internal fixation for distal radius fractures. *J Hand Surg* 17A: 745–755, 1992.
43. Müller ME, Nazarian S, Koch P, Schatzker J: *The Comprehensive Classification of Fractures of Long Bones*. Berlin: Springer-Verlag, 1990.
44. Nélaton A: *Eléments de pathologie chirurgicale*, Paris: Germer Ballière, 1844.
45. Nissen-Lie HS: Fractura radii "typica." *Nord Med* 1: 293–303, 1939.
46. Older TM, Stabler EV, Cassebaum WH: Colles' fracture: Evaluation of selection of therapy. *J Trauma* 5: 469–476, 1965.
47. Owen RA, Melton LJ, Johnson KA, Ilstrup DM, Riggs BL: Incidence of Colles' fracture in a North American community. *Am J Pub Health* 72: 605–607, 1982.
48. Peltier LF: Fractures of the distal end of the radius. An historical account. *Clin Orthop Rel Res* 187: 18–22, 1984.
49. Pilcher LS: Fractures of the lower extremity or base of the radius. *Ann Surg* 65: 1–25, 1917.
50. Ravitch M: Dupuytren's invention of the Mikulicz enterotome with a note on eponyms. *Perspect Biol Med* 22: 170, 1979.
51. Rayhack J: Symposium on distal radius fractures. Edited by William Cooney. *Contemp Orthop* 21: 75, 1990.
52. Roberts JB: A clinical, pathological, and experimental study of the fracture of the lower end of the radius with displacement of the carpal fragment toward the flexor or anterior surface of the wrist. *Am J Med Sci* 113: 10–80, 1897.
53. Rosenbach J: Ueber den Bruch des Radius am unteren Ende. *Klin Chir.* 66: 993, 1902.
54. Sarmiento A, Pratt GW, Berry NC, Sinclair WF: Colles' fracture: Functional bracing in supination. *J Bone Joint Surg [Am]* 57A: 311–317, 1975.
55. Sarmiento A, Zagorski JB, Sinclair WF: Functional bracing of Colles' fracture: A prospective study of immobilization in supination vs. pronation. *Clin Orthop Rel Res* 146: 175–183, 1980.
56. Schmalholz A: Closed reduction of axial compression in Colles' fracture is hardly possible. *Acta Orthop Scand* 60: 57–59, 1989.
57. Schurmeier HL: Mechanics of fractures of the wrist. *JAMA*, 77: 2119–2126, 1917.
58. Sennwald G: *The Wrist* Berlin, Heidelberg, New York: Springer-Verlag, 1987, pp. 136–138.
59. Solgård S: Classification of distal radius fractures. *Acta Orthop Scand* 56: 249–252, 1984.
60. Solgård S, Petersen VS: Epidemiology of distal radius fractures. *Acta Orthop Scand* 56: 391–393, 1985.
61. Stevens JH: Compression fractures of the lower end of the radius. *Ann Surg* 71: 594–618, 1920.
62. Taylor GW, Parsons CL: The role of the discus articularis in Colles' fracture. *J Bone Joint Surg [Am]* 20: 149–152, 1938.
63. Thomas FB: Reduction of Smith's fracture. *J Bone Joint Surg [Br]* 39B: 463–470, 1957.
64. von Linhart W: As quoted by Rolter H: Die Brüche der unteren Epiphyse des Radius durch Gegenstoss. *Z Gesellsch Ärzte*, 23, 1852.
65. Wilson PD: *Management of Fractures and Dislocations* Philadelphia: WB Saunders, 1928.

Chapter Three

Functional and Radiographic Anatomy

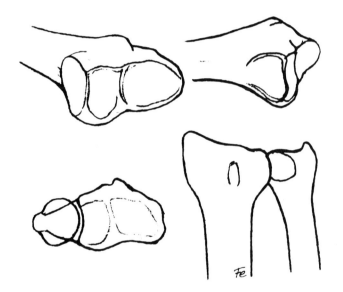

Nothing may inculpate or excoriate a surgeon more than a good x-ray.[3]

Carl Beck, M.D., 1898

Functional Anatomy

The distal end of the radius is appropriately considered the anatomic foundation of the wrist joint. It is dependent upon both the bony and the ligamentous integrity of this foundation for its mobility as well as its capacity to support axial load. Beginning 2 cm proximal to the radiocarpal joint at its metaphyseal flare, the end of the radius is uniquely designed to function as the anatomic bridge uniting the hand to the forearm.[20,21,34]

The wrist joint in man is distinguished from that in lower primates by having an exclusive radiocarpal joint. The development of the triangular fibrocartilage complex and loss of a well-defined articulation between the ulnar and carpus enhanced the ability of the upper limb to position the hand in space.[21,22]

The articular surface of the distal radius is biconcave and triangular in shape, with the apex of the triangle directed towards the styloid process while the base represents the sigmoid notch for articulation with the ulnar head (Fig. 3.1). The surface is divided into two hyaline cartilage-covered "facets" for articulation with the carpal scaphoid and lunate bones. A well-defined ridge traversing from the dorsal to the palmar surface separates the two facets. Both facets are themselves concave in both the anteroposterior and the radioulna directions.

The palmar surface of the distal end of the radius is relatively flat, extending volarly in a gentle curve. A tubercle is present midway, across from which arises the radioscapholunate ligament. In addition, a smooth impression is present on the styloid process which represents the site of origin of the stout radioscapholunate and radiotriquetral intrascapular ligaments (Fig. 3.2).

The dorsal aspect of the radius is convex. Lister's tubercle serves as a fulcrum around which passes the extensor pollicis longus tendon. A flattened

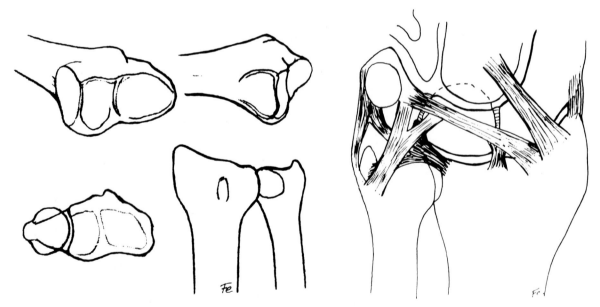

Figure 3.1. (*left* The articular surface of the distal radius is biconcave and triangular in shape. The surface is divided into two hyaline cartilage-covered "facets" from articulation with the scaphoid and lunate. The facets are concave in both the anteroposterior and the radioulnar directions.

Figure 3.2. (*right*) The volar radius and ulnar are the sites of origin of the restraining ligaments supporting the carpus. Stout radiocarpal and ulnocarpal ligaments maintain the normal kinematics of the radiocarpal articulation.

groove can be appreciated on the dorsal side of the radial styloid process which is the floor of the first dorsal extensor compartment. The anatomic relationships of the extensor retinaculum, six dorsal extensor compartments, and dorsal radial cortex are of extreme importance in the surgical approaches as well as the placement of internal fixation on the dorsum of the radius (Fig. 3.3).

The articular end of the radius slopes in an ulnar and palmar direction (see Radiology, below). The carpus will thus have a natural tendency to slide in an ulnar direction, resisted for the most part by the intracapsular and interosseous carpal ligaments arising from both the radius and the ulnar (Fig. 3.4).

Movements of the carpal bones on the distal radius occur in two axes when viewed with the hand resting in an anatomic position (Fig. 3.5). These include flexion and extension in the transverse plane and adduction and abduction in the horizontal plane.[20] The axis of flexion/extension passes between the proximal and distal carpal rows centered at the capitate-lunate articulation, while that of abduction/adduction lies more in the head of the capitate. The combination of these movements permits the hand to pass in a conical dimension described by Kapandji as the "cone of circumduction"[20] (Fig. 3.6).

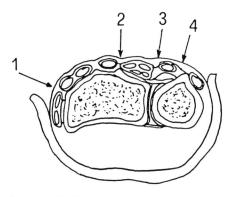

Figure 3.3. The six dorsal extensor compartments are strategically located for extensor function of the hand and wrist. The surgical approaches (1, 2, 3, 4) are based upon the orientation of these compartments (see Chapter 4).

Figure 3.4. The carpus will have a natural tendency to slide in an ulnar (a) and palmar (b) direction on the end of the radius. Reprinted with permission. Sennwald G: *The Wrist*. Berlin: Springer-Verlag, 1987, p. 15.

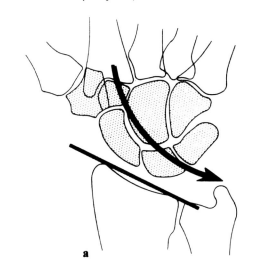

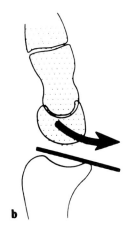

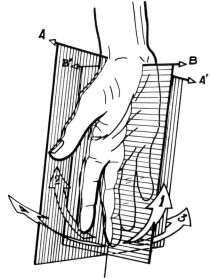

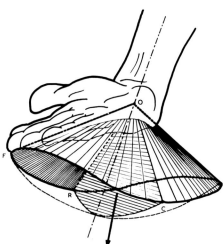

Figure 3.6. The combination of the movements of the wrist, including flexion, extension, adduction, and abduction, can be termed circumduction. The axis of the hand in space traces a conical surface described by Kapandji as the "cone of circumduction." The apex O is at the center of the wrist and a base is shown by points F, R, E, C which trace the path covered by the middle finger during maximal circumduction. Reprinted with permission. Kapandji IA: The Physiology of Joints. Edinburgh: Churchill Livingstone, 1982, p. 137.

Figure 3.5. The movements of the wrist as depicted by Kapandji occur around two axes when the hand is held in full supination. Transverse axis A → A' is in the frontal plane (vertically striped) and controls the movement of flexion (1) and extension (2) occurring in the sagittal plane (horizontally striped). The anteroposterior axis B → B' lies in the sagittal plane and controls the movements of adduction (3) and abduction (4) which take place in the frontal plane. Reprinted with permission. Kapandji IA: *The Physiology of Joints*. Edinburgh: Churchill Livingstone, 1982, p. 133.

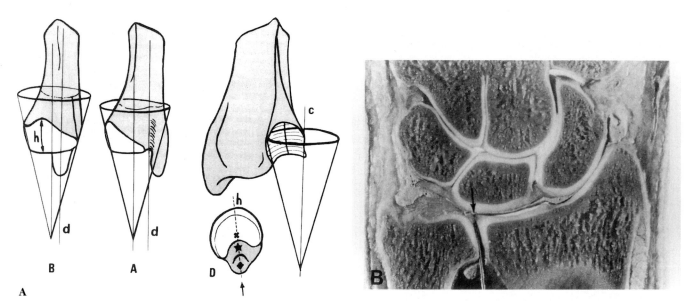

Figure 3.7. The inferior radioulnar joint is a trochoid (pivot) joint with cylindrical articular surfaces and only one degree of freedom, i.e., rotation about the axis of its interlocked surfaces. A. The distal radioulnar joint as depicted by Kapandji. The articular surface of the ulnar head, as seen from the head (B) and from the side (A), is at its widest anteriorly and laterally. The inferior surface of the ulnar head (D) is semilunar with its point of maximal width corresponding to the highest point (H) on the periphery. C and D depict the sphere of rotation of the radioulnar joint. B. An anatomic cross section of the radioulnar joint.

Axial compressive loads pass through the carpus into the radius and, to a considerably lesser degree, the ulnar head. Werner et al. suggested that when both the radius and distal ulnar are even (ulnar neutral), 80 percent of axial load is transmitted to the radius through the carpus.[48]

The other distinct articular surface of the end of the radius is the sigmoid notch. Semicylindrical in shape, it runs parallel to the "seat" of the ulnar head. The relationship of the articulating surface more closely resembles a cylinder and represents a trochoid joint (Fig. 3.7A and B). Rotation of the radius about the ulnar is accompanied by a translational movement, such that in supination the ulnar head is displaced anteriorly in the notch, whereas in pronation it moves dorsally.[20]

At the ulnar aspect of the lunate facet arises the triangular fibrocartilage, which extends onto the base of the ulnar styloid process, functioning as an important stabilizer of the distal radioulnar joint. It is situated between the ulnar head and carpal triquetrum. Its volar and dorsal margins are thickened, blending into the dorsal and volar radioulnar ligaments. The surfaces are biconcave and covered with hyaline cartilage.

Additional ("secondary") stabilizers of the distal radioulnar joint include the interosseous membrane of the forearm, the pronator quadratus muscle, and the tendons and sheaths of the extensor and flexor carpi ulnaris muscles.

Stability and mobility are ensured by the design and interactions of the radius with its carpal and ulnar articulations. Fractures that heal with deformity or disruption of these articulations will have a profound effect on the function of the entire wrist joint.

Radiology

Ever since Beck in 1898 demonstrated the capability of "roentgen-rays" to accurately display the skeletal disruptions associated with fractures of the distal end of the radius,[3] radiographic measurements have formed the foundation of evaluation of not only the injury but frequently also the outcome of treatment.

A number of radiographic measurements have come to be utilized in the anatomic evaluation of the distal end of the radius.[1,2,5,6,9,11,12,14,23,30,36,38–40,45,46] Variations in so-called normal values have reflected not only anatomic differences but also such factors as the position of the forearm and wrist in relationship to the x-ray beam.[8,11] Rotational malalignment will also have a direct effect on the radiographic reading.

Ulnar Inclination

In the frontal view, the slope or inclination of the distal end of the radius is represented by the angle formed by a line drawn from the tip of the radial styloid process to the ulnar corner of the articular surface of the distal end of the radius and a line drawn perpendicular to the longitudinal axis of the radius (Fig. 3.8A and B). The average inclination is between 22 and 23 degrees.[1,11,12,25,38] Here, too, the accuracy of measurement can be affected by a number of factors.[33] These include determination of the radiologic landmarks, particularly if the dorsomedial aspect of the radius is fractured and displaced (Fig. 3.9A–C). Castaing demonstrated the fact that measurement of the radial inclination may vary as much as 25 degrees in uninjured radii as the forearm is rotated from supination to pronation.[5] Rotational deformity of the distal fragment will also affect the measurement of the injured wrist.[11,12,17,26,28]

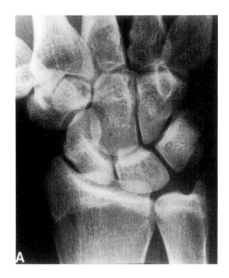

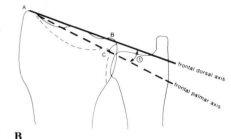

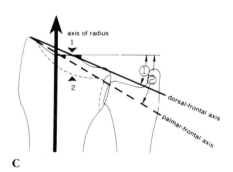

Figure 3.9. The angles of the ulnar inclination can be affected by whether or not the dorsal palmar lips of the distal radius are chosen. A. Standard anteroposterior radiograph of a normal wrist. B. The frontal dorsal axis (AB) and the frontal palmar axis (AC) are sketched. C. The angles of ulnar inclination can vary upwards of 7 degrees (1 and 2). With fracture and impaction, the dorsomedial aspect of the radius may become proximal to the apex of the palmar medial corner and can lead to underestimation of the dorsal impaction. Reprinted with permission from Sennwald G: *The Wrist.* Berlin: Springer-Verlag, 1987, p. 52.

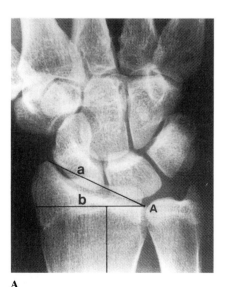

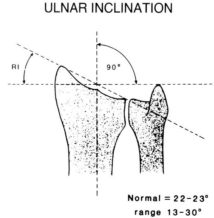

ULNAR INCLINATION

Normal = 22-23°
range 13-30°

Figure 3.8. In the frontal plane the average ulnar inclination is 22 to 23 degrees. A. The schematic depicts the measurement of ulnar. B. The ulnar inclination is measured the angle between a–A and a line inclination to the long axis of the radius.

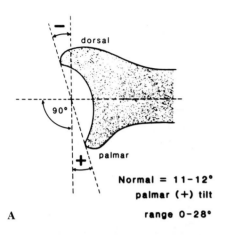

PALMAR TILT

Normal = 11–12°
palmar (+) tilt
range 0–28°

A

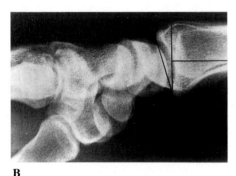

B

Figure 3.10A,B. In the sagittal plane the normal palmar tilt averages 11 to 12 degrees.

Palmar Inclination

To obtain the palmar inclination of the distal radius in the sagittal view, a line is drawn connecting the distalmost point of the dorsal and volar cortical rims. The angle that this line creates with a line drawn perpendicular to the longitudinal axis of the radius reflects the palmar inclination (Fig. 3.10A and B). Although most authors agree that this angle on average is between 10 and 12 degrees,[14,16,24] Friberg and Lundström observed a variability of normal subjects ranging from 4 to 22 degrees[11] (Table 3.1).

Radial Length

Radial length is also measured on the anteroposterior radiograph. This measurement (in millimeters) represents the distance between a line drawn at the tip of the styloid process, perpendicular to the long axis of the radius, and a second perpendicular line at the level of the distal articular surface of the ulnar head[5,14,15,32,38,46] (Fig. 3.11A and B). In Gartland and Werley's publication, the normal was 11 to 12 mm.[12]

Ulnar Variance

The vertical distance between a line parallel to the proximal surface of the lunate facet of the distal radius and a line parallel to the articular surface of the ulnar head has been referred to as the ulnar variance[18] (Fig. 3.12). As many distal radial fractures will involve the medial corner of the radius with or without the styloid process, there are some who believe this measurement may be more accurate for judging loss of radial length or height.[27,40] Comparison radiographs with the uninjured wrist ideally taken in the same manner with the shoulder abducted 90 degrees and elbow flexed 90 degrees will be necessary to determine normal length on an individual basis.[17,34,35] Hulten noted that in 61 percent of his cases, the ulnar head and the medial corner of the radius were at the same level bilaterally (neutral variance).[18] With fracture

Table 3.1. Results of the measurements Friberg and Lundström.

	Mean	SD (range)
Ulnar inclination		
Central ray perpendicular	25.4°	2.2° (20–30°)
Central ray directed 10° proximally	25°	2.2° (19–30°)
Volar inclination		
Central ray perpendicular	14.5°	4.3° (4–22°)
Central ray directed 15° proximally	9.3°	2.7° (4–15°)
Distance d between ulnar articular surface and a parallel plane through tip of radial styloid process.		
Central ray perpendicular	12.8 mm M 13.6 mm F 11.6 mm	2.3 mm (8–18 mm)
Central ray directed 10° proximally	12.8 mm M 13.3 mm F 12.0 mm	2.3 mm (9–18 mm)
Distance u between plane of ulnar articular surface and a parallel plane through the ulnar part of the radial articular surface		
Central ray perpendicular	0.32 mm	1.7 mm (+3 to −4 mm)
Central ray directed 10° proximally	0.13 mm	1.58 mm (+4 to −3 mm)

RADIAL LENGTH

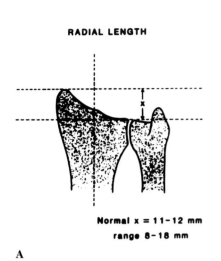

Normal x = 11-12 mm

range 8-18 mm

A

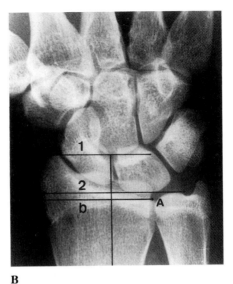

B

Figure 3.11A,B. In the frontal plane the radial length (height) averages 11 to 12 mm in reference to the distal radioulnar joint. A–b refers to the level of the ulnar corner of the distal radioulnar joint (volar). 1: line tangential to the top of the the radial styloid and perpendicular to the long axis of the radius 2. line perpendicular to the long axis of the and tangential to the ulnar head.

displacement, the ulnar head will commonly be in a distal relationship (positive variance).

Radial Width

The width of the distal radius has proven to be an important factor in evaluating outcome.[1,11,25,45] This width is the distance in millimeters, from the most lateral tip of the radial styloid process to the longitudinal axis through the center of the radius on the anteroposterior radiograph (Fig. 3.13).

Measurement of Deformity

When evaluating the extent of deformity associated with a distal radius fracture, comparison of the radiologic criteria outlined above to those of the opposite uninjured wrist will provide in most cases an accurate representation of the fracture.[7,11,12,14–16,23,26,36,38,43] These will also serve to control the adequacy of the reduction and anatomic position at the time of fracture union. It is noteworthy that Van der Linden and Ericson observed in their study of 250 consecutive cases of "bending type" fractures that only the loss of palmar inclination and change in radial width were independent of each other.[45] They

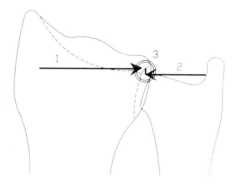

Figure 3.12. The vertical distance between the distal ends of the medial corner of the radius and the ulnar head represents the ulna variance. (See rest on Fig. 3.9)

RADIAL SHIFT

Normal d

d²

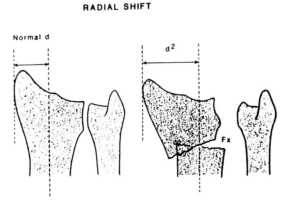

Fx

Figure 3.13. The radial shift represents the distance in millimeters between a longitudinal axis of the radius and the lateral tip of the radial styloid.

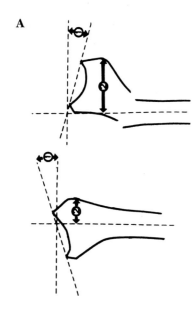

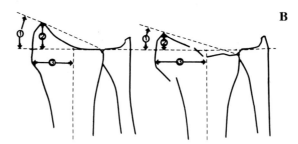

Figure 3.14. The measurement of deformity on the lateral radiograph as recommended by Van der Linden and Ericson. A. The dorsal angle (1) is the angle between a line perpendicular to the long axis and the articular surface indicated by a line joining its volar and dorsal margins of that surface. Dorsal shift is the increase in the distance from the long axis to the most dorsal point of the distal end of the bone (2). B. The measurement of radial shift as depicted by Van der Linden and Ericson. The radial angle (1) is the angle between a line perpendicular to the long axis and the radial articular surface, as indicated by a line joining its radial and ulnar margins. Shortening is the decrease in the distance that the styloid process projects distal to a perpendicular to the long axis drawn though the contour of the ulnar part of the wrist joint (2). Radial shift is the increase in the distance from the long axis to the most radial point of the styloid process (3). Reprinted with permission. Van der Linden W and Ericson R: Colles' fracture. How should its displacement be measured and how should it be immobilized? *J Bone Joint Surg* 43A: 1285–1288, 1981.

objectively measured these two deformities using two criteria which they termed "dorsal angle" and "radial displacement" (Fig. 3.14A and B).

Castaing et al. developed several radiographic measurements to quantitate deformity associated with fracture[5] (Fig. 3.15A–C)

1. Bascule frontale: this documents the change in the normal radial inclination as measured in the anteroposterior or frontal projection (Fig. 3.15A).

Figure 3.15. The radiographic measurement of Castaing. A. The "bascule frontale:" this documents the radial deviation of the distal fragment. B. The radioulnar index: this documents the change in ulnar variance. C. The "bascule sagittale:" this corresponds to the angle of the tilt of the distal fragment in the sagittal plane.

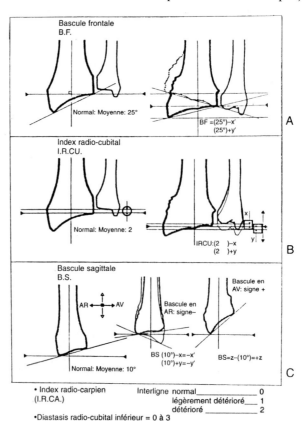

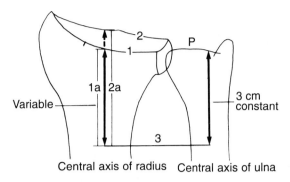

Figure 3.16. The measurement of impaction as defined by Sennwald. P is the fixed point representing the articular plateau of the ulna.1 is the palmar lip of the distal radius. 2 is the dorsal lip of the distal radius. 1a is the reference line for the distance of the palmar lip after fracture 2a is the reference line for the distance of the dorsal lip after fracture. 3 is the reference line that is measured from a point 3 cm from the end of the ulnar. Reprinted with permission from Sennwald G: *The Wrist.* Berlin: Springer-Verlag, 1987, p. 145.

2. Radioulnar index: this represents the change in the ulnar variance (Fig. 3.15B).
3. Bascule sagittale: this measurement corresponds to the angle of tilt of the distal fragment either in a dorsal or a palmar direction (Fig. 3.15C).

Sennwald, emphasizing the pitfalls that exist with accurately identifying the dorsal and palmar cortical rims in the frontal projection, developed a "measurement of impaction"[40] (Fig. 3.16). In this approach the ulnar serves as the fixed reference point. A straight line is drawn down its longitudinal axis, and 3 cm proximal to the articular surface a perpendicular is drawn to this line which crosses the radius. This intersection point will serve as the reference point from which the distance to the palmar or dorsal lip of the articular surface is measured. This measurement is always made on the line drawn along the longitudinal axis of the radius. Based upon similar measurement of the uninjured side, with the intact ulnar serving as a reference point, one can more accurately measure the degree of shortening throughout the course of treatment.

Abbaszadegan, Jonsson, and von Sivers added to the deformity measurements by changing the reference points for measuring radial displacement and dorsal displacement[1] (Fig. 3.17).

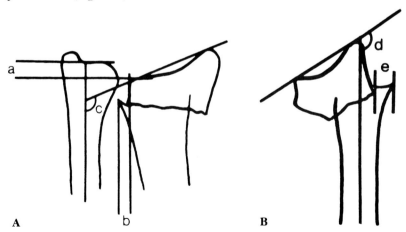

Figure 3.17. Abbaszadegan, Jonsson, and von Sivers method of measuring radiographic deformity. A. Anteroposterior radiographic parameters. Axial radial shortening (a): the difference in level between the distal ulnar surface and the ulnar part of the distal radial surface. Radial displacement (b): the dislocation of the distal fragment in relation and the radial shaft. Radial angle (c): the angle of the distal surface in relation to the long axis of the radius. B. Lateral radiographic parameters. Dorsal angle (d): the angle of the distal radial surface in relation to the long axis of the radius. Dorsal displacement (e): the distance between the distal radial fragment and the radial shaft. Reprinted with permission. Abbaszadegan H, Jonsson U, von Sivers K: Prediction of instability of Colles' fractures. *Acta Orthop Scand* 60: 646–650, 1989.

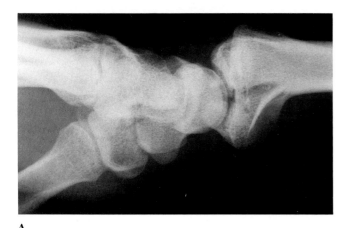

A

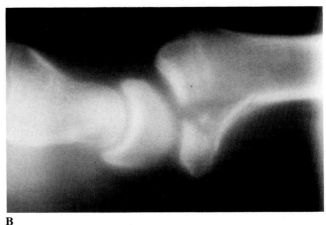

B

Figure 3.18. A shearing type fracture involved an element of impaction and displacement of the articular surface. A. The lateral radiograph suggests, but does not accurately depict, a detect in the articular surface. B. The lateral trispiral tomographic image accurately reveals an articular defect with impaction of the displaced articular fragment.

Trispiral Tomography

Although technological advances have ushered in the computed tomogram and magnetic resonance imaging, the trispiral tomogram remains the authors' most useful imaging technique for obtaining greater definition of complex fractures, particularly those involving impaction or rotation of the articular surface (Fig. 3.18A and B).

Anteroposterior and lateral trispiral tomograms will provide extremely useful images of even the most complex fracture morphology and should be considered in the preoperative planning of these injuries (Fig. 3.19A–D).

Figure 3.19. A combined Type V high-energy fracture is more accurately understood with trispiral tomographic images. A,B. The anteroposterior and lateral radiographs reveal a complex fracture pattern. C. The anterior trispiral tomogram shows clearly the volar aspect of the lunate facet to be displaced with the articular surface now facing proximally. D. The lateral trispiral tomogram shows the dorsal lunate facet displaced with impaction of the central aspect of the articular surface.

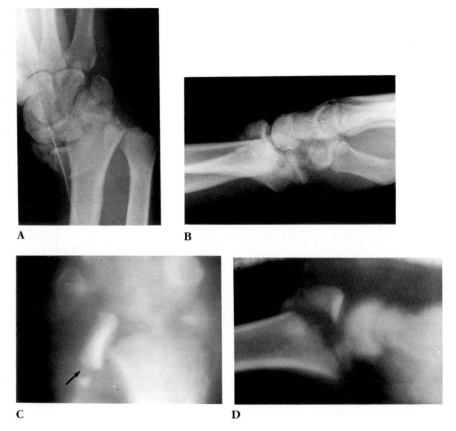

A

B

C

D

Computed Tomography

Although less frequently utilized or needed, computed tomography may be of use in the definition of complex articular injuries, the possibility of occult fractures, or injury to the distal radioulnar joint (Fig. 3.20A–D).[4,10,19,29,31,37,41,42,47]

The images in the axial plane prove useful in demonstrating the configuration of the articular injury as well as revealing the extent and location of displacement of the radioscaphoid and radiolunate fossa fragments.[37,42] These also allow for a greater appreciation of the metaphyseal comminution.

Projections in the sagittal and coronal planes can be useful for the evaluation of the metaphyseal comminution as well as the impaction of the articular surface.[42]

Disruption of the distal radioulnar joint as well as injury to either the sigmoid notch or the ulnar head is most clearly defined by the computed tomogram.[29]

Carpal Imaging

In the routine posteroanterior radiographs, the articular surfaces of the carpal bones should be parallel and the joint surfaces of similar width[13–15,44] (Fig. 3.21). A broken "arc" as described by Gilula[13] or overlapping of the normally

A   **B**

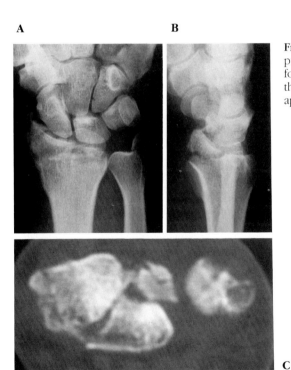

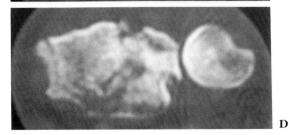

C

D

Figure 3.20. A four-part compression fracture is further defined using computed tomography (CT). A,B. Anteroposterior and lateral radiographs of the four-part compression fracture. C,D. The CT images reveal involvement of both the radial styloid and the lunate facets. The depth of involvement is not readily appreciated from single CT images.

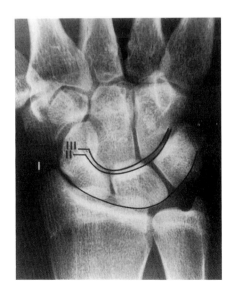

Figure 3.21. The normal carpal alignment as depicted by Gilula is represented by carpal arcs which are smooth with the joint spaces of similar widths and with parallel cortical margins.

equally spaced joint lines is highly suggestive of injury to either the supporting ligaments, the carpal bones, or both. When viewing the routine radiographs of any fracture of the distal end of the radius, the physician should be cognizant of the potential for an associated intercarpal ligamentous injury.

References

1. Abbaszadegan H, Jonsson U, von Sivers K: Prediction of instability of Colles' fractures. *Acta Orthop Scand* 60: 646–650, 1989.
2. Altissimi M, Antenucci R, Fiacca C, Mancini GB: Long-term results of conservative treatment of fractures of the distal radius. *Clin Orthop Rel Res* 206: 202–210, 1986.
3. Beck C: Colles' fracture and the roentgen rays. *Med News* (February) pp. 230–232, 1898.
4. Biondetti PR, Vannier MW, Gilula W: Wrist: Coronal and transaxial CT scanning. *Radiology* 163: 149–151, 1987.
5. Castaing J: Les fractures récentes de l'extrémité inférieure du radius chez l'adulte. *Rev Chir Orthop* 50: 581–696, 1964.
6. Cole JM, Obletz BE: Comminuted fractures of the distal end of the radius treated by skeletal transfixion in plaster cast: An end-result study of thirty-three cases. *J Bone Joint Surg [Am]* 48A: 931–945, 1966.
7. Dias JJ, Wray CC, Jones JM: The radiological deformity of Colles' fractures. *Injury* 18: 304–308, 1987.
8. DiBenedetto MR, Lubbers LM, Roff ME: Qualification of error in measurement of radial inclination angle and radiocarpal distance. *J Hand Surg* 16A: 399–400, 1991.
9. Dowling JJ, Sawyer B Jr: Comminuted Colles' fractures. Evaluation of a method of treatment. *J Bone Joint Surg [Am]* 43A: 657–668, 1961.
10. Frahm R, Drescher E: Radiologische Diagnostik nach komplizierter distaler Radiusfraktur inter besonder berücksichtigung der Computer-tomographie. *Fortschr Roentgenstr*, 148: 295, 1988.
11. Friberg S, Lundström B: Radiographic measurements of the radio-carpal joint in normal adults. *Acta Radiol Diag* 17: 249–256, 1976.
12. Gartland JJ, Werley CW: Evaluation of healed Colles' fractures. *J Bone Joint Surg [Am]* 33A: 895–907, 1951.
13. Gilula LA: Carpal injuries: Analytic approach and case exercises. *Am J Roentgenol* 133: 503–517, 1979.
14. Gilula LA: *The Traumatized Hand and Wrist: Radiographic and Anatomic Correlation Philadelphia*. WB Saunders, 1992.
15. Gilula LA, Destouet JM, Weeks PM: Roentgenographic diagnosis of the painful wrist. *Clin Orthop Rel Res* 187: 52–64, 1984.
16. Golden GN: Treatment and prognosis of Colles' fracture. *Lancet* 511, 1963.
17. Hardy DH, Totty WG, Reinus WR: Posteroanterior wrist radiography: Importance of arm positioning. *J Hand Surg* 12A: 509–513, 1987.
18. Hulten O: Ueber anatomische Variationen der Handgelenkenknochen. *Acta Radiol* 9: 155–168, 1928.
19. Johnston GH, Friedman L, Kriegler JC: Computerized tomographic evaluation of acute distal radial fractures. *J Hand Surg* 17A: 738–744, 1992.
20. Kapandji IA: Rotation (pronation and supination). In: *The Physiology of the Joints of the Upper Limb*. Edinburgh, London, Melbourne, and New York: Churchill-Livingstone, 1982, pp. 98–129.
21. Lewis OJ: The development of the human wrist joint during the fetal period. *Anat Rec* 166: 499–516, 1970.
22. Lewis OJ, Hamshere RJ, Bucknill TM: The anatomy of the wrist joint. *J Anat* 106: 539–552, 1970.
23. Lidström A: Fractures of the distal end of the radius. A clinical and statistical study of end results. *Acta Orthop Scand* 30 (Suppl 41): 1–118, 1959.
24. Mann FA, Kane SW, Gilula LA: Is dorsal tilting really normal? *J Hand Surg* (In Press).
25. Mann FA, Wilson AJ, Gilula LA: Radiographic evaluation of the wrist: What does the hand surgeon want to know? *Radiology* 184: 15–24, 1992.
26. Mayer JH: Colles' fractures. *Br J Surg* 27: 629–642, 1940.
27. Melone CP Jr: Articular fractures of the distal radius. *Orthop Clin No Am* 15: 217–236, 1984.
28. Milch H: Colles' fractures. *Bull Hosp Joint Disease* 11: 61–74, 1950.
29. Mino DE, Palmer AK, Levinsohn EM: The role of radiography and computerized tomography in the diagnosis of subluxation and dislocation of the distal radioulnar joint. *J Hand Surg* 8: 23–31, 1983.

30. Movin A, Karlsson U: *Skelettröntgen-undersökningar. Handbok för Röntgenpersonal.* Stockholm: Läromedelsförlagen, 1969.

31. Nakamura R, Horii E, Tanaka Y, Imaedo T: Three-dimensional CT imaging for wrist disorders. *J Hand Surg* 14B: 53–58, 1989.

32. Older TM, Stabler EV, Cassebaum WH: Colles' fracture: Evaluation of selection of therapy. *J Trauma* 5: 469–476, 1965.

33. Paley D, Axelrod TS, Martin C, Rubenstein J, McMurtry RY: Radiographic definition of the dorsal and palmar edges of the distal radius. *J Hand Surg* 14A: 272–276, 1989.

34. Palmer AK: Fractures of the distal radius. In: *Operative Hand Surgery*, edited by Green DP. New York: Churchill Livingstone, 1988, pp. 991–1026.

35. Palmer AK, Glisson RR, Werner FW: Ulnar variance determination. *J Hand Surg* 7: 376–379, 1982.

36. Porter M, Stockley I: Fractures of the distal radius. Intermediate and end results in relation to radiograph parameters. *Clin Orthop Rel Res* 220: 241–251, 1987.

37. Quinn SF, Murray W, Watkins T, Kloss J: CT scanning for determining the results of treatment of fractures of the wrist. *Am J Radiol* 149: 109–111, 1987.

38. Rubinovich RM, Rennie WR: Colles' fracture: End results in relation to radiologic parameters. *Can J Surg* 26: 361–363, 1983.

39. Scheck M: Long-term follow-up of treatment of comminuted fractures of the distal end of the radius by transfixation with Kirschner wires and cast. *J Bone Joint Surg [Am]* 44A: 337–351, 1962.

40. Sennwald G: *The Wrist*. Berlin,Heidelberg,New York: Springer-Verlag, 1987, pp. 136–138.

41. Space TC, Lovis DS, Francis I: Case report: CT findings in distal radioulnar dislocation. *J Comput Assist Tomogr* 10: 689, 1986.

42. Stewart HD, Innes AR, Burke PD: Factors influencing the outcome of Colles' fracture: An anatomical and functional study. *Injury* 16: 289–295, 1985.

43. Stewart NR, Gilula LA: CT of the wrist: A tailored approach. *Radiology* 183: 13–19, 1992.

44. Taleisnik J, Watson HK: Midcarpal instability caused by malunited fractures of the distal radius. *J Hand Surg* 9A: 350–357, 1984.

45. Van der Linden W, Ericson R: Colles' fracture. How should its displacement be measured and how should it be immobilized? *J Bone Joint Surg [Am]* 63A: 1285–1288, 1981.

46. Warwick D, Prothew D, Field J, Bannister GC: Radiological measurement of radial shortening in Colles' fracture. *J Hand Surg* 18B: 50–52, 1993.

47. Wechsler RJ, Wehbe MA, Rifkin MD: Computed tomographic diagnosis of distal radioulnar subluxation. *Skel Radiol*, 16: 1–8, 1987.

48. Werner FW, Palmer AK, Fortino MD, Short WH: Force transmission through the distal ulnar: Effect of ulnar variance, lunate fossa angulation, and radial and palmar tilt of the distal radius. *J Hand Surg* 17A: 423–428, 1992.

Chapter Four

Surgical Techniques

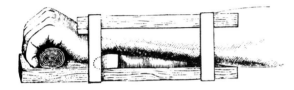

Acknowledging then the frequency of this fracture and the repeated failures attending its treatment, thus causing a partial, if not total loss of the use of the hand and fingers to a great number of our fellow-beings, it will be readily conceded that any rational plan, by which a more favorable result may be obtained is worthy the notice of the profession.

H.M. Shaw, Esq., 1847

Biomechanics of Fracture Reduction

Reduction of fractures of the distal radius will in most cases be obtained by applying a force opposite to that which produced the injury. Thus an understanding of the mechanism of injury proves extremely useful in deciding upon the appropriate reduction maneuvers. Dorsal bending-type fractures (Colles') exhibit increased dorsal angulation, shortening, and radial deviation and supination of the distal fragment. Palmar bending fractures (Smith's) have a reverse deformity pattern, with the distal fragment deviated in a palmar direction and with variable degrees of shortening and pronation with reference to the ulnar. Classically, dorsal bending fractures are reduced by applying longitudinal traction, palmar flexion, ulnar deviation, and pronation (Fig. 4.1).[12] Restoration of skeletal length in displaced and impacted fractures may be

Figure 4.1. The classic method of manipulative reduction of dorsal bending fractures (Colles') involves longitudinal traction and ulnar deviation, palmar flexion, and pronation of the hand and wrist.

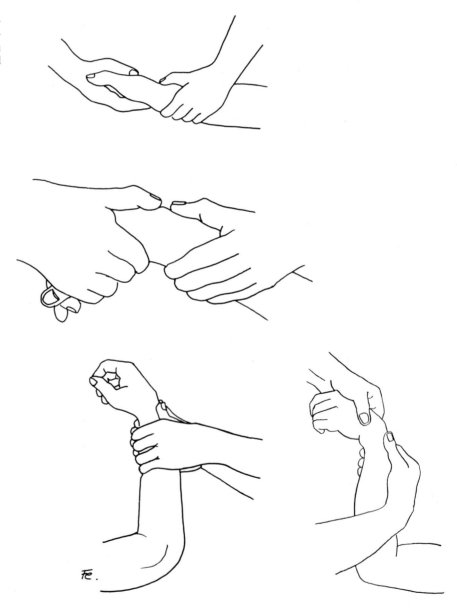

readily obtained by increasing the initial deformity until one cortex engages the other. This contact point is then used as a fulcrum to realign both fragments with a flexion maneuver. The principle of reduction is based upon the application of tension on the soft tissue hinges located on the concavity of the angulation.

Although immobilization in supination has been suggested, this position may not entirely prevent collapse of the fracture, particularly those that have metaphyseal comminution or articular compression fractures. Conversely, palmar bending fractures (Smith's) require extension and supination of the wrist to obtain a reduction.

One of the problems observed with longitudinal traction, particularly in comminuted fractures, is the failure to restore the anatomic palmar tilt of the distal articular surface.[1,2,4] Although extreme palmar flexion is effective in reproducing palmar tilt, it cannot be maintained due to the adverse effects on hand function and the risk of median nerve compression. Agee[1,2] has introduced the concept of "multiplanar ligamentotaxis" in which longitudinal traction is combined with palmar translation of the hand on the forearm. Palmar translation creates a sagittal moment of force in which the capitate will rotate the lunate palmarly. This in turn will produce a rotatory force that can effectively tilt the distal radial fragment in a palmar direction (Fig. 4.2). Agee further advocated radioulnar translation to realign the distal fragments with the radial shaft in the frontal plane.[2] This is successful by virtue of tension applied on the soft tissue hinge within the first and second dorsal compartments. Adequate reduction in the frontal plane is important to restore the anatomic relationship of the sigmoid notch and the ulnar head.

The principles of manipulative fracture reduction will apply primarily to those fractures which can be satisfactorily reduced. Impacted compression-type articular fractures, as well as those with extreme displacement, may not respond to reduction by ligamentotaxis and may require additional limited open reduction.

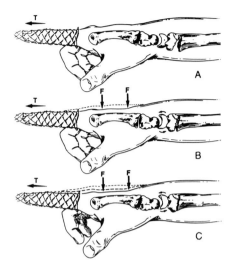

Figure 4.2. As depicted by Agee, palmar translation of the hand and carpus will create a sagittal moment of force in which the capitate will rotate the lunate in a palmar direction which, in turn, will effectively tilt the distal fragment in a palmar direction.

Surgical Approaches to the Distal Radius

A number of surgical options exist for approaching the distal end of the radius. As a general rule, the approaches should be extensile, offer sufficient exposure to accomplish the surgical goals, and heal with a limited degree of scarring.

Dorsal Approaches

The approaches to the dorsum of the end of the radius are performed through longitudinal straight incisions with the posterior surface of the radius and wrist exposed between extensor compartments (Fig. 4.3). The most radial incision is utilized for operative reduction of radial styloid fractures (Fig. 4.4A). This exposure develops the interval between the first and second extensor compartments. At risk in this surgical approach are the superficial radial nerve as it passes on to the dorsum of the hand as well as the dorsal radial artery, particularly if the incision is extended more distalward (Fig. 4.4B). Following incision of the extensor retinaculum, the underlying radial styloid can be easily approached and, if necessary, the wrist capsule opened to visualize the articular alignment (Fig. 4.5A–G).

Figure 4.3. The most common dorsal extensile approaches are illustrated with each approach demonstrating its location in relation to the extensor retinaculum.

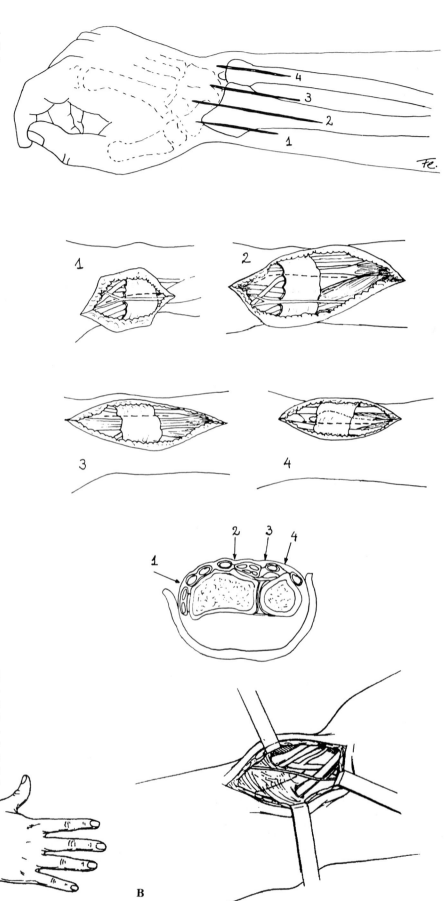

Figure 4.4. A dorsoradial incision is useful for approaching radial styloid fracture fragments. A. The incision is marked out on the skin. B. The approach is between the second and third extensor compartments. Care must be taken to avoid injury to the dorsal branch of the radial sensory nerve and artery should the incision extends more distally to the dorsal radial artery branch.

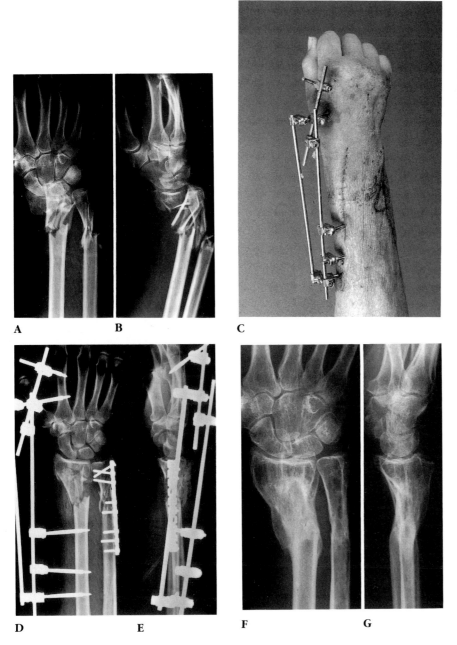

A   B   C

D   E   F   G

Figure 4.5. The dorsoradial incision is illustrated in this complex high-energy fracture of both the radius and the ulnar. A,B. The initial anteroposterior and lateral radiographs reveal the degree of complexity of this fracture. C. An external fixator was applied and the fracture was manipulated and bone was grafted through the dorsoradial incision. D,E. Anteroposterior and lateral radiographs at 4 weeks following fixation and bone grafting of the metaphyseal defect of the distal radius. F,G. Anteroposterior and lateral radiographs at 1 year following treatment. Although there is metaphyseal deformity, the radiocarpal alignment proved to be very functional, and the patient gained nearly full forearm rotation.

The second incision to the dorsum of the radius lies between the third and fourth extensor compartments (Fig. 4.6a). This exposure is chosen for complex articular fractures involving both the scaphoid and the lunate facets of the distal radius. The fourth compartment can be elevated subperiosteally leaving the inferior surface of the compartment intact, which will help minimize contact irritation of the extensor tendons over a dorsally placed implant. The extensor pollicis longus tendon is mobilized and is left above the retinaculum at the time of wound closure to avoid tendon injury either by subsequent ischemia or by direct contact with an implant (Fig. 4.6B). The dorsal wrist capsule can be opened through a longitudinal arthrotomy should added visualization of the radial articular surface or the carpus be required. Repair of this arthrotomy is performed prior to closure (Fig. 4.7A–D).

The fixation of the fractures through this approach involves initial reduction and stabilization of the radial styloid fragment. The reduction can be carefully checked by looking toward the anatomic realignment of the fracture at the metaphyseal level. Once this is secured, it is pinned obliquely to the proximal

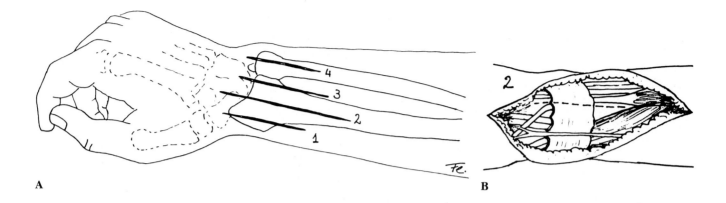

A   B

Figure 4.6. The extensile second dorsal incision is useful for most complex impacted articular fractures that require extensive exposure. A. The incision is marked out in the are a between the second and third or between the third and fourth extensor compartments. B. The incision is made between the third and fourth extensor compartments, bringing the approach to the distal radius.

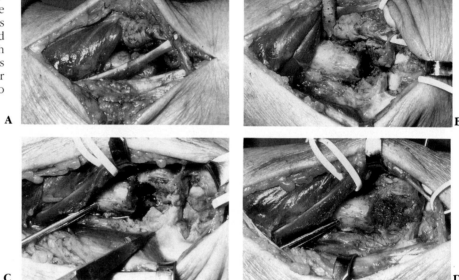

A   B

C   D

Figure 4.7. The extensile dorsal incision for complex articular fractures between the second and third extensor compartments is illustrated. A. The extensor pollicis longus is separated from the fourth compartment. B. The displaced articular fracture fragments are readily visible. The carpus is exposed through a transverse capsulotomy of the dorsal wrist capsule. C. The fracture fragments are anatomically reduced using a pointed awl. Note the metaphyseal defect that is now present. D. The metaphyseal defect is filled with autogenous iliac crest cancellous graft, and the fracture fragments are pinned using a kirschner wire percutaneously placed transversely through the radial styloid across the scaphoid and lunate facet fragments of the distal radius.

radial metaphysis. The dorsal rim fracture is then reduced against the scaphoid and lunate correcting dorsal subluxation of the carpus. Intraarticular congruity is checked through a dorsal transverse arthrotomy or with the imagine intensifier (Fig. 4.7B and C). The articular fragments can be pinned into the intact volar corner of the radius, or, depending upon the size of the dorsal rim fracture, small T or L plates or screws can be used for fixation (Fig. 4.8A–F). If possible, implants should be avoided, to reduce the risk of tenosynovitis created by the implant with the overlying extensor tendons. Following fracture stabilization, we close the retinaculum, leaving the extensor pollicis longus outside the retinaculum, and a suction drain is applied.

A third approach lies between the fourth and fifth extensor compartments.

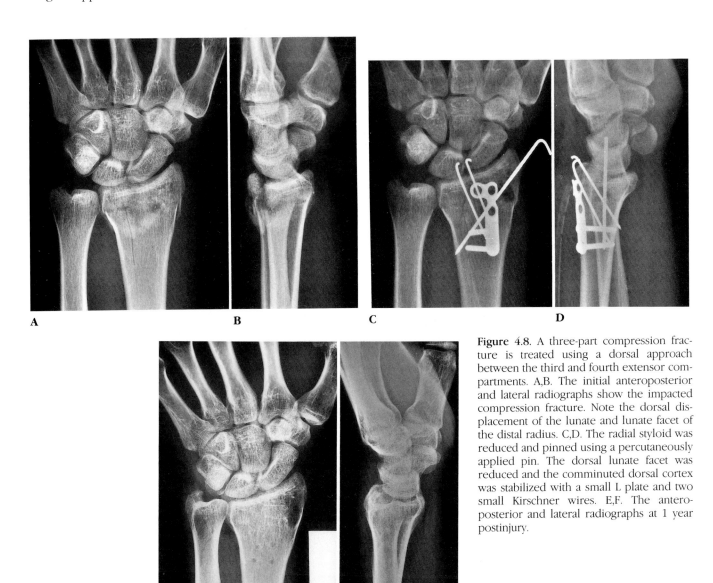

A B C D

E F

Figure 4.8. A three-part compression fracture is treated using a dorsal approach between the third and fourth extensor compartments. A,B. The initial anteroposterior and lateral radiographs show the impacted compression fracture. Note the dorsal displacement of the lunate and lunate facet of the distal radius. C,D. The radial styloid was reduced and pinned using a percutaneously applied pin. The dorsal lunate facet was reduced and the comminuted dorsal cortex was stabilized with a small L plate and two small Kirschner wires. E,F. The anteroposterior and lateral radiographs at 1 year postinjury.

This approach is prefered when limited open reduction of fractures affecting the lunate facet (die-punch fragments) is required (Fig. 4.9A–C). Percutaneous manipulation of the lunate facet fractures can be accomplished through this site (Fig. 4.10A and B). Once the interval between the fourth and fifth extensor compartments has been developed, the distal portion of the capsule of the distal radioulnar joint may be opened for direct evaluation of the reduction of the lunate facet or sigmoid notch of the radius.

The final dorsal incision lies between the fifth and sixth dorsal extensor compartments and is useful for the open reduction of fractures affecting the distal ulnar or for the primary reattachment of the ulnar styloid and/or repair of the triangular fibrocartilage (Fig. 4.3). Some caution must be exercised to search for and protect any branches of the dorsal cutaneous ulnar nerve.

Figure 4.9. Dorsal incision No. 3 is primarily applicable for fractures of the dorsoulnar aspect of the radius and/or those involving the sigmoid notch and ulnar head. A. The incision is drawn out over the dorsoulnar aspect of the radius. B. The incision is noted between the fourth and fifth extensor compartments. C. When the fourth and fifth compartments are elevated, the approach is directly to the dorsoulnar aspect of the radius and sigmoid notch.

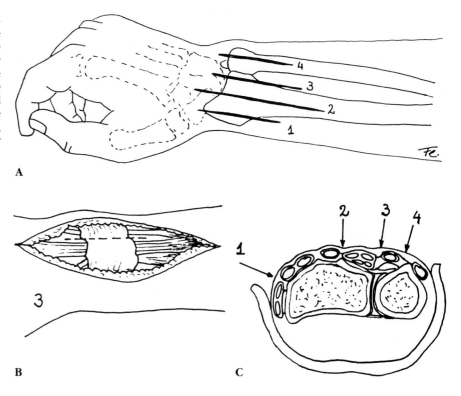

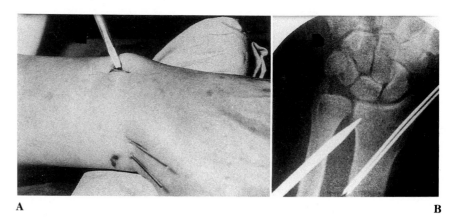

Figure 4.10. Percutaneous manipulation of a lunate facet fracture can be accomplished through a small incision between the fourth and fifth extensor compartments. A. A small pointed awl is introduced into the incision. B. The radiograph shows the location of the pointed awl.

Volar Approaches

For fractures affecting the volar rim of the distal radius, such as volar shearing fractures, the surgical approach is that of the terminal part of the classic Henry approach for the anterior exposure to the distal radius (Fig. 4.11A and B).[18] An incision is made between the flexor carpi radialis tendon and the radial artery (Fig. 4.12A). This interval is developed, revealing the flexor pollicis longus muscle belly at the more proximal extent of the wound and the pronator quadratus muscle more distally (Fig. 4.12B). The radial artery is carefully retracted in a radialward direction while the tendons of the flexor carpi radialis and flexor pollicis longus are retracted ulnarwards. The pronator quadratus is divided at its most radial aspect, leaving a small cuff of muscle for later reattachment (Fig. 4.12C). Any elevation of the muscle belly of the flexor pollicis longus should be performed at its most radial aspect, as it receives its innervation from the anterior interosseous nerve on its ulnar side. After the pronator quadratus has been divided and elevated, the fracture is readily visualized (Fig. 4.12D), and reduction maneuvers can be accomplished under direct vision (Fig. 4.12E). The pronator should be repaired upon closure, particularly if a volar buttress plate has been applied.

After careful exposure of the fracture site and clearing of the fracture hematoma, reduction can be most readily obtained by hyperextending the

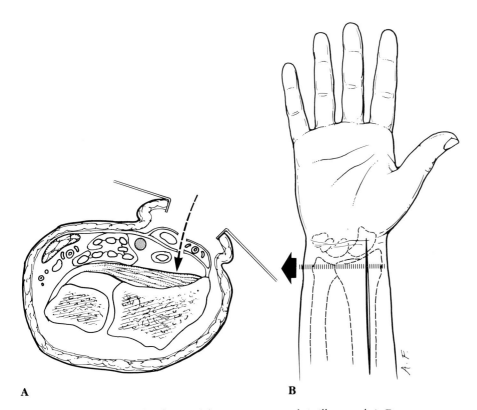

A   **B**

Figure 4.11. The classic distal part of the Henry approach is illustrated. A. Demonstrates the skin incision. B. Demonstrates the surgical approach between the tendon of the flexor carpi radialis and the radial artery.

Figure 4.12. The anterior Henry approach is illustrated in this patient who underwent an osteotomy for a palmar-displaced, malunited distal radius fracture. A. The cutaneous incision is marked out bordering the interval between the tendon of the flexor carpi radialis and the radial artery. B. This schematic and operative photo illustrates the radial artery (ar) and the tendon of the flexor carpi radialis (fcr) identitified following opening of the skin. C. This schematic and clinical illustration demonstrates elevation of the pronator quadratus (PQ) from its attachment on the radial side of the distal radius. The muscle of the flexor pollicis longus (FPL) is identified but does not require elevation. *(Figure continues on facing page.)*

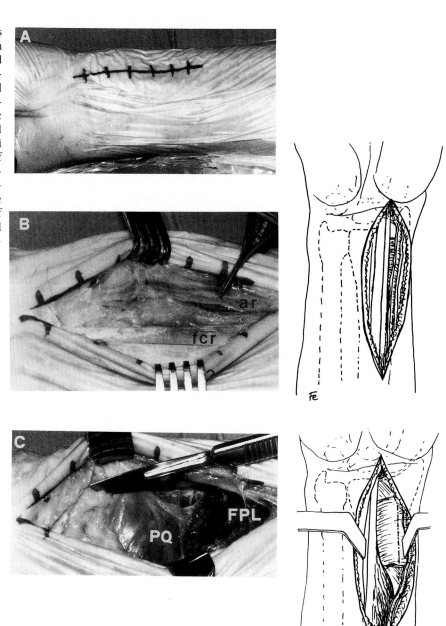

wrist over a rolled towel with the forearm held in full supination (Fig. 4.13). Fracture reduction can then be held temporarily with volar to dorsal Kirschner wires (Fig. 4.14A and B). One technique that can be useful is to place the provisional fixation wire into the fracture fragment in such a way that the distal hole of a small T plate can be placed over the wire in an appropriate position to buttress the fracture. The buttress plate is pre-bent so that there is a small gap between the mid-portion of the plate and the bone just proximal to the fracture site (Fig. 4.15A–C). This gap will help to create the buttressing effect after application of the screws. After the definitive position of the plate has been checked, the most proximal screw is inserted first (Fig. 4.15A). The introduction of the second screw firmly compresses the plate against the radial shaft, obtaining a buttress effect over the distal fragment (Fig. 4.15B). Intra-

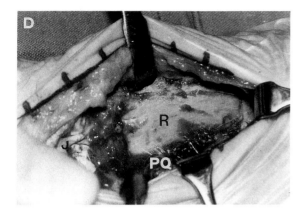

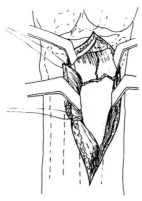

D. This schematic and clinical photo demonstrates the exposure following elevation of the pronator quadratus (PQ) illustrating the metaphyseal aspect of the distal radius (R). E. Following osteotomy and placement of the bone graft (G), an excellent exposure allows for the placement of a buttress plate and screws (P).

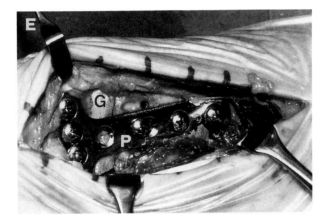

articular congruity should be checked with the image intensifier. Should an articular step-off be identified, the second screw of the plate can be removed and the volar fragment again reduced using a periosteal elevator or sharp awl to adjust its position under the plate. The second screw can then be replaced to secure the reduction. If the volar fragment has a sagittal split, the fracture line can be reduced and held with fixation of the screws in the T plate placed eccentrically at the outer edges of the hole. This will create a compression effect to the sagittal fracture lines with tightening of the screws (Fig. 4.15C).

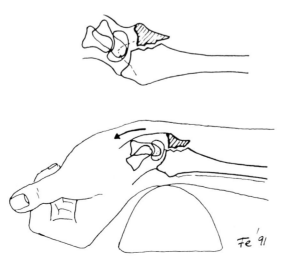

Figure 4.13. The technique of manipulative reduction of palmar shearing fractures is facilitated using longitudinal traction and extension of the wrist over a rolled towel.

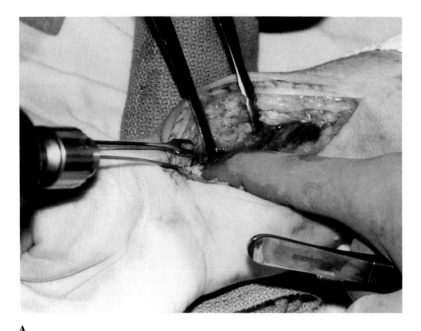

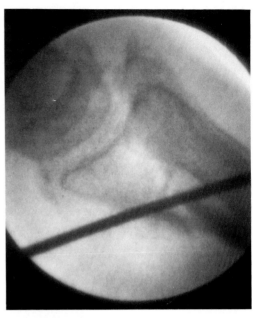

A   **B**

Figure 4.14. A palmar fracture can be provisionally fixed with a smooth Kirschner wire. A. A smooth Kirschner wire is introduced obliquely from volar to dorsal. An oscillating drill is used to avoid injury to soft tissue structures. B. The lateral intraoperative image confirms the position of the wire.

The buttressing effect of the plate without additional screw fixation to the distal part of the plate may suffice for single fragments of the articular rim. If absolute stability is not achieved with the buttress plate alone, two or three screws may be inserted into the distal holes (Fig. 4.15C). Volar rim fractures or more extensive comminution may have independent fragment instability and require separate initial fixation with screws or Kirschner wires before applying the plate.

Once fracture fixation is secured, the tourniquet is released, hemostasis is obtained, and the wound is closed over a suction drain. The pronator quadratus is reattached prior to closure of the skin. Ordinarily, we apply a volar splint

Figure 4.15. The techniques of buttress plating of palmar shearing fractures. A. Initially the plate is slightly straightened from its natural bend and the most proximal screw is applied. By applying the second screw with the plate bent slightly off the bone, tightening the plate will enhance the buttressing effect and, in turn, push the distal fragment dorsally. B. With the second screw tightened, the plate is applying contact pressure on the palmar fragment. C. With sagittal split fractures, screws can be placed in the distal holes to hold the split fracture fragments.

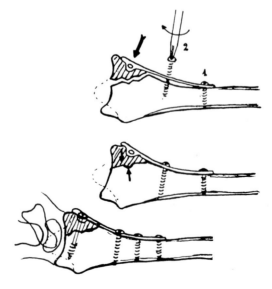

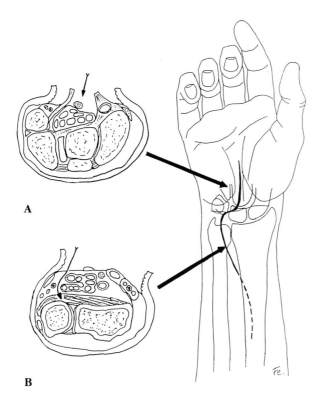

Figure 4.16. The extensile approach to the ulnar side of the distal radius and carpal tunnel illustrated. A. The level of the approach is demonstrated at the proximal margin of the carpal tunnel. The median nerve is identified and the flexor tendons and median nerve can be retracted in a radial direction. B. The surgical approach at the level of the ulnar side of the distal radius demonstrates the ability to retract the flexor tendons and median nerve in a radial direction, providing direct exposure to the palmar ulnar side of the radius.

with the wrist in a neutral position for the first 2 postoperative weeks, at which time the skin sutures are removed and a removable splint is applied for the next 2 weeks. The patient is encouraged to use his or her hands for activities of daily living, but manual work or sports are forbidden until 6 or 8 weeks, at which time fracture consolidation is complete.

A more extensile approach is preferred when exposure is needed for displaced fragments involving the ulnar aspect of the distal radius as well as release of the transverse retinacular ligament and distal antebrachial fascia (Fig. 4.16A and B). The flexor tendons are mobilized radialward and the ulnar nerve and artery in an ulnar direction (Fig. 4.16A). In this approach, the pronator quadratus is partially divided at its more distal aspect overlying the distal radioulnar joint to provide exposure to this area. Whenever possible, care should be taken not to disturb the volar radioulnar ligaments as well as the volar aspect of the triangular fibrocartilage. It is ordinarily not necessary to fully elevate the pronator quadratus from its bony attachment onto the ulnar. The more distal part of this incision represents the standard incision for carpal release (Fig. 4.16B) The transverse retinacular ligament in young individuals may be repaired by Z-lengthening of the ligament.

A third incision can be made between the extensor carpi ulnaris and flexor carpi ulnaris which provides a direct approach for internal fixation of fractures of the distal part of the ulnar shaft. The ulnar lies subcutaneously in this region, facilitating its direct exposure. However, care should be taken to minimize periosteal stripping, and the close proximity of the ulnar nerve and artery and the ulnar dorsal sensory nerve branch must be borne in mind.

Percutaneous Pin Fixation

Percutaneous pin fixation represents an important treatment modality for a number of unstable fracture patterns. These include not only dorsal bending fractures, but also some three- and four-part intraarticular compression fractures. Percutaneous pins are combined with either a plaster cast or an external skeletal fixator, depending upon the fracture type and associated soft tissue problems.

The basic requirements for this technique include an image intensifier, power drill, and smooth Kirschner wires. With the image intensifier properly draped, a closed manipulative reduction is done by combining longitudinal traction, palmar flexion, and ulnar deviation. The quality of the reduction can be accurately determined using fluoroscopic control while traction is maintained. Although some prefer longitudinal traction using sterile finger traps with 2.5 to 5 kg of counterweight across the upper arm, emphasis should be placed upon obtaining an anatomic reduction, which will often require angulation and rotation of the distal fragment. At times, restoration of the palmar tilt of the distal radius can be achieved only by palmar translation of the hand and wrist in conjunction with the longitudinal traction.[1,2]

When combined with external skeletal fixation in articular compression fractures or those fractures associated with soft tissue swelling, an external fixator is applied prior to the placement of the percutaneous pins.

A number of techniques of percutaneous pin fixation have been described. These include pins placed through the radial styloid;[29,41] two pins crossing into the radius;[5,24,39] intrafocal pinning within the fracture site;[17,22,23,33] ulnar to radial pinning without transfixation of the distal radioulnar joint;[10,11,25] one radial styloid pin and a second across the distal radioulnar joint;[31] and pins from the ulnar to the radius with transfixation of the distal radioulnar joint[3] (Fig. 4.17A–F).[35]

For the most part, with unstable extraarticular bending fractures, the authors have preferred the placement of pins, either through the radial styloid alone or in combination with an additional pin directed through the dorsoulnar aspect of the radius (Fig. 4.18A–M). With the fractures reduced manually and controlled using the image intensifier, a smooth 0.062-inch (1.6-mm) Kirschner wire is directed from the tip of the radial styloid just dorsal to the first extensor compartment at an angle of approximately 45 degrees to cross the fracture and enter the dorsoulnar cortex of the radius proximal to the fracture (Fig. 4.18G and H). These pins are best placed using a power drill. At least two pins should be placed through the radial styloid, and it is helpful to bear in mind that the tip of the styloid lies volar to the midlateral line of the radius (Fig. 4.18H). If the wire is placed so that it exits at the fracture site or dose not obtain satisfactory purchase of the cortical bone of the radius more proximally to the fracture fixation of the were and, ultimately, fracture reduction will be last (Fig. 4.18J and K).

The authors frequently place an additional wire into the fracture fragment inserted into the dorsoulnar corner of the radius between the fourth and fifth extensor compartments and directed from dorsoulnar to palmar radial in a distal to proximal direction (Fig. 4.19A and B).

With the fracture reduced and wire placement confirmed on radiographic control, the tips of the wire are bent and left just outside the skin (Fig. 4.18I). If a below-elbow cast is applied, a window should be cut over the pins to offset the possibility of local irritation by the overlying cast. We generally remove the pins between 6 and 8 weeks following placement.

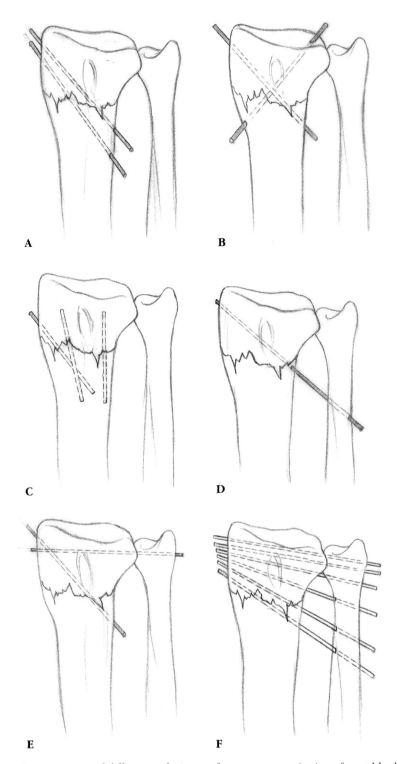

Figure 4.17. A variety of different techniques of percutaneous pinning of unstable distal radius fractures have been described. A. Pins placed primarily through the radial styloid. B. Crossing pins from the radial and ulnar sides of the distal fragment into the distal shaft. C. The intrafocal technique advocated by Kapandji. D. Ulna to radius pinning without transfixation of the distal radioulnar joint. E. A radial styloid pin and one across the distal radioulnar joint. F. Multiple pins from the ulnar to the radius including transfixation of the distal radioulnar joint.

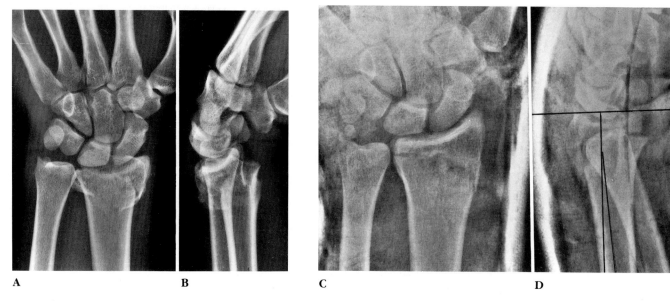

A   **B**   **C**   **D**

Figure 4.18. An unstable compression fracture treated with percutaneous pins. A,B. The initial anteroposterior and lateral radiographs of the unstable compression fracture. C,D. A closed reduction and short arm plaster was applied. The initial radiographs reveal an acceptable reduction. E,F. Radiographs taken 7 days postreduction reveal displacement of the fracture. (*Figure continues on facing page.*)

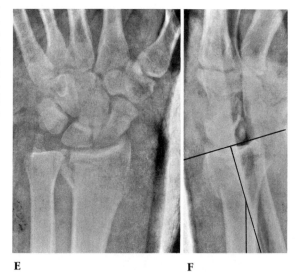

E   **F**

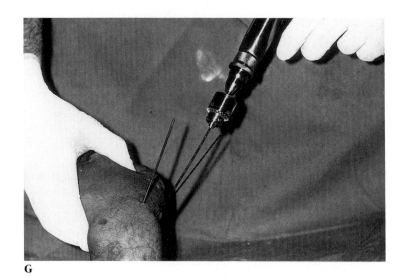

G

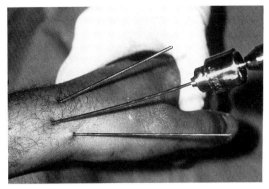

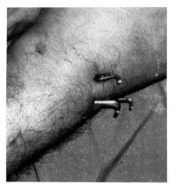

G,H. A remanipulation was performed with the surgeon's hand maintaining the reduction while 1.6-mm (0.62-inch) smooth Kirschner wires were placed from the radial styloid across the fracture site. I. The pins are cut outside of the skin. J,K. Anteroposterior and lateral radiographs following fracture remanipulation, percutaneous pinning, and application of a below-elbow plaster cast. L,M. Anteroposterior and lateral radiographs 6 weeks following the percutaneous pinning. The pins have been removed and the reduction maintained.

H   **I**

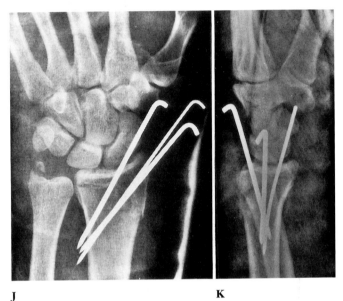

J   **K**

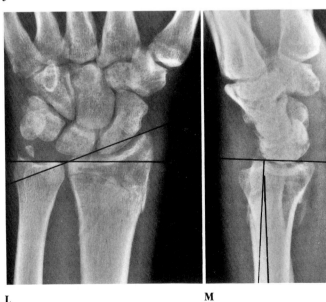

L   **M**

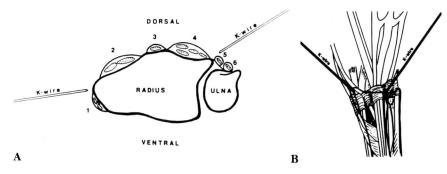

Figure 4.19. The technique of percutaneous pin fixation a illustrated by Clancey.[5] A. The radial styloid pin is passed from volar radial to dorsoulnar. B. A dorsoulnar pin goes between the fourth and fifth compartments. Reprinted with permission. Clancey G: Percutaneous Kirschner wire fixation of Colles' fracture. *J Bone Joint Surg* 66A: 1008–1014, 1984.

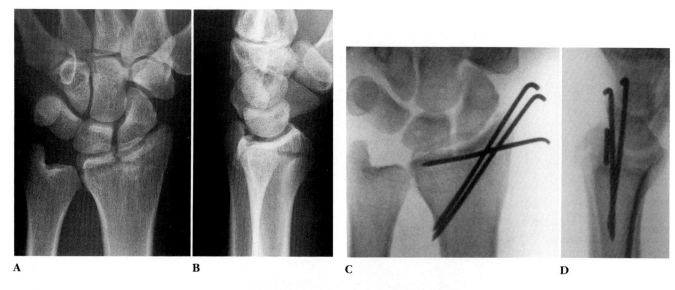

A   **B**   **C**   **D**

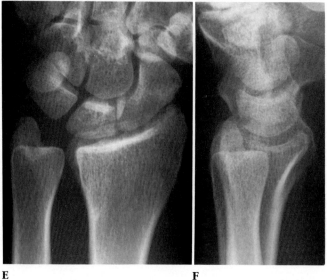

E   **F**

Figure 4.20. An impacted, three-part articular compression fracture represents an excellent illustration of the technique of manipulative reduction and percutaneous pin fixation. A,B. The initial anteroposterior and lateral radiographs of the impacted articular fracture. C,D. Following a closed manipulative reduction, the radial styloid fragment was pinned using two stout smooth Kirschner wires. A transverse smooth Kirschner wire from radial to ulnar supported the reduced dorsoulnar lunate facet. Note that the transverse wire is nearly subchondral as it supports the reduced fragment. E,F. Anteroposterior and lateral radiographs 2 years postinjury. Note the anatomic restoration.

The above technique of percutaneous pinning represents the authors' most commonly applied tactic (Fig. 4.20A–F). Other primary techniques, including the intrafocal techniques of Kapandji, will be discussed in some detail in Chapter 5.

Closed Reduction and Percutaneous Pinning with Arthroscopic

The introduction of the small-diameter arthroscope has offered the possibility of manipulating articular fracture fragments under direction vision.[7,40] An initial reduction is performed by manipulation and traction with control using the image intensifier. Alternatively, an external fixator can be applied, maintaining the length of the radius and additionally providing continuous distraction while arthroscopy is performed.

Prior to using the arthroscope, a compressive elastic bandage is wrapped around the forearm to retard fluid extravasation into the muscle compartments. Additionally, it may be preferable to perform the arthroscopic-assisted reduction 3 or 4 days following the fracture to minimize the problem of obscuring of visualization of the articular surfaces by active bleeding.

The usual landmarks for a wrist arthroscopy are identified with a marking pen; the landmarks, however, may be distorted by swelling associated with the injury. Small incisions with blunt dissection to the wrist capsule are recommended to avoid cutaneous nerve injury.[40] In many cases, visualization of the distal articular surface is obtained with the arthroscope in a No. 3 or 4 portal with the inflow cannula placed in the 6U portal. The entire joint, including the distal radius, triangular fibrocartilage, and intracapsular and intracarpal ligaments, should be inspected for associated injury. Scapholunate dissociation is not uncommon with radial styloid fractures, and the arthroscope can be extremely useful in visualizing this region.

Fracture fragments can be disimpacted using a small dissector introduced percutaneously. Each fragment to be reduced is manipulated under direct vision with percutaneous insertion of a 0.5-inch (1.2-mm) smooth Kirschner wire introduced into the fragment proximal to the level of the joint. This Kirschner wire can be used to help reduce the fragment into position under direct visualization through the arthroscope. Larger fragments should be reduced initially, followed by smaller fragments, each with the own Kirschner wire as a "joy stick" helping to reduce the fragment. Once all of the fragments are reduced, compression can be applied using a pointed reduction clamp and the pins advanced into adjacent fragments.

The reduction must also be checked by radiographic control (Fig. 4.21A–H).

External Skeletal Fixation

External skeletal fixation remains an important tactic in the management of fractures of the distal end of the radius.[3,8,9,13,21,37] Attention to detail is important not only in the recognition of indications and functions of the external fixator but also in its specific application.

Most wrist external fixators in current use are applied as unilateral frames.[15,16,20] Transarticular frames are applied with pins in the distal radial diaphysis crossing the wrist to pins into the second and sometimes third

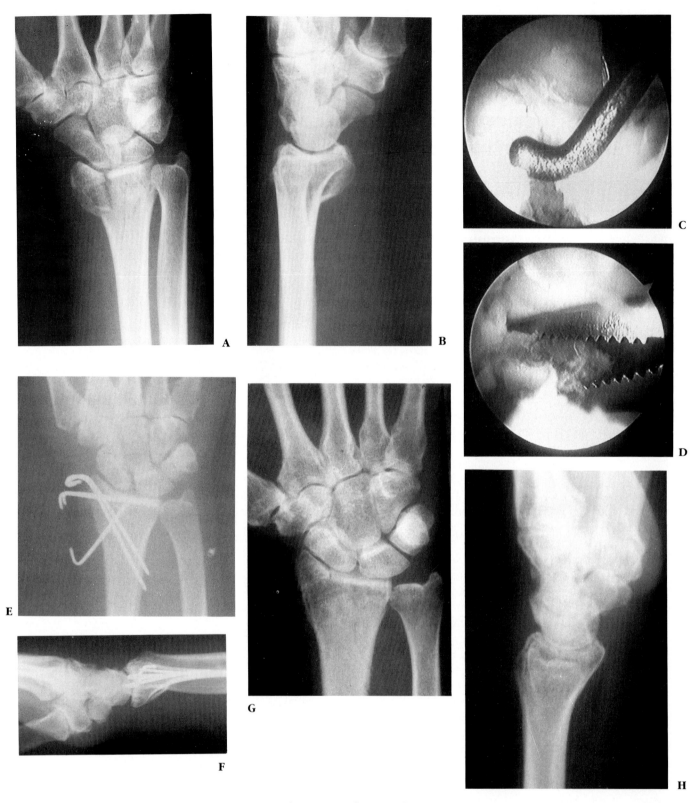

Figure 4.21. A complex articular fracture reduced under arthroscopic control. Case courtesy of Dr. William Geissler. A,B. Anteroposterior and lateral radiographs of an intraarticular fracture in a 25-year-old tennis player. C. Arthroscopic view of the displaced styloid fragment. A 1-mm arthroscopic probe palpates the fracture site. D. A loose body is removed from the radiocarpal joint space. E,F. Anteroposterior and lateral radiographs following reduction and percutaneous pin fixation. G,H. Anteroposterior and lateral radiographs at 2 years. Excellent function was obtained.

metacarpal. Half-threaded pins of variable sizes are used, depending in part on the size and quality of the underlying bone as well as the specific frame design (Fig. 4.22A–F). However, for certain indications, the fixator can be used to stabilize the distal end of the radius without crossing the radiocarpal joint. These include those fractures without comminution, especially in younger patients. This technique can be utilized as alternative treatment of distal radial osteotomies or even intraoperatively to help reduce complex fractures and/or malunions (Fig. 4.23A and B).[27,28,30]

Circular or semicircular frames have been applied in cases of distraction osteogenesis or progressive correction for congenital, developmental, or post-traumatic deformities of the forearm (Fig. 4.24A–E).

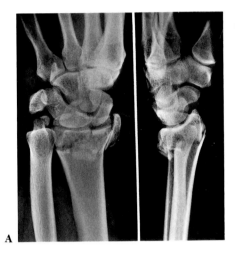
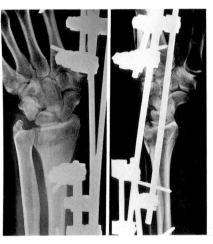
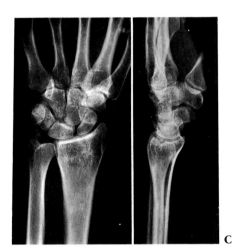

A   B   C

Figure 4.22. A dorsal bending fracture with metaphyseal comminution was anatomically reduced and held using external fixation. A,B. The anteroposterior and lateral radiographs show the complex dorsal bending fracture. C,D. The fracture was anatomically reduced by longitudinal traction with some ulnar deviation and palmar translation of the carpus. The reduction was maintained using external fixation alone. E. Anteroposterior and lateral radiographs 3 years following injury demonstrating the maintenance of the anatomic alignment. Full and pain-free function was achieved.

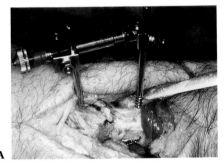

A

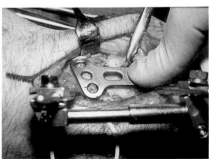

B

Figure 4.23. In certain instances, an external fixator can be used without crossing the radiocarpal joint. A. A malunited fracture treated 8 weeks postinjury. The fixator is applied as a mini distractor to allow for gentle reduction. B. The fixator is used temporarily to hold the reduction while plate fixation is applied.

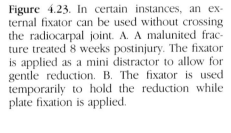

Figure 4.24. A circular frame is useful for correction of severe congenital or post-traumatic deformities. A. The antero-posterior radiograph of a severe forearm deformity following childhood infection of the radius in a 30-year-old woman. B. The clinical appearance of deformity. C. A circular frame was applied to slowly bring the hand and wrist into an acceptable position. A resection of the distal ulnar was also performed. D,E. Following realignment, a plate and bone graft spanned the defect in the radius. Excellent function resulted.

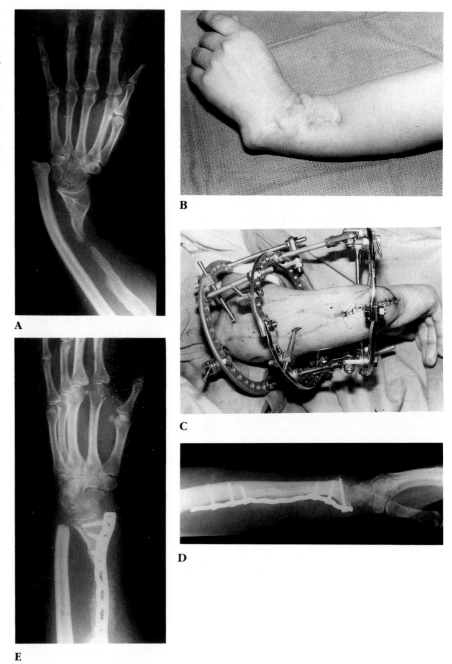

External Fixator Function

Depending upon the specific mechanical features inherent in the specific fracture pattern, external fixation may act as a joint distractor, neutralization frame, buttress, or even to compress the fracture.

With joint distraction, the device in reality has two roles. The first is that of obtaining an indirect reduction of comminuted intraarticular fractures through tension on the capsuloligamentous attachments and, in some cases, through a change in the intraarticular joint pressure due to distraction; the latter may produce a "vacuum effect" that would help explain how successful reduction of fracture fragments without capsular attachments may occur.[36] A second role of the external fixator frame in joint distraction is to maintain fracture fragment alignment when the device is statically locked (Fig. 4.25A–J). The distraction

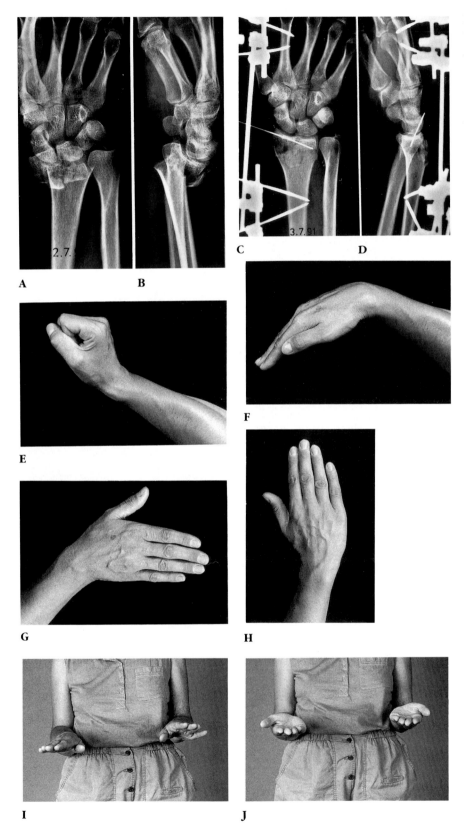

Figure 4.25. The technique of converging external fixator pins is demonstrated in this complex articular fracture in a young woman. A,B. The initial anteroposterior radiographs show the complex compression displaced multifragmented articular and metaphyseal fracture. C,D. Following manipulative reduction, external fixation was applied. Note the convergence of the pins in the second metacarpal and distal radius. A percutaneous pin was used to support the articular reconstruction. At a 6-year follow-up E,F. satisfactory wrist extension and flexion were noted. G,H. At a 6-year follow-up, satisfactory radial and ulnar deviation was maintained. I,J. At a 6-years followup, forearm rotation was maintained.

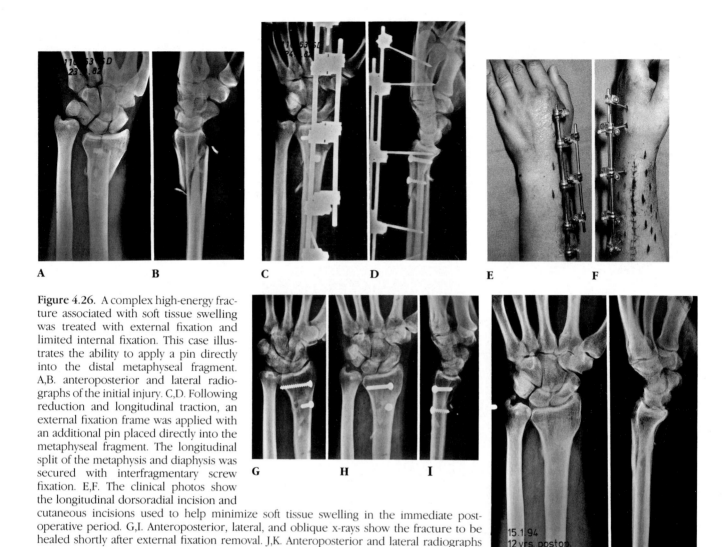

Figure 4.26. A complex high-energy fracture associated with soft tissue swelling was treated with external fixation and limited internal fixation. This case illustrates the ability to apply a pin directly into the distal metaphyseal fragment. A,B. anteroposterior and lateral radiographs of the initial injury. C,D. Following reduction and longitudinal traction, an external fixation frame was applied with an additional pin placed directly into the metaphyseal fragment. The longitudinal split of the metaphysis and diaphysis was secured with interfragmentary screw fixation. E,F. The clinical photos show the longitudinal dorsoradial incision and cutaneous incisions used to help minimize soft tissue swelling in the immediate postoperative period. G,I. Anteroposterior, lateral, and oblique x-rays show the fracture to be healed shortly after external fixation removal. J,K. Anteroposterior and lateral radiographs 12 years following the injury. Note the maintenance of the near-anatomic reduction. (*Figure continues on facing page.*)

maintained by the frame is of particular use in the setting of complex carpal dislocations[15,20,21] and in certain reconstructive procedures in which restoration of normal carpal height is required. The adverse effects of untoward or prolonged longitudinal joint distraction may be the creation of extrinsic extensor tightness with metacarpophalangeal joint hyperextension[1] and possible loss of radiocarpal and intercarpal mobility.

An external fixation frame can function as a neutralization device. Here also two possible applications exist. In the first place, the external fixator will unload and protect a fracture which has internal fixation in which the overall rigidity of the fixation is insufficient to prevent secondary displacement under functional loading (Fig. 4.26A–Q).

A second situation in which neutralization occurs with an external fixator is the protection of bending, torsional, and shearing forces acting upon a realigned extraarticular bending fracture (Fig. 4.22A–F).

When an external fixation frame is utilized to temporarily bridge large skeletal defects, it is now acting in a buttress fashion. The frame itself will represent a means of carrying functional loading between the proximal and

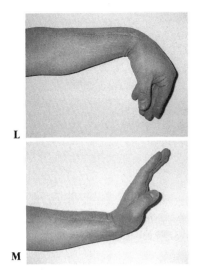

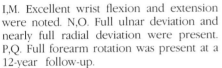

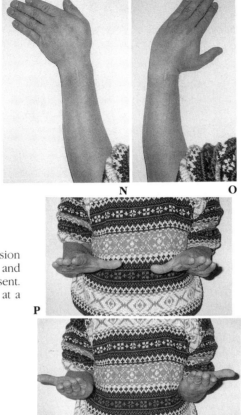

I,M. Excellent wrist flexion and extension were noted. N,O. Full ulnar deviation and nearly full radial deviation were present. P,Q. Full forearm rotation was present at a 12-year follow-up.

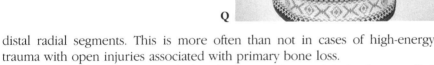

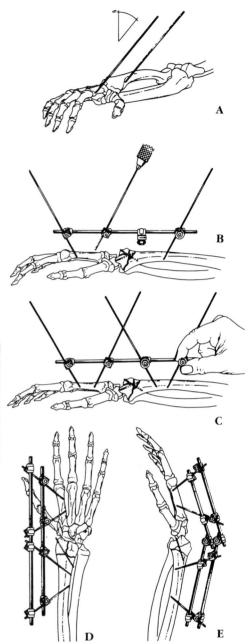

distal radial segments. This is more often than not in cases of high-energy trauma with open injuries associated with primary bone loss.

An additional situation in which a frame can be used is in the so-called dynamic fashion. These fixators are designed to permit some mobility of the radiocarpal joint with the fixator in place and joint distraction maintained. The exact positioning of the fixator, with the center of rotation of the wrist being maintained in the head of the capitate, is critical so that bending moments during functional motion occur at the carpal level and not at the fracture site.[6,26,32,34]

Technique of Application

The application of external fixation requires adequate anesthesia, ideally an image intensifier, and appropriate equipment for small bone surgery (Fig. 4.27A–E).[19]

A pneumatic tourniquet should be applied on the upper arm but not inflated unless absolutely necessary. Prior to application of the external fixator, the major displacement of the distal radius fracture should be reduced by longitudinal traction and manipulation. The adequacy of the reduction is controlled under image intensification (Fig. 4.28A and B). In fact, if the reduction is acceptable, percutaneous pins can be placed into the radial styloid prior to the application of the external fixator.

As the authors have had the bulk of their experience with the AO/ASIF external fixation frame, this device will be used to illustrate the technique of application. Once the gross fracture malalignment is reduced, the arm and the

Figure 4.27. The techniques of external fixation application in conjunction with cutaneous pin fixation are illustrated in this schematic. A. The pins are placed at an angle of 45 degrees from the horizontal. B. One technique is to achieve longitudinal traction using two pins—one in the metacarpal and one in the radius—and stably secure the fracture with percutaneous pins. The remaining two external fixation pins can be placed using the pin to bar clamps keeping the wrist in a neutral position. C. Once the four pins have been placed, subtending an angle of 30 to 60 degrees between the two sets of pins, the pin bar clamps can be tightened. D. A second bar is applied keeping the hand and wrist in neutral. E. Should palmar flexion or deviation be required, the two pin clusters can be connected to each other using bar-to-bar clamps.

Figure 4.28. The technique of external fixation is illustrated in a step-by-step fashion. A. Both the arm and the iliac crest should be sterile and draped. B. The use of image intensification is extremely important in the technique of external fixation and percutaneous pin fixation. C. The strategic location of the pins can be controlled by marking the specific locus on the skin using image intensification. D. The more distal metacarpal pin is to be placed at the junction of the mid and distal third metacarpals. E. The placement of the metacarpal pin can be controlled with image intensification. F. The two radial pins are placed to avoid the muscles of the abductor pollicis longus and extensor pollicis longus. G. All the pins should be placed through small incisions with dissection to the bone and freeing the soft tissues from the area for the pin placement. H. A drill guide with a serrated end should be used in all instances. I. The radial pin can be controlled as well by the use of image. J,K. One technique for facilitating reduction is to apply a small mini distractor *(Figure continues on facing page.)*

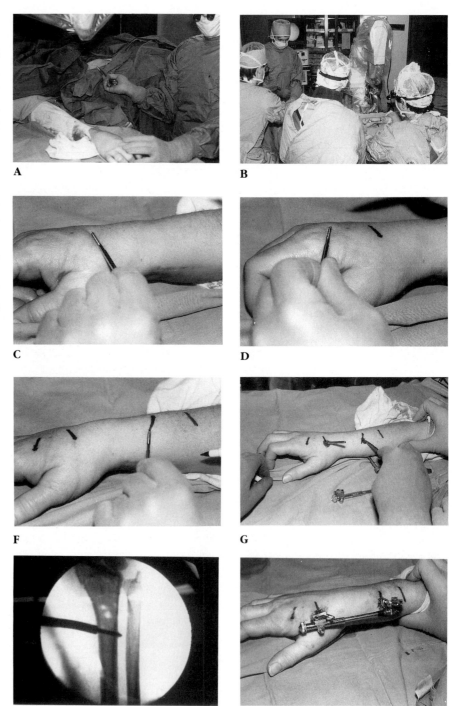

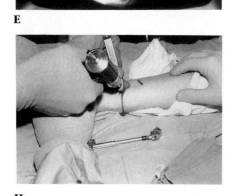

ipsilateral iliac crest are prepared in a sterile manner and draped for the possible need for more extensive surgical manipulation and even autogenous iliac crest bone graft (Fig. 4.28B).

The technique of pin insertion remains very much the same regardless of the type of pin utilized. Pin insertion should be performed through small incisions following soft tissue dissection to identify the underlying bone. A hemostat or dissecting scissor is used to spread the soft tissues, following which a protective drill sleeve is placed through the opening directly onto the bone. Precise location of pin application is enhanced by using the image

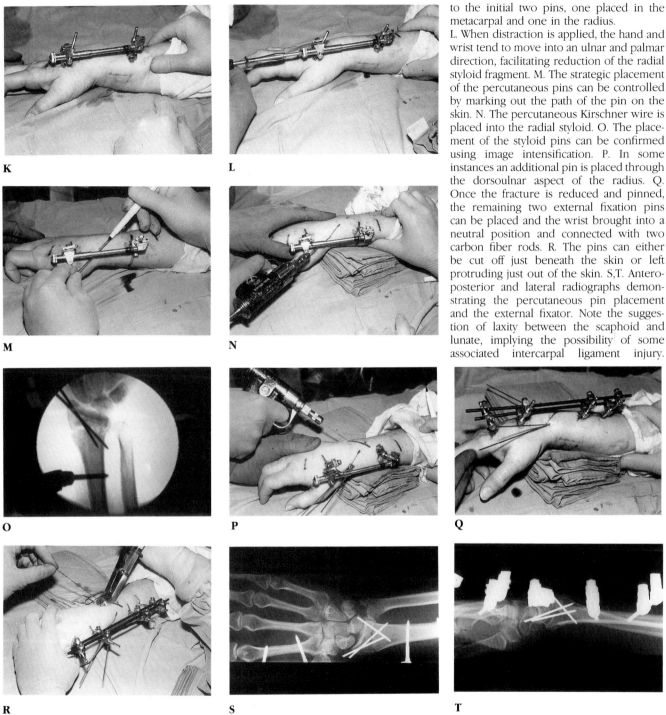

K

L

M

N

O

P

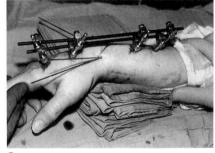

Q

R

S

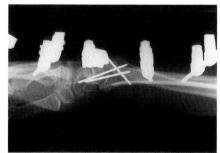

T

to the initial two pins, one placed in the metacarpal and one in the radius.

L. When distraction is applied, the hand and wrist tend to move into an ulnar and palmar direction, facilitating reduction of the radial styloid fragment. M. The strategic placement of the percutaneous pins can be controlled by marking out the path of the pin on the skin. N. The percutaneous Kirschner wire is placed into the radial styloid. O. The placement of the styloid pins can be confirmed using image intensification. P. In some instances an additional pin is placed through the dorsoulnar aspect of the radius. Q. Once the fracture is reduced and pinned, the remaining two external fixation pins can be placed and the wrist brought into a neutral position and connected with two carbon fiber rods. R. The pins can either be cut off just beneath the skin or left protruding just out of the skin. S,T. Antero-posterior and lateral radiographs demonstrating the percutaneous pin placement and the external fixator. Note the suggestion of laxity between the scaphoid and lunate, implying the possibility of some associated intercarpal ligament injury.

intensifier prior to making the skin incision to precisely identify the location of the pin placement into the metacarpal and distal diaphysis of the radius (Fig. 4.28C and D). In the metacarpal it is our preference to place one pin at the base of the second metacarpal and one in the more distal aspect of the metacarpal. The first dorsal interosseous muscle, extensor tendons, and branches of the radial sensory nerve must be spared with the placement of the pin which can be accomplished by using protective drill sleeves. In harder bone, a 2.0-mm drill bit is used to predrill a hole for the 2.5-mm Schanz pins. In the second metacarpal, pins are placed approximately 45 degrees from the transverse axis of the palm in a converging fashion, creating an angle of 45 to 60 degrees between the two pins in the metacarpal. The placement can be confirmed using the image intensifier and the accuracy of the pin placement enhanced by rotating the hand to obtain a three-dimensional picture of the pin placement and extent of pin penetration into the opposite cortex of the metacarpal (Fig. 4.28E).

Placement of the pins into the distal third of the radius will in most cases be at a point approximately 10 to 12 cm proximal to the radial styloid.[38] This point is preferably just proximal to the muscle bellies of the abductor pollicis longus and extensor pollicis brevis. Again through small incisions and utilizing a serrated drill guide, one can avoid injury to the overlying tendons, muscle bellies, or branches of the radial sensory nerve. In the radius we currently are using 4.0-mm Schanz pins and predrilling with a 2.5-mm drill bit. Again, the position of the pins and their depths can be confirmed by image control (Fig. 4.28F–I).

An alternative method for obtaining distraction and aid in the reduction of complex articular injuries is with the use of a small distractor applied to one Schanz pin placed at the base of the second metacarpal and one placed into the distal radius (Fig. 4.28J and K). By distraction using these two pin placements, there is a natural tendency for the hand and wrist to move into ulnar deviation and a modest degree of palmar flexion. This, in turn, will help reduce the radial styloid part of the articular fracture and will be most beneficial for extraarticular dorsal bending-type fractures (Fig. 4.28L). The distractor will also serve to free up the surgeon's hands for subsequent placement of percutaneous Kirschner wires or limited open reduction (Fig. 4.28M). With the fracture reduction confirmed, the Kirschner wires can be placed under image control (Fig. 4.28N–P). At this juncture the remaining two external fixation pins can be applied and the frame constructed (Fig. 4.28Q and R). It is preferable to maintain the wrist in a neutral position rather than the position maintained while traction was applied. Thus the fixator should be readjusted to keep the hand and wrist in a neutral position, which will enhance overall digital articular and tendon function (Fig. 4.28S and T).

The stability of the external frame and pins can be increased by a number of features. In the first place, predrilling holes prior to pin placement will eliminate the possibility of "toggling" occurring when the pin is asked to cut its own hole in both the near and the opposite cortex. Secondly, having pins with a smooth shank filling the near cortex hole, with the diameter of the shank slightly larger than the hole in the near cortex, will in effect create a radial preload, providing increased contact pressure in a circumferential manner, minimizing bone resorption due to motion. By increasing the pin-to-pin distance on the same side of the fracture and decreasing the pin-to-pin distance across the fracture, enhanced stability will result. Finally, placing the connecting rod closer to the radius and metacarpals will also increase the stability of the frame. For most situations, we have used two connecting rods, one placed fairly close to the skin and the other approximately 1 to 1½ cm away from the first connecting bar. When the hand and wrist are placed in a position other than a neutral position with reference to the distal radius, the connecting bars will be required to have bar-to-bar connecting clamps to provide this freedom of positioning (Fig. 4.27A–E).

At the conclusion of the case, the external fixator pins are wrapped with sterile gauze. If skin tension has changed, with the skin appearing taut around the base of the pins, a small incision should be made to release the tension prior to leaving the operating room. A volar splint is applied and it is maintained for the first 3 postoperative weeks.

The external fixator allows for free motion of the digits and even for forearm rotation. It is critical to have the patient begin active digital exercises as early as the first postoperative day. Supervision should be maintained by both the treating surgeon and by a trained therapist to monitor the patient's progress, provide instruction and encouragement, and provide antiedema measures such as Coban wraps.

Manipulative Reduction of Displaced Articular Fractures with Percutaneous Pinning

Three-part, as well as some four-part compression fractures of the distal end of the radius with dorsoulnar and radial styloid fracture fragments can often be treated by a combination of longitudinal traction with external fixation and percutaneous pin fixation.[14] External fixation in these cases is preferable, to help control both radial shortening and metaphyseal angulation of the distal fragments.

The initial reduction of these types of fracture patterns can be obtained either by longitudinal traction and fracture manipulation by the surgeon or by using longitudinal traction with a small distractor (Fig. 4.29A–D). The tactic involves initial stabilization of the radial styloid with percutaneous Kirschner wires followed by manipulative reduction of the dorsoulnar fragment using external longitudinal traction with the hand and wrist now in radial deviation,

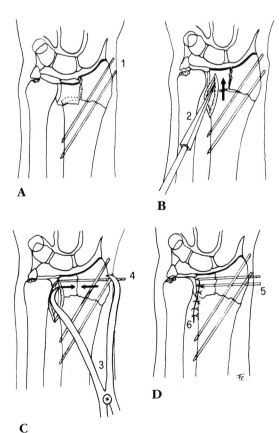

Figure 4.29. The tactics of percutaneous pin fixation of simple three-part compression articular fractures. A. The radial styloid fragment (1) is initially reduced and stabilized with two or three smooth Kirschner wires. B. The dorsoulnar facet fragment may require a limited skin incision and elevation using a pointed awl (2) C. Closure of the sagittal gap between the articular fragments is facilitated by the placement of a pointed bone reduction clamp (3) applying interfragmentary compression (4). D. The dorsoulnar fragment is pinned by two smooth Kirschner wires introduced across the radial styloid (5) into the dorsoulnar fragment. Care is taken to avoid entrance of the pins into the distal radioulnar joint (6).

Figure 4.30. A compression-type fracture with displacement of the radial styloid and dorsoulnar facet of the distal radius. A,B. The anteroposterior and lateral radiographs reveal displacement of the articular fragment. C. A closed manipulative reduction of the radial styloid was performed using longitudinal traction, palmar flexion, and ulnar deviation of the hand and wrist. This was followed by the placement of two smooth Kirschner wires through the radial styloid obliquely into the more proximal radius. D. The dorsoulnar fragment did not reduce with longitudinal traction and radial deviation of the hand and wrist. Therefore a small incision was made between the fourth and fifth extensor compartments, and a pointed awl was used to elevate the fragment. E. The pointed awl is ideal for pushing the fragment under image control. F. The fracture reduction is controlled under the image intensifier. G. Using a pointed reduction clamp, interfragmentary compression can be achieved between the articular fragments in order to reduce the sagittal space between the two fragments while pins are placed transversely across the radial styloid into the dorsoulnar fragment. H. Three smooth Kirschner wires are placed transversely through the styloid into the dorsoulnar fragment. I,J. Anteroposterior and lateral radiographs of the fractures at 5 weeks postpinning. K,L. Four months following pin removal, excellent reduction is maintained.

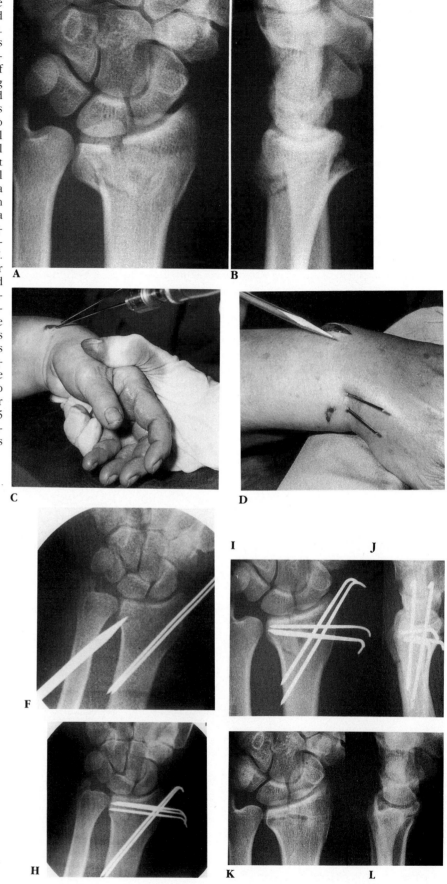

or using a small pointed awl placed through a small incision within the vicinity of the fourth and fifth extensor compartments just proximal to the lunate facet (Fig. 4.30A–L). Once this fracture fragment is elevated, a pointed bone reduction forceps is carefully placed on the medial fragment through the dorsoulnar incision and on the skin overlying the radial styloid fragment to help close any sagittal separation between the articular fragments (Fig. 4.30G). The forceps are left in place while one or two small Kirschner wires are introduced transversely from the radial styloid toward the sigmoid notch. Particular attention must be taken not to enter the distal radioulnar joint (Fig. 4.30H).

If there are no soft tissue problems, a short below-elbow cast can be used, although in most cases an external fixation device is left in place for 6 weeks, at which time it is removed along with the percutaneously placed pins.

Closed and Limited Open Reduction Techniques for Displaced Volar Articular Fragments

In complex four-part articular compression fractures in which the lunate facet is split into dorsal and volar fragments, the volar fragment, if displaced and rotated, may not be capable of being reduced by manipulative or even percutaneous means alone.

The technique for this particular fracture pattern is once again based upon the concept of identification of the distal radial articular fragments as distinct entities. These include the distal radial metaphysis, radial styloid, dorsoulnar aspect of the lunate facet, and palmar half of the lunate facet (Fig. 4.31A–D).

Length and gross alignment can be obtained with longitudinal traction alone and maintained by the application of an external skeletal fixation device. The radial styloid fragment, once reduced, can be secured with percutaneously placed smooth Kirschner wires (Fig. 4.32A–J).

With a displaced and rotated volar lunate facet fragment that cannot be accurately reduced by longitudinal traction, it is advisable to secure at this

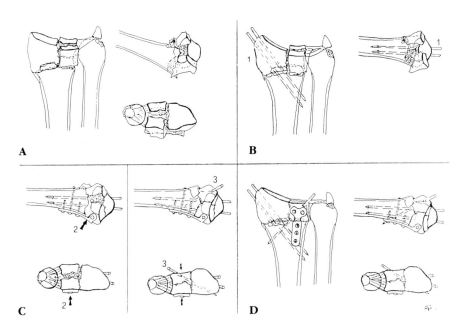

A

B

C

D

Figure 4.31. The surgical tactics and illustrated for complex four-part articular fractures in which the lunate facet is split and the volar fragment rotated. A. Pictorial presentation of a complex four-part articular fracture. B. The radial styloid fragment (1) is reduced and percutaneously pinned. C. Through a volar approach, the volar lunate facet fragment is reduced and supported with a small plate (2). The dorsal lunate facet fragment is reduced and pinned (3). Schematic of the entire surgical construct.

Figure 4.32. A four-part compression intra-articular fracture is treated with a combination of percutaneous and limited open reduction of the volar fragment. A,B. Initial anteroposterior and lateral radiographs demonstrating the articular compression fracture. C,D. Following ligamentotaxis and application of an external fixator, the radial styloid was effectively reduced. E,F. Following pinning of the radial styloid, a limited volar approach was made, and the small displaced volar lunate facet fracture fragment was reduced under direct vision and pinned, with the pins retrieved through the dorsal skin. The dorsal lunate facet fragment was then manipulated using a pointed awl and pinned with transverse, smooth Kirschner wires. G,H. Anteroposterior and lateral radiographs at 5 weeks following removal of the external fixator and all but one of the Kirschner wires. This later had to be removed under regional anesthesia. I,J. Anteroposterior and lateral radiographs 4 years postinjury. The patient experienced minimal if any symptoms.

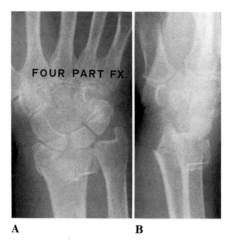

A   B

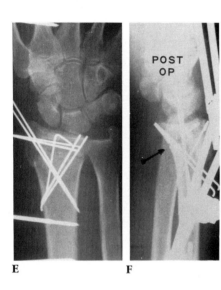

E   F

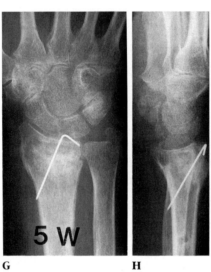

G   H

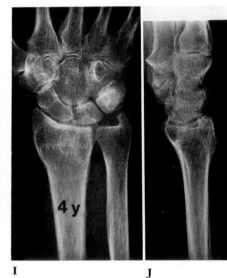

C   D

I   J

point a reduction of the anterior displaced fragment. Once this is accomplished, the dorsoulnar lunate facet fragment can be more readily reduced by closed or percutaneous techniques onto the reduced volar fragment. A longitudinal incision is made along the ulnar-volar side of the distal forearm. The ulnar nerves and arteries are identified and protected. The flexor tendons are retracted radialward, and the distal portion of the pronator quadratus is incised and the distal part of this muscle elevated from the vicinity of the displaced volar ulnar articular fragment. The soft tissue attachments to the small fragment should be preserved, and the surgeon should take heed to avoid opening the volar capsular ligaments of the radiocarpal joint for the purpose of directly observing the articular surface. The adequacy of reduction can be based upon its realignment with the radial styloid fragment as well as the distal radial metaphysis. Furthermore, by displacing this fragment initially, the surgeon can visualize the articular surface from within the metaphysis, thereby observing displaced, impacted articular fragments that may not have been apparent on the initial radiographs.

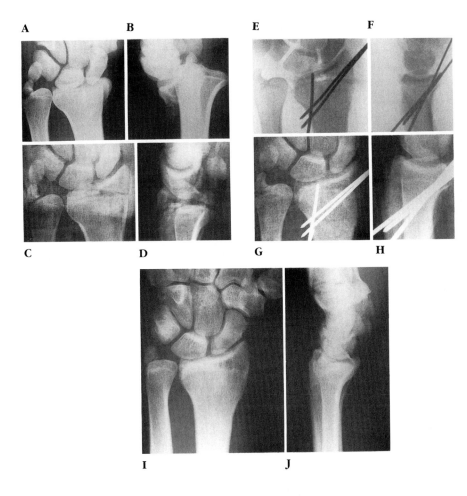

Figure 4.33. A complex articular fracture treated with combined percutaneous and open reduction. A,B. Initial anteroposterior and lateral radiographs. C,D. Closed treatment demonstrated major articular malalignment. E,F. Limited open and closed reduction and percutaneous pinning with a near anatomic result. G,H. At 6 weeks, fracture union. I,J. Follow-up radiographs at 1 year reveal maintenance of anatomic reduction.

In the event that the volar fragment is small, fixation can be effectively achieved with a single smooth Kirschner wire introduced obliquely from the volar surface of the fragment across the metaphysis and retrieved through the dorsal skin of the forearm (Fig. 4.32E and F). For larger fragments, screw fixation alone, or even a small L or T plate, can be used to provide an effective "buttress" for this reduced fragment. Screws should not be placed in the distal portion of the small plate, as these can interfere with reduction of the dorsoulnar lunate fragment (Fig. 4.31A–E).

At this juncture, the case can proceed as described for the closed manipulative reduction of three- and four-part fractures, using either a pointed awl or a pointed reduction forceps to help reduce the dorsoulnar fragment, which can then be pinned in a transverse starting from the radial styloid across into the dorsoulnar fragment (Fig. 4.33A–J).

Techniques of Distal Ulna Stabilization

The unstable distal ulnar may be associated with soft tissue disruption, including the triangular fibrocartilage complex (Type IIA), a large ulnar styloid fracture (Type IIB), or a complex fracture involving the ulnar head or neck (Type IIIB).

The recommended surgical approach for the complex distal ulnar fracture or ulnar styloid disruption is that between the extensor carpi ulnaris and flexor

Figure 4.34. A complex ulnar neck fracture is stabilized with a third-tubular plate.

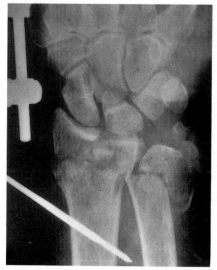
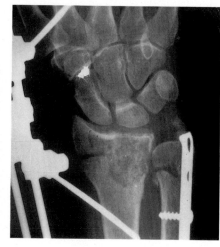

Figure 4.35. Ulnar styloid fractures can be stabilized in several ways. A. The tension band technique of ulnar styloid stabilization. B. Ulnar styloid fixation with a cannulated screw.

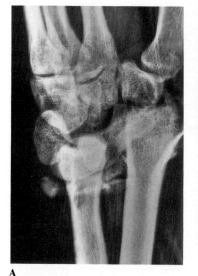
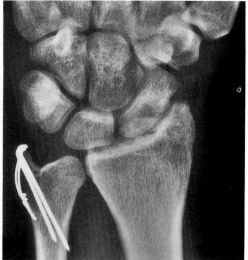

A

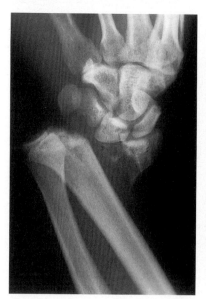
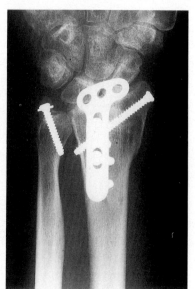

B

carpi ulnaris along the ulnar border of the forearm. The dorsal sensory branch of the ulnar nerve must be visualized to protect it from direct injury during the surgical approach.

For complex fractures of the ulnar head and/or neck, a 2.7-mm condylar plate or a small-fragment 2.7-mm DC plate is preferably placed directly along the ulnar border (Fig. 4.34).

The ulnar styloid, in fact, tends to be more palmar in its anatomic position and thus may effectively be reached through this approach rather than a dorsal approach. A number of options exist for fixation of this styloid, including a tension band technique (Fig. 4.35A), Herbert screw, or cannulated screw (Fig. 4.35B). The tension band technique is quite straightforward and does not require complex equipment. Two 0.045-inch (1.2-mm) Kirschner wires are driven obliquely across the styloid into the more proximal dorsal aspect of the ulnar neck. The points of the wires are allowed to protrude slightly from the bone, around which a thin stainless steel wire can be looped, with the loops extending along the ulnar styloid over the ends of the pin, which are then bent off and driven into the bone.

The unstable ulnar that remains displaced despite anatomic reduction of the distal radius fracture, including the dorsoulnar aspect of the lunate facet, is approached dorsally between the fifth and sixth extensor compartments. More often than not, this injury has disrupted the retinacular sheath supporting the extensor carpi ulnaris, the dorsal radioulnar collateral ligament, and the triangular fibrocartilage. The triangular fibrocartilage, if disrupted from the base of the ulnar styloid, can be reapproximated with intraosseous sutures placed through the triangular fibrocartilage, passed through drill holes, and tied over the outer border of the ulnar. The dorsal radioulnar ligament is then repaired with closure of available capsule if present. The extensor carpi ulnaris is brought back over the end of the ulnar and secured in place with a flap created from the extensor retinaculum. Postoperatively the limb is immobilized for 4 weeks in approximately 30 to 45 degrees of supination.

References

1. Agee JM: External fixation. *Orthop Clin North Am* 24: 265–274, 1993.
2. Agee JM: Distal radius fracture: Multiplanar ligamentotaxis. *Hand Clin* 9: 577–586, 1993.
3. Anderson R, O'Neil G: Comminuted fractures of the distal end of the radius. *Surg Gynecol Obstet* 78: 434–440, 1944.
4. Bartosh RA, Saldaña MJ: Intraarticular fractures of the distal radius. A cadaveric study to determine if ligamentotaxis restores palmar tilt. *J Hand Surg* 15A: 18–21, 1990.
5. Clancey G: Percutaneous Kirschner wire fixation of Colles' fracture. *J Bone Joint Surg [Am]* 66A: 1008–1014, 1984.
6. Clyburn TA: Dynamic external fixation for comminuted intraarticular fractures of the distal end of the radius. *J Bone Joint Surg [Am]* 69A: 248–254, 1987.
7. Cooney WP, Berger RA: Treatment of complex fractures of the distal radius: Combined use of internal and external fixation and arthroscopic reduction. *Hand Clin* 9: 603–612, 1993.
8. Cooney WP: External fixation of distal radius fractures. *Clin Orthop Rel Res* 180: 44–49, 1983.
9. Cooney WP, Linscheid RL, Dobyns JH: External pin fixation for unstable Colles' fractures. *J Bone Joint Surg [Am]* 61A: 840–845, 1979.
10. DePalma AF: Comminuted fractures of the distal end of the radius treated by ulnar pinning. *J Bone Joint Surg [Am]* 34A: 651–662, 1952.
11. Dowling JJ, Sawyer B, Jr: Comminuted Colles' fractures. Evaluation of a method of treatment. *J Bone Joint Surg [Am]* 43A: 657–668, 1961.
12. Dupuytren B: *Injuries and Diseases of Bone*. London: 1847.
13. Edwards GS: Intraarticular fractures of the distal part of the radius. Treatment with the small AO external fixator. *J Bone Joint Surg [Am]* 73A: 1241–1250, 1991.

14. Fernandez DL: Fractures of the distal radius. Operative treatment. *AAOS Instructional Course Lectures* 42: 73–88, 1993.
15. Fernandez DL, Jakob RP, Büchler U: External fixation of the wrist. Current indications and techniques. *Ann Chir Gyn* 72: 298–302, 1983.
16. Frykman GK, Tooma GS: Comparison of 11 external fixators for treatment of unstable wrist fractures. *J Hand Surg* 14: 247–254, 1989.
17. Greatting MD, Bishop AT: Intrafocal (Kapandji) pinning of unstable fracture of the distal radius. *Orthop Clin of North Am* 24: 301–307, 1993.
18. Henry WA: *Extensile Exposures* 2nd edition. Edinburgh: Churchill Livingstone, 1973.
19. Hertel R, Jakob RP: Static external fixation of the wrist. *Hand Clin* 9: 567–576, 1993.
20. Jakob RP, Fernandez DL: The treatment of wrist fractures with the small AO external fixation device. In: *Current Concepts of External Fixation of Fractures*, edited by Uhthoff HK. Berlin: Springer-Verlag, 1982, pp. 307–314.
21. Jupiter JB: External skeletal fixation of the upper extremity. *AAOS Instructional Course Lectures* 39: 209–218, 1990.
22. Kapandji A: L'embrochage intrafocal des fractures de l'extrémité inférieure du radius: Dix ans après. *Ann Chir Main* 6: 57, 1987(Abstract).
23. Kapandji A: L'ostéosythèse par double embrochage intrafocal. Traitement fonctionnel des fractures non articulaires de l'extrémité inférieure du radius. *Ann Chir* 30: 903–908, 1976.
24. Kwasny O, Hertz H, Schabus R: Percutaneous drill wire fixation for treating distal radius fractures at dislocation risk [German]. *Arch Traumatol* 20: 97, 1990.
25. Ledoux A, Ravis A, van der Ghinst M: Pinning of fractures of the inferior extremity of the radius [French]. *Rev Chir Orthop* 59: 427–438, 1973.
26. Lennox JD, Page BJ, Mandell RM: Use of the Clyburn external fixator in fractures of the distal radius. *J Trauma* 29: 326–331, 1989.
27. Leung KS, Shen WY, Leung PC: Ligamentotaxis and bone grafting for comminuted fractures of the distal radius. *J Bone Joint Surg [Br]* 71B: 838–842, 1989.
28. Leung KS, Shen WY, Tsang HK, Chiu KH, Leung PC, Hung LK: An effective treatment of comminuted fracture of the distal radius. *J Hand Surg* 15A: 11–17, 1990.
29. Mah E, Atkinson R: Percutaneous Kirschner wire stabilization following closed reduction of Colles' fractures. *J Hand Surg* 17B: 55–61, 1992.
30. Melendez EM, Mehne DK, Posner PC: Treatment of unstable Colles' fractures with a new radius minifixator. *J Hand Surg* 14A: 807–811, 1989.
31. Mortier JP, Kuhlmann JN, Richet C: Baux S: Brochage horizontal cubito-radial dans les fractures de l'extrémité inférieure du radius comportent un fragment postero-interne. *Rev Chir Orthop* 72: 567–571, 1986.
32. Nakata RY, Chand Y, Matiko JD, Frykman GK, Wood VE: External fixators for wrist fractures: A biomechanical and clinical study. *J Hand Surg* 10A: 845–851, 1985.
33. Nonnemacher J, Neumeier K: Intrafokale Verdrantung bei Handgelenkfrakturen. *Hand Chir* 19: 67, 1987.
34. Pennig DW: Dynamic external fixation of distal radius fractures. *Hand Clin* 9: 587–602, 1993.
35. Rayhack J: The history and evolution of percutaneous pinning of displaced distal radius fractures. *Orthop Clin North Am* 24: 287–300, 1993.
36. Schuind FA, Burny F, Chao EYS: *Biomechanical Properties and design considerations in upper extremity external fixation*. Hand Clinics 9: 543–553, 1993.
37. Sanders RA, Keppel FL, Waldrop JI: External fixation of distal radius fractures. Results and complications. *J Hand Surg* 11A: 385–390, 1991.
38. Seitz WH, Jr, Putnam MD, Dick HM: Limited open surgical approach for external fixation of distal radius fractures. *J Hand Surg* 15A: 288–293, 1990.
39. Stein A, Katz S: Stabilization of comminuted fractures of the distal inch of the radius: Percutaneous pinning. *Clin Orthop Rel Res* 108: 174–181, 1975.
40. Whipple TL: *Arthroscopic Surgery: The Wrist*. Philadelphia: JB Lippincott Co, 1992.
41. Willenegger H, Guggenbuhl A: Zur operativen Behandlung bestimmter Fälle von distalen Radius Frakturen. *Helv Chir Acta* 26: 81–87, 1959.

Chapter Five

Extraarticular Bending Fractures

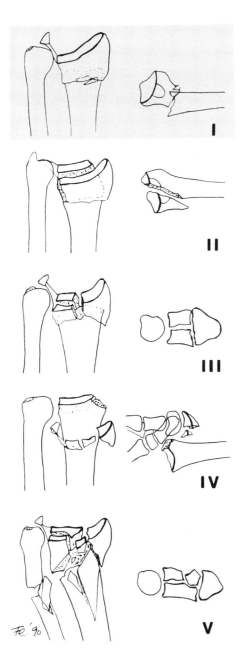

No fractures perhaps require more careful examination than those of the carpal extremity of the radius, for neither is their precise nature clearly defined, nor yet are their unsatisfactory after consequences sufficiently, as a rule, impressed upon the patients.[27]

G.W. Callender, 1865

I

II

III

IV

V

A Practical, Treatment Oriented Classification of Fractures of the Distal Radius and Associated Distal Radioulnar Joint Lesions.
Diego L. Fernandez, M.D. PD

FRACTURE TYPES (ADULTS) BASED ON THE MECHANISM OF INJURY	CHILDREN FRACTURE EQUIVALENT	STABILITY/ INSTABILITY: high risk of secondary displacement after initial adequate reduction	DISPLACEMENT PATTERN	NUMBER OF FRAGMENTS	ASSOCIATED LESIONS carpal ligament, fractures, median, ulnar nerve, tendons, ipsilat., fx upper extremity, compartment syndrome	RECOMMENDED TREATMENT
TYPE I BENDING FRACTURE OF THE METAPHYSIS 	DISTAL FOREARM FRACTURE SALTER II	STABLE UNSTABLE	NON-DISPLACED DORSALLY (Colles-Pouteau) VOLARLY (Smith) PROXIMAL COMBINED	ALWAYS 2 MAIN FRAGMENTS + VARYING DEGREE OF METAPHYSEAL COMMINUTION (instability)	UNCOMMON	CONSERVATIVE (stable fxs) PERCUTANEOUS PINNING (extra- or intrafocal) EXTERNAL FIXATION (exceptionally BONE GRAFT)
TYPE II SHEARING FRACTURE OF THE JOINT SURFACE 	SALTER IV	UNSTABLE	DORSAL RADIAL VOLAR PROXIMAL COMBINED	TWO-PART THREE-PART COMMINUTED	LESS UNCOMMON	OPEN REDUCTION SCREW-/PLATE FIXATION
TYPE III COMPRESSION FRACTURE OF THE JOINT SURFACE 	SALTER III, IV, V	STABLE UNSTABLE	NON-DISPLACED DORSAL RADIAL VOLAR PROXIMAL COMBINED	TWO-PART THREE-PART FOUR-PART COMMINUTED	COMMON	CONSERVATIVE CLOSED, LIMITED, ARTHROSCOPIC ASSISTED, OR EXTENSILE OPEN REDUCTION PERCUTANEOUS PINS COMBINED EXTERNAL AND INTERNAL FIXATION BONE GRAFT
TYPE IV AVULSION FRACTURES, RADIO CARPAL FRACTURE DISLOCATION 	VERY RARE	UNSTABLE	DORSAL RADIAL VOLAR PROXIMAL COMBINED	TWO-PART (radial styloid ulnar styloid) THREE-PART (volar, dorsal margin) COMMINUTED	FREQUENT	CLOSED OR OPEN REDUCTION PIN OR SCREW FIXATION TENSION WIRING
TYPE V COMBINED FRACTURES (I - II - III - IV) HIGH-VELOCITY INJURY 	VERY RARE	UNSTABLE	DORSAL RADIAL VOLAR PROXIMAL COMBINED	COMMINUTED and/or BONE LOSS (frequently intraarticular, open, seldom extraarticular)	ALWAYS PRESENT	COMBINED METHOD

Fracture of the distal radius: a associated distal radioulnar joint (DRUJ) lesions.

	Patho-anatomy of the lesion	Degree of joint surface involvement	Prognosis	Recommended treatment
Type 1 Stable (following reduction of the radius the DRUJ is congruous and stable)	A Avulsion fracture tip ulnar styloid B Stable fracture ulnar neck	None	Good	A+B Functional aftertreatment Encourage early pronation-supination exercises Note: Extraarticular <u>unstable</u> fractures of the ulna at the metaphyseal level or distal shaft require stable plate fixation
Type II Unstable (subluxation or dislocation of the ulnar head present)	A Substance tear of TFCC and/or palmar and dorsal capsular ligaments B Avulsion fracture base of the ulnar styloid	None	• Chronic instability • Painful limitation of supination if left unreduced • Possible late arthritic changes	A <u>Closed treatment</u> Reduce subluxation, sugar tong splint in 45° of supination four to six weeks A+B <u>Operative treatment</u> Repair TFCC or fix ulnar styloid with tension band wiring Immobilize wrist and elbow in supination (cast) or transfix ulna/radius with k-wire and forearm cast
Type III Potentially unstable (subluxation possible)	A Intraarticular fracture of the sigmoid notch B Intraarticular fracture of the ulnar head	Present	• Dorsal subluxation possible together with dorsally displaced die punch or dorso-ulnar fragment • Risk of early degenerative changes and severe limitation of forearm rotation if left unreduced	A Anatomic reduction of palmar and dorsal sigmoid notch fragments. If residual subluxation tendency present immobilize as in type II injury B Functional aftertreatment to enhance remodelling of ulnar head If DRUJ remains painful: partial ulnar resection, darrach or sauvé-kapandji procedure at a later date

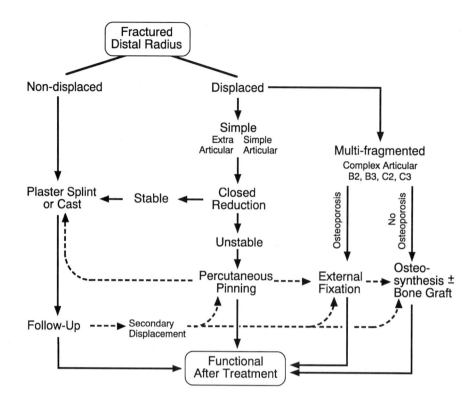

Extraarticular Bending Fractures

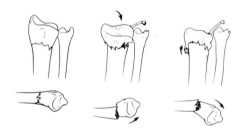

The rationale of developing an approach to understanding and treating fractures of the distal end of the radius based upon their mechanism of injury will become evident in the discussion of the "bending fracture." Given the fact that the vast literature on the subject of distal radius fractures has more often than not combined numerous different fracture patterns under eponymic descriptions, ("Colles," "Pouteau," "Goyrand"), it is no wonder that there continues to exist so much disagreement regarding optimal treatment and expected outcome. By subdividing these fractures on the basis of specific anatomic patterns, it is the authors' hope that the reader will appreciate the specific features inherent in each fracture type. This will facilitate the formulation of effective treatment plans based upon both the needs of the fracture and those of the patient.

In this chapter we will focus on the issues that continue to be of importance to the clinician when faced with the common extraarticular bending fracture—very much the same ones that have frustrated physicians over the past two centuries (see Chapter 1). These include the optimal means of fracture classification, distinguishing stable from unstable fracture patterns; techniques of fracture reduction; type, position, and duration of immobilization; management of unstable fractures; indications for interventional treatment; identification and approach to complications; and expected outcome.

Incidence

Given the fact that epidemiologic studies have combined many patterns of distal radius fractures, it would be difficult, if not impossible, to document the incidence of extraarticular bending fractures. Yet the commonplace nature of fractures of the distal end of the radius is clearly apparent in both historical and contemporary studies (see Chapter 2).[57,81,85,96,156,228] Frykman identified the extraarticular bending fracture (Types I and II) in 36.3% of all the fractures in his series.[76]

Mechanism

Most injuries to the wrist and lower end of the radius are the result of a fall on the outstretched hand. The specific injury pattern will be based upon a number of factors, among which are the velocity and position of the hand and wrist at impact, the degree of rotation of the forearm, and the quality of the underlying bone (Fig. 5.1).

With a forward fall, one might expect the hand to hit the ground in a hyperextended position with the forearm pronated and the elbow flexed (Fig. 5.2). Two distinct forces will be concentrated at the level of the wrist. These are the thrust of the torso transmitted along the long axis of the radius, counteracted by the ground reaction force acting in a proximal direction across the carpal bones. The latter can, in certain cases, induce bending stresses at the level of the metaphyseal bone. This, in turn, will result in failure of the volar cortex due to tensile stress and impaction of the dorsal cortex due to compression forces. A certain degree of impaction and collapse of the cancellous bone of the distal metaphysis will occur, due in large part to the penetration of the harder cortical edge of the proximal diaphyseal fragment.

Conversely, with a similar forward or backward thrust with the forearm supinated, one might expect to see a palmarly displaced bending fracture (Fig. 5.3). Tension forces are now located on the dorsal aspect of the metaphysis, with the volar cortex failing under compression load.

The torsional component of the injury should not be underestimated. This will produce a variable degree of disruption of the distal radioulnar joint. With dorsally displaced bending fractures, the distal fragment will be seen to supinate with respect to the diaphysis of the radius, while the reverse will be the case with the palmarly displaced bending fracture (Fig. 5.4).[128,146]

Castaing identified a fracture of the ulnar styloid in 50 percent to 60 percent of distal radius fractures, with a fracture, of the head or neck of the ulnar in 1.5 percent—all reflecting an injury pattern which has extended from the distal end of the radius across the supporting structures of the joint.[229] Furthermore,

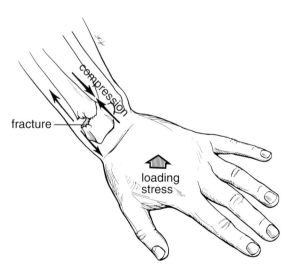

Figure 5.1. The extraarticular bending fracture is the result of a fall on the outstretched hand. The specific pattern will be the result of the velocity of the fall and the position of the hand and forearm.

Figure 5.2. When landing with the wrist hyperextended, forward displacement of the torso pronating the forearm will result in a dorsally displaced fracture pattern.

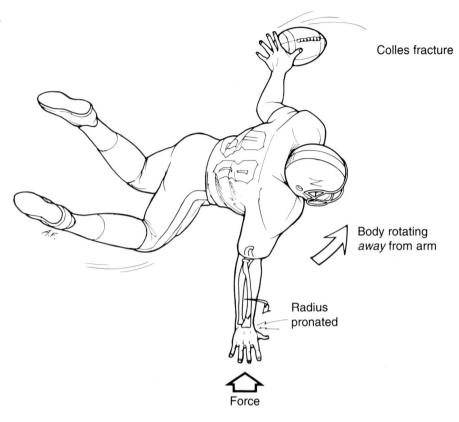

Colles fracture

Body rotating *away* from arm

Radius pronated

Force

Figure 5.3. With a fall causing the torso to be thrust backwards and the forearm supinated, a palmarly displaced fracture will result.

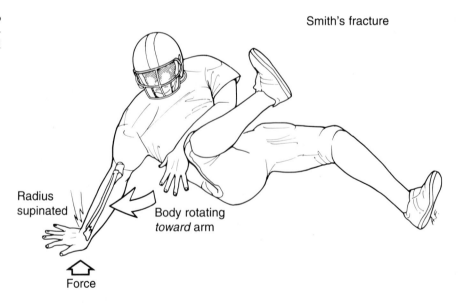

Smith's fracture

Radius supinated

Body rotating *toward* arm

Force

in many instances, the triangular fibrocartilage complex has been injured with or without associated fracture of the ulnar styloid process. This will be commonplace in those extraarticular bending fractures which are widely displaced on presentation. The ulnar-sided component of these fractures will play a fundamental role not only in treatment methods but also in expected outcomes.[76]

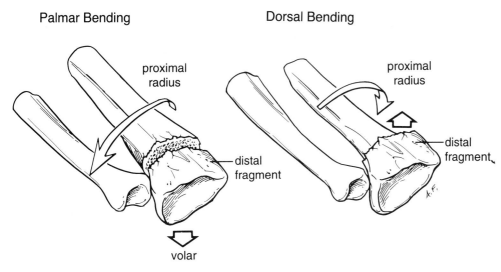

Palmar Bending

Dorsal Bending

proximal
radius

proximal
radius

distal
fragment

distal
fragment

volar

Figure 5.4. Extraarticular bending fractures feature displacement in multiple directions including rotational deformity.

Treatment Considerations

A number of factors will enter into the decision-making process in the treatment of bending fractures of the distal end of the radius. These will include the fracture pattern, the presence of absence of comminution, the intrinsic fracture stability and its initial displacement, and the condition of the underlying bone (Table 5.1).

In addition, individual patient-related factors such as lifestyle, associated medical conditions, psychological outlook, anticipated functional loading compliance, and condition of the soft tissues will be of equal importance.[148]

Classification

The numerous classification systems for fractures of the distal end of the radius are highlighted in Chapter 2. Several of these are particularly useful for extraarticular bending fractures.[159,164,198] The awareness and application of more detailed classifications of the extraarticular bending fractures will prove extremely important not only for more accurate fracture documentation but also in consideration of treatment. Without question, a good deal of the difficulty in interpreting the experience in the literature stems from a lack of a unified system of fracture classification.

There exist several more contemporary classifications which are specifically designed to differentiate patterns of extraarticular bending fractures and thereby prove extremely useful. It will become evident that the presence or absence of comminution of the metaphyseal region is the critical feature in identifying specific responses to treatment—specifically, inherent stability following manipulative reduction and cast application.

Older, Stabler, and Cassebaum in 1965 published a useful classification for metaphyseal dorsal bending fractures.[159] Four groups were established ranging from essentially nondisplaced (Group I) to displaced fractures with extensive metaphyseal comminution, shortening relative to the ulnar, and extension into the radiocarpal joint (Group IV) (Fig. 5.5).

Figure 5.5. The classification of dorsally displaced extraarticular fractures by Older, Stabler, and Cassebaum.

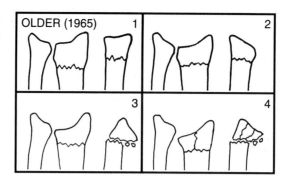

Type I — Nondisplaced.
Type II — Displaced with minimal comminution.
Type III — Displaced with comminution of the dorsal radius.
Type IV — Displaced with severe comminution of the radial head.

Jenkins in 1989 proposed a classification of dorsally displaced bending fractures based entirely upon the presence and extent of comminution (Fig. 5.6).[105]

Group I — No radiographically visible comminution.
Group II — Comminution of the dorsal radial cortex without comminution of the fracture fragment.
Group III — Comminution of the fracture fragment without significant involvement of the dorsal cortex.
Group IV — Comminution of both the distal fragment and the dorsal cortex. As the fracture line involves the distal fracture fragment in Groups III and IV, intraarticular involvement is very common within these groups. Such involvement is not, however, inevitable, nor does it affect the fracture's placement within the classification.

The Comprehensive Classification of fractures not only identifies the direction of displacement and the presence and extent of comminution, but also provides a means of documenting the specific nature of the ulnar-sided involvement. It also serves to more accurately identify and subclassify volar bending fractures (Fig. 5.7).[156]

Figure 5.6. Jenkins' classification for dorsally displaced bending fractures is based specifically on comminution.

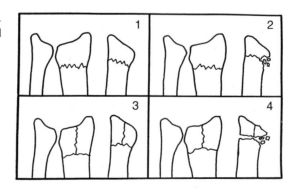

Ulnar Injury Classification (Fig. 5.8)

1—Tear triangular fibrocartilage and/or distal radioulnar ligament
2—Fracture ulnar styloid (and/or distal radioulnar ligament)
3—Fracture neck of ulnar
4—Metaphyseal comminuted fracture of the distal ulnar
5—Fracture through the head of the ulnar
6—Comminuted articular fracture of the distal ulnar

A1 EXTRAARTICULAR: Fractures neither affect the articular surface of the radiocarpal nor the radio-ulnar joints.

Figure 5.7. The Comprehensive Classification identifies the presence and extent of comminution as well as the direction of displacement of the distal fragment.

A1 Extra-articular fracture, of the ulna, radius intact

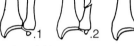

1 styloid process
2 metaphyseal simple
3 metaphyseal multifragmentary

A2 Extra-articular fracture, of the radius, simple and impacted

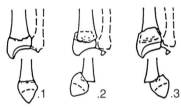

1 without any tilt
2 with dorsal tilt (Pouteau-Colles)
3 with volar tilt (Goyran-Smith)

A3 Extra-articular fracture, of the radius, multifragmentary

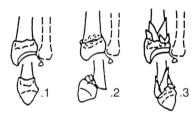

1 impacted with axial shortening
2 with a wedge
3 complex

Figure 5.8. The Comprehensive Classification of ulnar side injury.

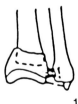
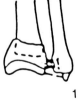

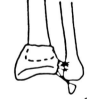

1   2

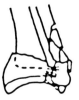

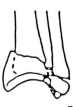

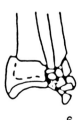

3   4   5   6

	Patho-anatomy of the lesion	Degree of joint surface involvement	Prognosis	Recommended treatment
Type 1 **Stable** (following reduction of the radius the DRUJ is congruous and stable)	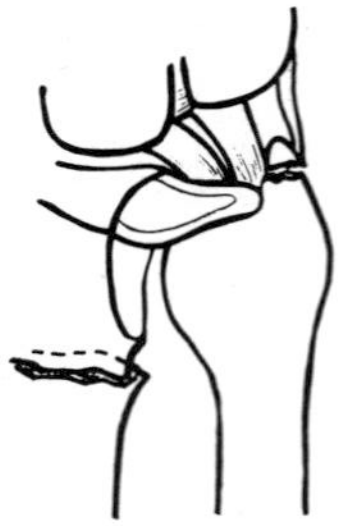 A Avulsion fracture tip ulnar styloid 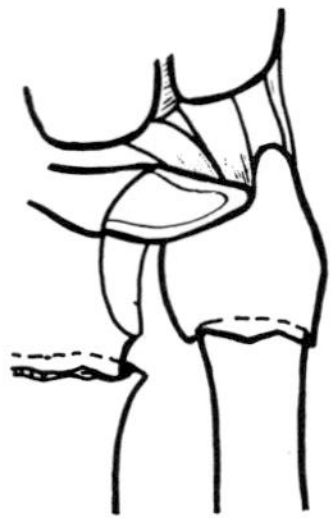 B Stable fracture ulnar neck	None	Good	A+B Functional aftertreatment Encourage early pronation-supination exercises Note: Extraarticular <u>unstable</u> fractures of the ulna at the metaphyseal level or distal shaft require stable plate fixation
Type II **Unstable** (subluxation or dislocation of the ulnar head present)	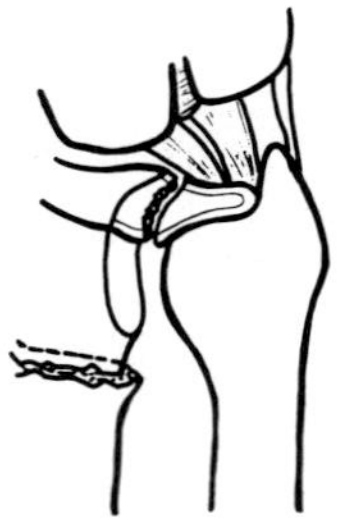 A Substance tear of TFCC and/or palmar and dorsal capsular ligaments 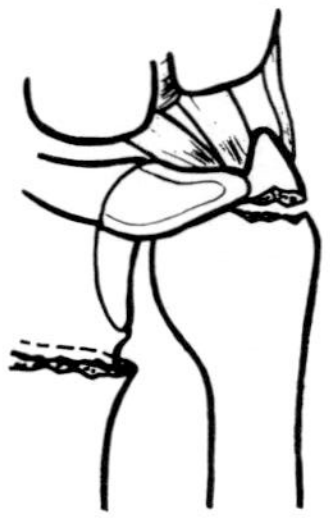 B Avulsion fracture base of the ulnar styloid	None	• Chronic instability • Painful limitation of supination if left unreduced • Possible late arthritic changes	A <u>Closed treatment</u> Reduce subluxation, sugar tong splint in 45° of supination four to six weeks A+B <u>Operative treatment</u> Repair TFCC or fix ulnar styloid with tension band wiring Immobilize wrist and elbow in supination (cast) or transfix ulna/radius with k-wire and forearm cast
Type III **Potentially unstable** (subluxation possible)	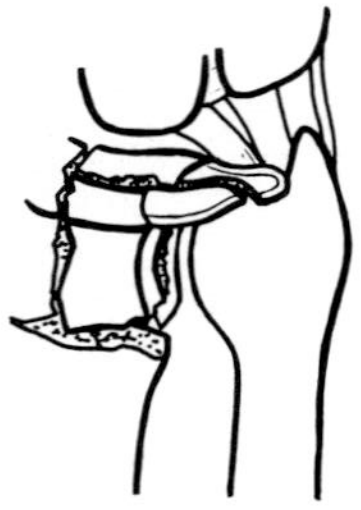 A Intraarticular fracture of the sigmoid notch 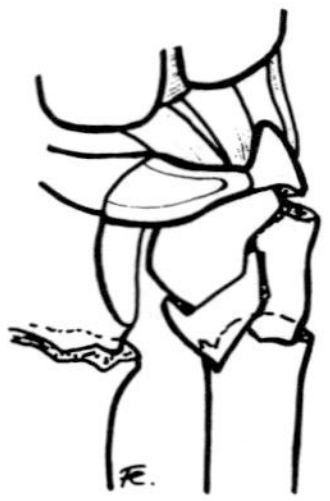 B Intraarticular fracture of the ulnar head	Present	• Dorsal subluxation possible together with dorsally displaced die punch or dorso-ulnar fragment • Risk of early degenerative changes and severe limitation of forearm rotation if left unreduced	A Anatomic reduction of palmar and dorsal sigmoid notch fragments. If residual subluxation tendency present immobilize as in type II injury B Functional aftertreatment to enhance remodelling of ulnar head If DRUJ remains painful: partial ulnar resection, darrach or sauvé-kapandji procedure at a later date

Figure 5.9. Fernandez classification of associated distal radioulnar joint injuries.

Fernandez Classification of Distal Radioulnar Joint Lesions (Fig. 5.9)

Type I: Stable — Following reduction of the radius fracture, the distal radio-ulnar joint is congruous and stable.
   a. Avulsion fracture tip of styloid
   b. Stable ulnar neck fracture
Type II: Unstable — Following reduction of the radius fracture, there is sub-luxation or dislocation of the ulnar head.
   a. Substance tear TFCC and/or palmar and dorsal capsular ligaments
   b. Avulsion fracture base of ulnar styloid
Type III: Potentially unstable — Subluxation possible.
   a. Intraarticular fracture of the sigmoid notch
   b. Intraarticular fracture of the ulnar head

Palmar Displaced Bending Fracture (Thomas Classification) (Fig. 5.10)[212]

Type I — An extraarticular fracture with palmar displacement
Type II — An intraarticular fracture with volar and proximal displacement of the distal fragment along with the carpus
Type III — An extraarticular fracture with volar displacement of the distal fragment and carpus

Fernandez Classification of Extraarticular Palmar Displaced Bending Fractures (Fig. 5.11)[65]

Type A — Transverse metaphyseal fracture
Type B — Oblique metaphyseal fracture
Type C — Metaphyseal comminution

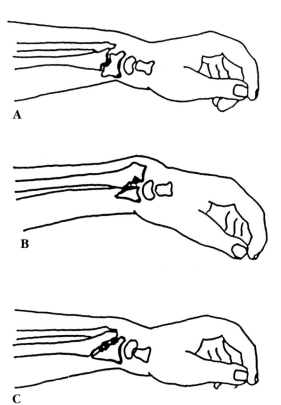

Figure 5.10. Thomas classification of palmarly displaced fractures.

Figure 5.11. Fernandez classification of palmarly displaced extraarticular bending fractures.

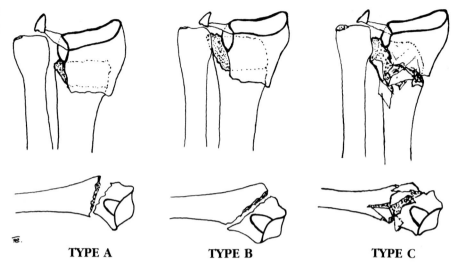

Figure 5.11. Fernandez classification of palmarly displaced extraarticular bending fractures.

TYPE A   **TYPE B**   **TYPE C**

Stability

The stability of a bending fracture is best defined as the ability of the fracture to resist displacement once it has been manipulated into an anatomic position.[148] A number of factors will interact to influence fracture stability. These include the extent of the initial displacement,[47,53,97,198,199,215,216] the presence and degree of metaphyseal comminution,[5,6,30,35,37,39,51,81,88,91,105,106,111,127,159,184,205,224,225] and/or the presence of localized osteoporosis.[164,199]

Lafontaine, Hardy, and Delince studied 112 consecutive fractures of the distal radius treated conservatively and suggested five factors that could relate to instability following fracture reduction.[127] These included:

1. Initial dorsal angulation greater than 20 degrees
2. Dorsal comminution
3. Intraarticular radiocarpal fracture
4. Associated ulnar fractures
5. Patient age greater than 60 years

They noted that fractures associated with three or more factors were unstable following closed reduction and plaster immobilization (Fig. 5.12A–D].

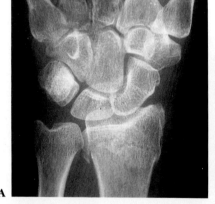

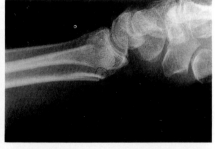

Figure 5.12. An unstable extraarticular bending fracture in a 60-year-old woman. A,B. Anteroposterior and lateral radiograph of the initial fracture demonstrates displacement and extensive metaphyseal comminution. C. Displacement is readily visible 2 weeks after fracture reduction and cast application. D. The fracture united, having redisplaced to its original position.

A

B

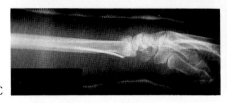

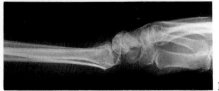

C

D

On the other hand, stable fractures are those that will not displace either at the time of presentation or following manipulative reduction.[75,96,171,181] Abbaszadegan, Jonsson, and von Sivers defined these as bending fractures presenting with minimal displacement with dorsal angulation less than 5 degrees and axial shortening less than 2 mm (Fig. 5.13A–F).[5]

Definition of stability of bending fractures

Stable	Unstable
Minimal displacement	Widely displaced
Minimal or no comminution	Metaphyseal commununiton
Low energy of injury	High energy of injury
Impaction at fracture site	Defect postfracture reduction

Displacement

Direction of Displacement

A number of radiographic measurements have been used to document the direction and degree of displacement of bending fractures (see Chapter 3). For the more commonplace dorsally displaced fractures, most have relied upon the measurement of dorsal displacement of the distal fragment measured in degrees, the amount of shortening of the distal radial fragment in relationship to the distal ulnar measured in millimeters, and the loss of the normal ulnar inclination of the distal articular surface measured in degrees.[33,76,81,136,159,222] It is of interest that in many cases these measurements are interrelated, i.e., when the dorsal angulation is improved, so are the shortening and loss of ulnar inclination.

Van der Linden and Ericson in 1981 demonstrated that radial shift of the distal fragment is also an important radiographic feature to be measured.[215] Furthermore, they observed that a large radial shift does not imply that the dorsal angulation is also large and that, in fact, these two measurements can be independent of each other. This will be important not only in comparing results from series to series but also in the recognition that a closed reduction will be satisfactory only if both of these displacements are reduced. If that were to occur, i.e., the distal fragment was pushed ulnarward and palmarly, radial length and restoration of the ulnar inclination would also return.

One should also be aware that the distal fragment in dorsally displaced bending fractures will be supinated in reference to the proximal radius, with the reverse being the case with volar displaced fractures. This feature may be more difficult to accurately assess radiographically (Fig. 5.4).

A careful scrutiny of the literature supports the authors' own experience that immobilization of dorsal bending fractures with casts or splints, with or without a manipulative reduction, has its primary place in treatment of those fractures which are inherently stable. These, for the most part, are nondisplaced or are displaced but without metaphyseal comminution (Table 5.1).

Extent of Displacement

While evidence continues to accumulate suggesting a strict parallel between the quality of the anatomic result and the residual functional capacity of the wrist,[72,73,84,149,217] it is well recognized that adequate wrist function and absence of pain can coexist with radiographic deformity following an extraarticular metaphyseal bending fracture.

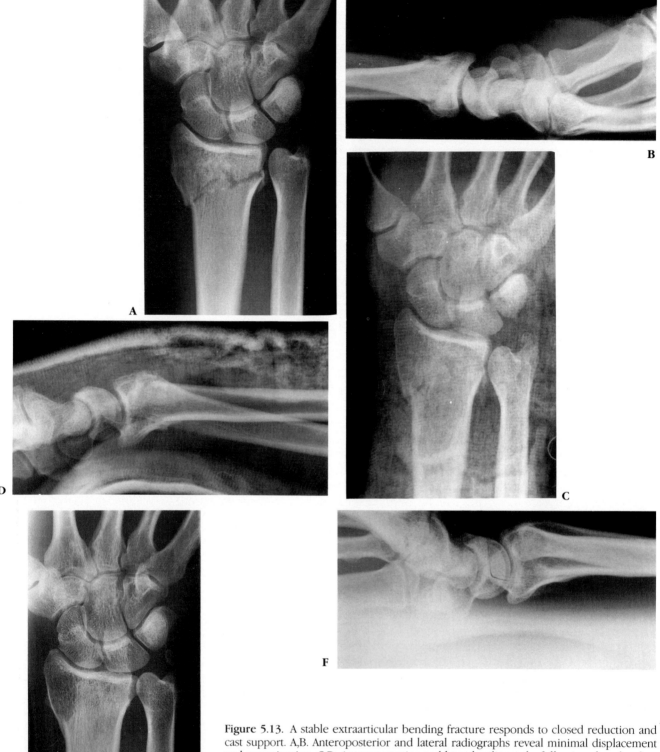

Figure 5.13. A stable extraarticular bending fracture responds to closed reduction and cast support. A,B. Anteroposterior and lateral radiographs reveal minimal displacement and comminution. C,D. Anteroposterior and lateral radiographs following closed reduction and cast. Anatomic restoration was gained. E,F. One year postfracture, an anatomic result is seen on the anteroposterior and lateral radiograph.

Many have concluded that uncorrected dorsal angulation beyond 20 degrees with radial shortening, or radial shift of the distal fragment with or without shortening and disruption of the distal radioulnar joint, will more likely than not impair wrist and/or forearm function.[66,73,149,154,177,217] These radiographic parameters, although not as carefully documented, will be of equal significance with palmar displaced fractures. Therefore, we believe that it is important, with those fractures whose initial displacement is equal to or greater than the above parameters, to consider manipulative reduction for those patients whose functional needs would require a more anatomic reposition.

Nondisplaced Fractures

Functional Treatment

Bending fractures of the distal radius which present with little or no displacement offer a favorable long-term prognosis.[2,49–52,136,139,159,162,174,203,226] This fact was recognized early on by a number of investigators who suggested that these fractures should not be immobilized in circumferential plaster casts, but rather should be supported, if at all, with a sling, with the hand and wrist permitted to hang in an ulnar direction encouraging functional exercises (Fig. 5.14).[9,50,139,162]

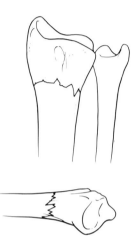

We would concur with Abbaszadegan, Conradi, and Jonsson who defined "minimal" displacement as dorsal angulation less than 5 degrees and axial shortening less than 2 mm.[2] They observed such fractures to be stable, even when supported with elastic bandages rather than plaster casts. This situation is not to be confused with a fracture which is stable on presentation but malaliqued which when reduced will result in a metaphyseal defect leading to a loss of reduction when immobilized in a cast or brace (Fig. 5.15A–H).

The management of the nondisplaced or minimally displaced bending fractures will depend on a number of factors. Among these are the patient's activity level, functional needs, and associated medical conditions and expectations, as well as the condition of the soft tissues. For the younger patient or the more active older patient, it is our preference to immobilize the limb in a well-molded below-elbow cast for 4 weeks, followed by a removable thermoplast splint for an additional 2 weeks. Control radiographs within 7 to 10 days postinjury are recommended, as displacement would be more likely to occur at this juncture.[199]

In the event that associated soft tissue swelling would preclude the application of a circular cast at the time of initial treatment, a plaster or thermoplast volar splint in conjunction with elevation, elastic wraps, and hand therapy will be sufficient to provide comfort and limit the possibility of fracture displacement. Once swelling has diminished, a circular cast can be more safely applied.

In geriatric patients and those with "hairline" fractures, the duration of immobilization can be reduced to 3 or 4 weeks. The decision to discontinue the immobilization should be based upon clinical findings of tenderness at the fracture site as well as radiographic evidence of healing. With geriatric patients in particular, careful follow-up is essential to make certain that they are not only exercising the digits but also mobilizing the ipsilateral elbow and shoulder.

An additional subset of stable bending fractures that may receive functional treatment is that of the displaced but impacted fracture in the geriatric patient with advanced osteoporosis. Reduction of this type of fracture would lead to the creation of a metaphyseal bony defect and most assuredly an unstable situation (Fig. 5.16A–D). In these instances, the radioulnar length discrepancy can be addressed later with a resection of the distal ulnar if this condition

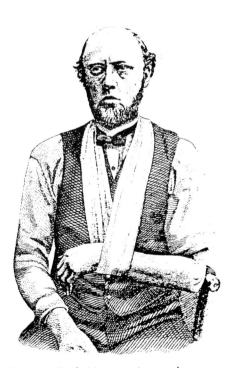

Figure 5.14. Many nineteenth-century surgeons suggested that stable, impacted dorsal bending fractures be supported with a sling with the hand and wrist permitted to hang in an ulnar direction.

Figure 5.15. A displaced but impacted dorsal bending fracture with extensive metaphyseal comminution is "stable" upon presentation but unstable postreduction. A,B. Anteroposterior and lateral radiograph of the comminuted metaphyseal fracture upon presentation. C,D. Anteroposterior and lateral radiograph postmanipulative reduction and cast. E,F. Six weeks postreduction and cast, fracture displacement has occurred. Note also the subluxation of the distal radioulnar joint. G,H. Six months postfracture, the patient experienced functional difficulties with forearm supination.

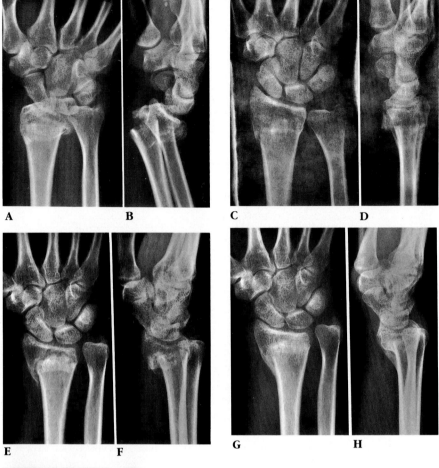

Figure 5.16. An unstable fracture in an 81-year-old male redisplaced and healed with deformity. Little functional disability was noted. A,B. The anteroposterior and lateral radiographs show a major deformity. C,D. Excellent forearm rotation was retained in spite of the complete disruption of the distal radioulnar joint.

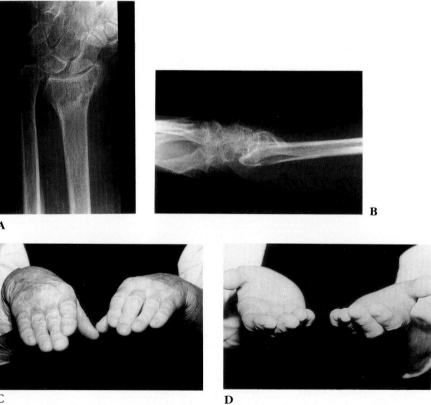

proves sufficiently symptomatic to interfere with the individual's quality of life as well as his or her ability to perform the basic requirements of daily living.

Complications

The nondisplaced or impacted minimally displaced bending fracture in most instances will result in an excellent symptomatic and functional outcome. The patient should be cautioned, however, that some discomfort and limitations of function are to be expected for the initial 6 to 9 months postinjury. In addition, some patients may note discomfort specific to the distal radioulnar joint area even in the face of anatomic restoration of the joint. This, too, will be seen to resolve in the vast majority of cases.

One complication that appears uniquely to be associated with nondisplaced fractures is that of spontaneous rupture of the extensor pollicis longus tendon.[32,46,95,108,195,214] The vast majority of these ruptures will occur within the first 8 weeks after fracture, although some cases have been reported years postinjury.[61,144] Although this problem is discussed in detail in Chapter 11, it is important to be aware of this potential complication with a nondisplaced fracture. Prodromal symptoms, including tenderness, swelling, or crepitus about Lister's tubercle, should raise suspicion of an impending tendon disruption. Decompression at this stage could offset a complete rupture.[98,124]

Neurologic complications, particularly involving the median nerve, can also complicate these fractures. The surgeon should take heed to carefully assess the neurologic function both at the time of initial treatment and during the early period of follow-up (see Chapter 11).

Displaced but "Stable" Bending Fractures

Displaced Fracture—"Stable" Pattern

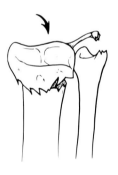

Although some have suggested that careful restoration of the skeletal anatomy may not be essential for the recovery of hand and wrist function,[17,32,56,102,145,147,159,182,194,204,213] there remains overwhelming support for the relationship of anatomic restoration and a functional outcome.[10,12,13,19,25,33,37,39,41,44,49,85,88,111,131,136,143,149,152,164,187,193,200,208,215,217]

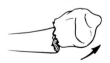

Those extraarticular fractures which present with little radiographic evidence of comminution, less than 5 to 10 degrees of either dorsal or volar angulation of the distal fragment, and less than a few millimeters of radial shortening represent stable fracture patterns. Once reduced, these will have a high likelihood of the reduction being held in place by cast immobilization (Fig. 5.17A–H). Despite the extensive experience in the management of bending fractures, both stable and unstable, there remain a number of issues which continue to evoke controversy. These include the type of anesthesia, the method of fracture reduction, and the type, position, and duration of immobilization.

Anesthesia

Three basic forms of anesthesia have been widely used in the management of displaced distal radius fractures that require reduction: local anesthesia or "hematoma block," regional anesthesia with either Bier or brachial plexus block, and general anesthesia.

Figure 5.17. A displaced but "stable" dorsal bending fracture. A,B. Anteroposterior and lateral radiographs of the displaced fracture. Comminution involves only the dorsal cortex. C,D. The postreduction radiographs reveal an anatomic reduction. E,F. Control radiographs 4 weeks post reduction. A well-molded cast has been applied. Note the dorsal molding. G,H. Fracture union and anatomic restoration seen at 6 weeks.

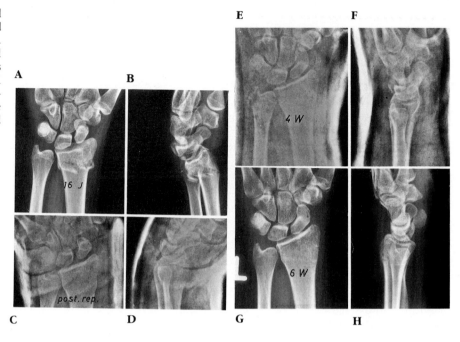

Local infiltration of the fracture hematoma can be effective, especially in these displaced but intrinsically stable fractures in which the reduction is anticipated to be uncomplicated. With dorsally displaced fractures, we prefer to infiltrate the fracture site with 5 to 7 cc of 1 or 2 percent xylocaine without epinephrine, with the point of entrance of the needle being from the volar side. This is in contrast to most descriptions in the literature, which report that infiltration is done through a dorsal needle puncture. One may find, however, that the impacted dorsal cortex may not permit the needle to enter the fracture site easily. A second injection, also of approximately 5 cc of xylocaine, is introduced into the area of the distal radioulnar joint and ulnar styloid.[141] With a volarly displaced fracture, the hematoma is better infiltrated from the dorsal aspect.

The effectiveness of local anesthetic agents in providing sufficient analgesia to perform a fracture reduction has been well supported in the literature.[19,31,54,76,137] Although concern has been raised by some regarding the potential systemic toxicity of the local anesthetic agents if absorbed into the blood stream,[167] this would be an extremely rare circumstance.

In view of the concern that hematoma block will provide neither sufficient analgesia nor adequate muscle relaxation,[221] we prefer either Bier block with intravenous lidocaine or brachial plexus block.[4,39,92,94,166] These forms of anesthesia would be especially indicated in those instances in which local skin or soft tissue contusions or edema contraindicate the use of local anesthesia. Given that complications, including fatalities, have been reported using regional anesthetic techniques,[93] it is advisable, whenever possible, that the regional anesthetic be administered by an anesthesiologist with a second physician nearby.

For the most part, general anesthesia should be reserved for specific instances such as the pediatric patient, patients with known allergies to local anesthetic agents, or situations in which the fracture is associated with other injuries requiring operative intervention.

Fracture Reduction

Closed manipulative reduction and cast immobilization remains the treatment of choice today, just as it has over the past 150 years. Ford and Key stated, "There are as many methods of reduction as there are fracture surgeons."[71] However, the reduction of displaced dorsal bending fractures has been based on two approaches: direct manipulation of the fracture fragment, as contrasted to indirect reduction of the fragment via longitudinal traction of the hand and carpus.

Fracture Manipulation

Too little stress has been laid on reduction. Some authors...trusted to the continued pressure of pads. This plan is now recognized as the fruitful source of the melancholy termination of the accident in a hand and wrist deformed and incapable of respectably performing their physiological functions.

T.K. Cruse, 1874[48]

The technique of direct manipulation of the distal fracture fragment featuring "disimpaction" of the distal fragment prior to reduction has usually been attributed to Robert Jones.[110] Yet this technique may well have had its origins in the writings of Colles, who pointed out that longitudinal traction would correct the fracture deformity and rocking back and forth would confirm the diagnosis of fracture by the palpable crepitation.[42] Jones's influence on the English-speaking Orthopaedic world persists even today, as his carefully described technique of manipulative reduction continues to be taught (see Chapter 1).[36]

The technique described by Robert Jones requires an assistant to provide countertraction on the arm above the elbow. The surgeon places the thenar eminence of one hand dorsally over the lower radius at the level of the wrist and the other hand over the lower forearm in line with the radial shaft. The deformity of the fracture is then increased by extension of the distal fragment (Fig. 5.18). With traction still maintained, the surgeon manipulates the distal fragment into a volar and ulnar direction, all the while with the opposite hand applying counterpressure against the proximal radius. The final maneuver is to "lock" the fracture fragment by placing the patient's hand and the distal fracture fragment into pronation.

With the manipulative reduction completed, the hand should be allowed to rest naturally without support to clinically assess the stability of the reduced fracture.

Longitudinal Traction

Although the reduction technique based upon longitudinal traction was initially popularized by Böhler in the 1920s,[23,24] Lidström attributes an extension type of device to achieve fracture reduction to Bardenheur as early as the late nineteenth century.[136] Böhler's technique is based upon application of a strong longitudinal traction to the patient's thumb and digits against a fixed and flexed upper arm while the fracture is directly manipulated by the surgeon.

The original technique required at least one but more often two assistants. The assistants' and patient's hands were coated with an adhesive, as the traction required was at times prolonged. This proved a limiting factor with this technique, as success was often dependent upon the strength and attentiveness of the assistants.[26]

Figure 5.18. The technique of manipulative reduction of dorsally displaced extra-articular bending fractures. *Top:* The surgeon uses both hands to stabilize the forearm and the hand and wrist while the fracture deformity is increased by extending the wrist. *Middle:* While traction is maintained, the distal fragment is manipulated in a volar and ulnar direction. *Lower:* The fracture is locked in place and the patient's hand and fracture fragment is rotated.

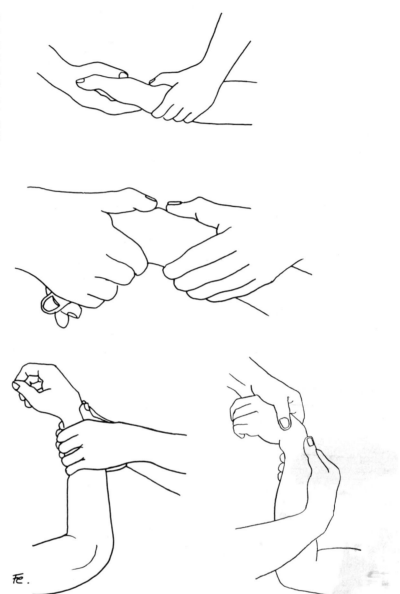

Caldwell in 1931 introduced metallic "finger traps," which, along with counterweight suspended over the upper arm, could provide continuous longitudinal traction without the need for assistants. This soon became well accepted worldwide (Fig. 5.19).[16,29,39,51,56,181]

Although longitudinal traction will effectively restore longitudinal alignment of the distal fragment, its ulnar inclination, the relationship of the distal radioulnar joint, and restoration of the normal volar tilt of the articular surface of the distal radius may not be as easily achieved. There are several explanations for this. In the first place, as shown by Bartosh and Saldaña, the dorsal capsular ligaments of the wrist will tighten before their counterpart on the volar aspect, thereby limiting the ability of the dorsal soft tissue hinge to further reduce the distal fragment into its palmar inclination.[14] Secondly, as suggested by Agee, continued longitudinal traction may actually lead to an increase in the dorsal inclination of the distal fragment, as the distal fragment will tend to pivot on the taut dorsal soft tissue hinge (Fig. 5.20).[8] Agee goes on

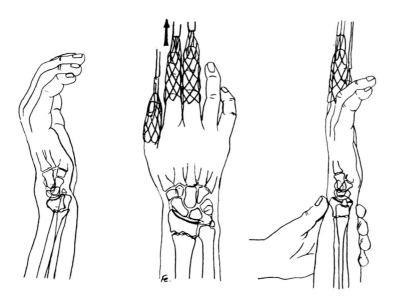

Figure 5.19. Since the introduction of metallic "finger traps," longitudinal traction can be provided without the need for assistants.

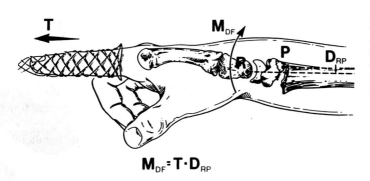

$$M_{DF} = T \cdot D_{RP}$$

Figure 5.20. As presented by John Agee, M.D., excessive longitudinal traction will actually accentuate the dorsal tilt of the distal fragment. (Reproduced with permission. Hand Biomechanics Lab, Inc., Sacramento, CA.)

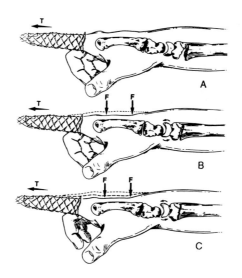

Figure 5.21. The longitudinal length can be restored by longitudinal traction. Palmar (volar) tilt of the distal radius articular surface can be obtained and maintained by a palmar translating force. Note that progressive palmar translation transmits this force through the carpus to the distal radius, hinging the distal fragment about the attached dorsal soft tissue hinge. (Reproduced with permission. Hand Biomechanics Lab, Inc., Sacramento, CA.)

to point out that although increasing flexion on the wrist will aid in bringing the distal fragment into a more anatomic position, this is a less optimal position for immobilization. Rather, he suggests that the same effect can be achieved by palmarly translating the hand. This in turn will provide a subluxation of the midcarpal joint, which will in effect help to restore the palmar inclination of the articular surface (Fig. 5.21).

Immobilization

However unusual the case, all indications will be met and the injured part given the best possible chance of resulting respectably, if we do not hurry our reduction but take time to study the sound wrist and forearm; and then after having brought the maimed parts to as close correspondence with the uninjured as time and patient manipulation will admit, apply the splints so stuffed and packed as to present an accurate cast of the surface on which they are to lie. Thus will the splints supply the place of the surgeon's hands, the best of all retentive apparatuses.

T.K. Cruse, 1874[48]

In spite of the widespread application of cast treatment for bending fractures, a number of questions remain regarding this approach. These include the specific form of immobilization, the position of the hand and wrist as well as the forearm, and the duration of the confinement. Answers to these questions may not be forthcoming from previous literature. Given that, for the most part, studies have tended to include a variety of fracture patterns grouped together under eponymic descriptions, specific experience applied to displaced extraarticular bending fractures alone—both intrinsically stable and unstable—is not readily available. This is further complicated by the wide variation in the duration of follow-up, evaluation of outcome, and age and functional requirements of the patients.

The direction and types of immobilization virtually parallel the history of the literature on this subject (see Chapter 1). Although various types and forms of splints have been in use since Colles' description of dorsal and volar wooden splints, encircling plaster casts have become the standard worldwide in the twentieth century. While some disagreement continues to exist as to whether or not the cast should extend above the elbow (see below), for the most part authors have stressed leaving the metacarpophalangeal joints free to encourage digital motion.[11,19,22,36,63,74,75,81,85,136,137,143,173,194,223]

Some authors have expressed a strong opinion that the forearm should be immobilized in supination in an above-elbow cast,[15,63,64A,138,146,211] particularly with evidence of instability of the distal radioulnar joints, whereas others have equally as confidently recommended that the forearm be kept in pronation.[43,59,128,220]

The fact remains that a number of comparative studies, notwithstanding the heterogeneous nature of the fracture patterns and variability of evaluation, have shown no convincing evidence to support a specific need for immobilization of the forearm in any position.[25,97,163,175,206,215,220] Rather, their studies would suggest that the maintenance of fracture reduction is more dependent upon not only the accuracy of the initial reduction but also the inherent stability of the fracture patterns.

It has been the authors' preference that displaced but intrinsically stable extraarticular dorsal bending fractures can be effectively maintained initially in a sugar tong splint followed by a below-elbow immobilization, provided care is taken to apply appropriate molding of the cast.

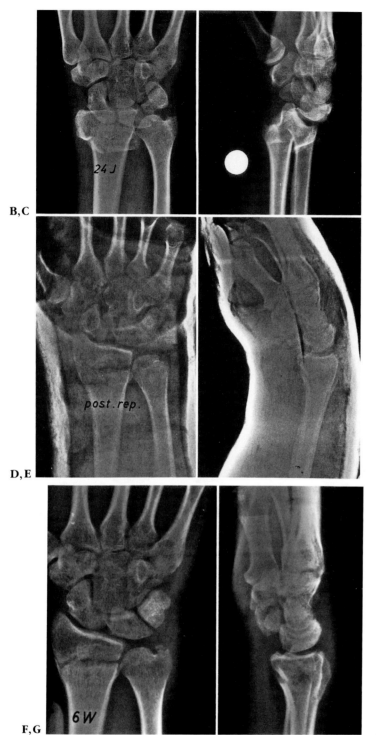

B,C

24 J

post.rep.

D,E

6W

F,G

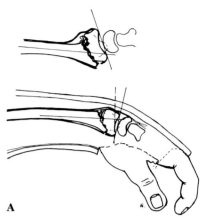

A

Figure 5.22. The authors believe the hand and wrist should be held for the first 2 to 3 weeks postfracture reduction in some ulnar deviation as well as a modest amount of flexion. A. The ulnar deviation and a small amount of palmar flexion will help maintain the soft tissue hinge surrounding the dorsal and radial side of the fracture fragment. B,C. A displaced extraarticular bending fracture. D,E. Anteroposterior and lateral radiographs postreduction with the hand and wrist supported in a molded splint. F,G. The splint was changed to a molded short arm cast 3 weeks postreduction, and at 6 weeks the anteroposterior and lateral radiographs show the near-anatomic reduction.

There continues to be some difference of opinion on the position of the hand and wrist during fracture immobilization. Although the position of more extreme flexion and ulnar deviation, known today as the Cotton-Loder position, has been recognized to put the hand and wrist in jeopardy of median nerve compression as well as inhibiting hand function,[83,140] many still prefer some degree of palmar flexion and ulnar deviation (Fig. 5.22A–G).[19,28,36,70,81,85,137,143,173,194,218] Many of these authors stress, however, that the position of the wrist should be changed at 10 to 14 days posttreatment to one of neutral or slight extension but continuing the ulnar deviation, which in fact was the position originally recommended by Zuppinger in 1910 and Böhler in 1929.[24,28,76,136,146,209,211]

In a prospective study, Gupta in 1991,[90] utilizing a careful molding technique in the application of a plaster cast, suggested that good results could likewise be obtained by immobilizing the wrist in extension. He initially molded the fracture itself in a palmar direction. Then, while the surgeon is maintaining this position, an assistant moves the patient's wrist into extension. Finally, as the plaster is hardening, the wrist is also moved into some ulnar deviation. The final position assumes almost an S shape. When compared to other methods, the author demonstrated this position to have the lowest incidence of redisplacement.

The authors support the observations of Stewart et al.[208] who concluded that in these displaced but stable fractures the position of splintage is not the sole influence on the anatomic end result.

Given that the vast majority of displaced but inherently stable dorsal extra-articular bending fractures can be effectively managed by closed reduction and plaster support, it is interesting to review the principles espoused by Charnley.[36] Although he notes that a circular cast is mechanically more ready ideal, a molded three-point system can equally control most fractures. Local plaster molding, rather than the position of the hand and wrist, proves to be the most reliable and direct means of preventing displacement of the fracture. His "splint" application is based upon a plaster support applied to the radial side of the wrist and forearm, which must extend at least to the midline of the forearm on the palmar surface. The plaster on the palmar side should be thick enough to "take a permanent impression from the surgeon's thenar eminence while the plaster is setting." Curving the splint on the radial side will help to negate the tendency of the fracture to radially deviate (Fig. 5.23). A dorsal molding will also be of fundamental importance to prevent redislocation dorsally of the fracture fragment.

Although Charnley's recommendation would seem to many to represent the fundamental principles of fracture immobilization with external plaster support, the authors strongly believe that they are worth highlighting, as they continue to abide by his recommendations.

Cast immobilization has carried with it concerns regarding restricted range of motion, muscle weakness, and long-term disability (see Chapter 1).[1,3,12,183,207,208] Several alternatives to functional splinting have been proposed. A traditional method, undoubtedly having its origins countless decades ago, is used in China and many other civilizations.[192] Most displaced but stable dorsal bending fractures are well supported by this method, which is based upon the use of strategically placed "pressure pads" and wooden splints. Futami and Yamamoto in 1989 published their experience with this method, suggesting it to be extremely useful, particularly for the elderly patient.[79] One pad is placed dorsally over the distal fracture fragment, one palmarly proximal to the fracture, and one along the radial aspect of the fracture fragment. Four wooden splints are placed around the distal limb and supported with encircling bandages. The patients are seen twice weekly, the bandages are secured and control radiographs are performed, and the fixation is maintained for 5 to 6 weeks (Fig. 5.24).

Functional fracture bracing using more modern materials, as promoted by Sarmiento and co-workers, has also been applied to the distal radius fracture.[129,182,183] These investigators suggested that although the functional brace would effectively stabilize the fracture, the early digital and wrist motion

Figure 5.23. The immobilization technique developed by Charnley is based upon the concept of a three-point splint. Three-point molding at the sites of the arrows as well as ulnar deviation and slight palmar flexion of the wrist will provide sufficient stability for the displaced but not excessively comminuted bending fracture.

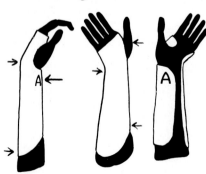

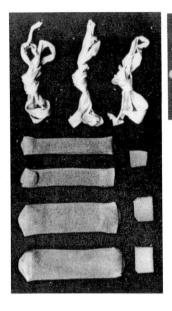

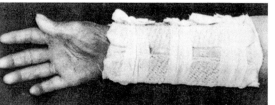

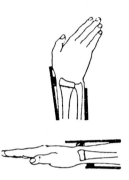

Figure 5.24. The traditional Chinese medicine treatment of distal radius fractures includes the use of pressure pads and wooden splints. Reprinted with permission from Futami T, Yamamoto M. Chinese external fixation treatment for fractures of the distal end of the radius. *J Hand Surg* 14A: 1028–1032, 1989.

would enhance osteogenesis, facilitate return of muscle strength and tone, and allow for a more rapid resolution of soft tissue swelling.

Sarmiento and co-workers established two phases of treatment.[182,183] In the first week following closed fracture reduction, an above-elbow plaster splint was applied, maintaining the forearm in supination, the elbow flexed, and the wrist in some palmar flexion and ulnar deviation. Following that, the splint would be removed and an isoprene fracture brace applied which permitted flexion of the elbow from a 45-degree block to full extension, holding the forearm in supination and allowing full flexion of the wrist from a neutral position (Fig. 5.25).

The concept of functional bracing has been used by others, with some noting enhanced outcome when compared to the plaster support[18,25,68,130] and others noting no significant difference.[49,206] It is clear from an analysis of prior experience with these functional braces that they require experience in the application of braces made from thermoplastic materials and may not be suitable without such experienced personnel.

The authors have had little experience with functional braces but recognize their potential usefulness, particularly if they can be provided "off-the-shelf," thereby making their application more universal.

Duration of Immobilization

Most well-reduced extraarticular dorsal bending fractures will heal by 4 to 5 weeks postinjury. Wählstrom and colleagues, using ^{99}Tc bone scans, observed well-advanced new bone formation by 28 days postinjury and suggest that little additional immobilization will be required beyond this point.[220] This observation has been supported by others.[75,171] However, the authors stress that this deviation of immobilization applies primarily to minimally displaced or displaced fractures without underlying metaphyseal comminution. Longer immobilization will be necessary when the latter is present (see below).

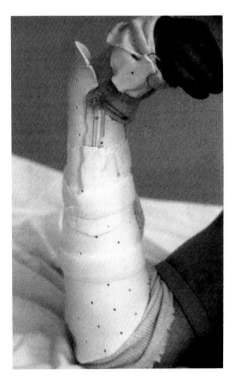

Figure 5.25. The fracture brace advocated by Sarmiento and colleagues holds the forearm in supination allowing flexion of the wrist from a neutral position.

Displaced—Unstable Dorsal Bending Fracture

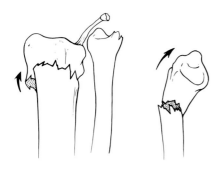

Dorsally displaced extraarticular bending fractures that are either widely displaced at presentation, have metaphyseal comminution extending volarly to involve the anterior cortex, occur in the older patient, have already redisplaced in plaster, or have an associated large ulnar styloid or ulnar head or neck fracture—all will more likely than not redisplace following closed reduction and cast application.[5,21,39,44,48,49,51,56,64,72,81,91,106,111,119,121,123,136,147,159,164,169,185,199,208,215]

The value of remanipulation and repeat cast application has been addressed by several investigators.[41,136,147,150,185] Schmalholz attempted remanipulation and cast in 146 unstable fractures and achieved a successful outcome in only 7 of 105 fractures, which featured both dorsal angulation and metaphyseal comminution.[185] In contrast, re-reduction and plaster support maintained the position in 11 of 27 fractures in which dorsal angulation was the only deformity. His conclusion, confirmed by Collert and Isacson[41] and by McQueen, MacLaren, and Chalmers,[150] was that there will be limited chances for a remanipulation to hold its position in the presence of axial compression of the metaphysis, in an older age patient, or with dorsal displacement and dorsal impaction of the metaphyseal bone.[185,186]

This has been the authors' experience as well. We believe that redisplacement in plaster support would define the fracture as unstable, thereby suggesting that an alternative approach to maintain the reduction be considered.

A number of alternative treatment options have proven effective in maintaining fracture reduction in the presence of an unstable fracture pattern. These include the placement of percutaneous Kirschner wires,[37,51,55,62,80,82,872,103,116,117,131,155,161,178,205,227,229] metal external fixation,[7,8,10,14,38,47,48,58,72,77,1002,101,104,106,122,123,133–135,151,157,172,179,185–187,189,190,210,216,225] and, on occasion, operative reduction with or without external fixation.[135]

The decision to proceed with these more interventional approaches must take into account a number of factors in addition to the fracture pattern. These include local factors, such as soft tissue conditions, as well as individual patient needs. It has become quite clear that the anticipated functional requirements of the individual patient should influence the method of fracture stabilization to a far greater extent than the chronologic age of the patient.

Percutaneous Pinning

The percutaneous placement of smooth Kirschner wires to stabilize the complex extraarticular bending fracture was described as early as 1908 by Lambotte.[170] A variety of techniques of pin placement have been described. These include pins placed through the radial styloid (Fig. 5.26A),[55,142,227] two pins crossing into the radius (Fig. 5.26B),[37,125,126,205] "intrafocal" pinning within the fracture site (Fig. 5.26C),[87,116,117,158] ulnar to radius pinning without transfixation of the distal radioulnar joint (Fig. 5.26D),[51,56,80,132] one radial styloid pin and a second across the distal radioulnar joint (Fig. 5.26E),[155] and pins ulnar to radius with transfixation of the distal radioulnar joint. (Fig. 5.26F).[170]

With the exception of the intrafocal pinning technique advocated by Kapandji,[116,117] in most cases the pins are to be protected by a circular, below-elbow plaster cast. When faced with soft tissue swelling or the need to consider median nerve release, it is our preference to apply a metal external fixation device along with the percutaneous pins (Fig. 5.28).

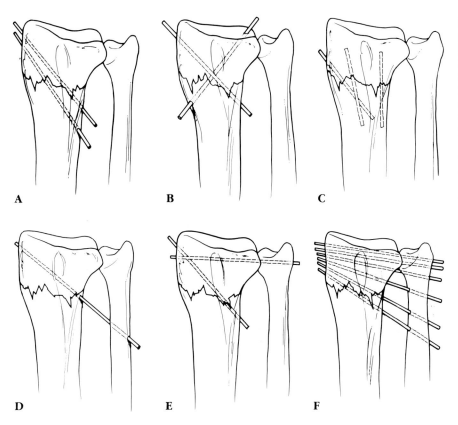

Figure 5.26. A number of different techniques of percutaneous pinning of unstable bending fractures have been described. A. Pins placed primarily through the radial styloid. B. Crossing pins from the radial and ulnar sides of the distal fragment into the distal shaft. C. The intrafocal technique advocated by Kapandji. D. Ulnar to radius pinning without transfixation of the distal radioulnar joint. E. A radial styloid pin and one across the distal radioulnar joint. F. Multiple pins from the ulnar to the radius including transfixation of the distal radioulnar joint.

For the majority of these unstable fractures, we have found that placement of the pins either through the styloid alone or with a second pin directed through the dorsoulnar aspect of the radius will provide adequate stability. The image intensifier is extremely useful in these cases. In the two-pin techniques advocated by Clancey,[37] once the fracture has been manipulated into a reduced position, the forearm is supported on an arm board while the hand is permitted to hang free. The initial smooth 0.062-inch Kirschner wire is directed, using a power wire driver, into the tip of the radial styloid just dorsal to the first extensor compartment. The pin is introduced across the fracture site at an angle of approximately 45 degrees to the long axis of the radius (Fig. 5.27). The second smooth Kirschner wire is inserted into the dorsolulnar corner of the radius between the fourth and fifth extensor compartments. This is directed from dorsal to palmarward in a distal to proximal direction (Fig. 5.28A–F). It is essential that both Kirschner wires penetrate the intact cortex of the radius proximal to the fracture. Inadvertent placement of the wire into the fracture site will lead to loss of reduction and migration of the wires (see Chapter 4).

Once the position of the wires has been confirmed by radiographic control, the tips of the wires are either bent and left just outside the skin or cut off to lie just beneath the skin. A window is preferably made in the cast over the site of the pins to avoid local irritation. Usually the cast or external fixateur can be removed 6 weeks postapplication, while the Kirschner wires are kept in place for an additional 2 weeks to reduce the chance of late fracture collapse (Fig. 5.29A–H).

Mention should be made of the "intrafocal pinning" technique initially described by Kapandji in 1976.[116] Kapandji's initial indications were centered

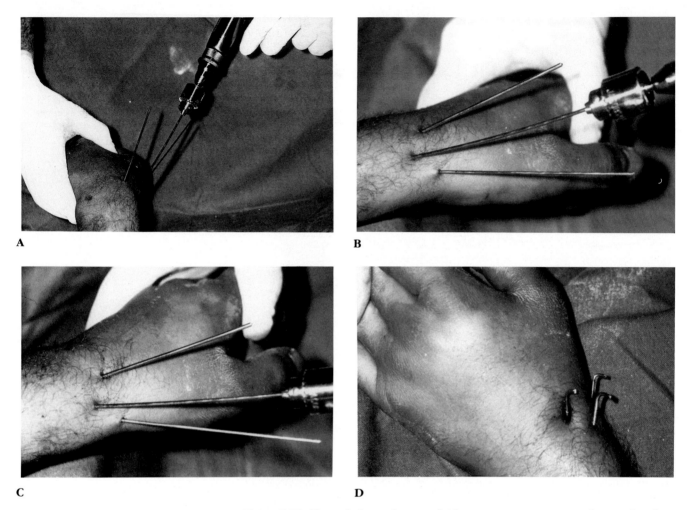

A

B

C

D

Figure 5.27. The technique of trans-styloid percutaneous pinning is illustrated in these pictures. Stout smooth pins are preferred which are either cut below the skin or bent and left outside.

primarily around unstable extraarticular fractures in younger patients. Although others have extended this technique towards older patients,[62,80,158] it remains most effective in those unstable fractures without substantial volar comminution or focal osteopenia. Fracture reduction has proven more difficult to maintain in the elderly patient using this technique.

Although the specific number of pins and their placement will vary, the Kapandji technique is fundamentally based upon placing one or more 0.062-inch smooth Kirschner wires directly into the fracture, functioning to help reduce the fracture as well as to provide an internal splint. The initial pin should be introduced radially between the first and second extensor compartments parallel to the fracture line. A second pin is introduced between the third and fourth dorsal extensor compartments—also initially parallel to the fracture line. Both pins are next directed obliquely at approximately a 45-degree angle to the long axis of the radius and driven with a power wire driver across to the intact proximal cortex. By doing so, the surgeon is able to better achieve and maintain both the restoration of radial length and the volar tilt of the distal radial articular surface (Fig. 5.26C).

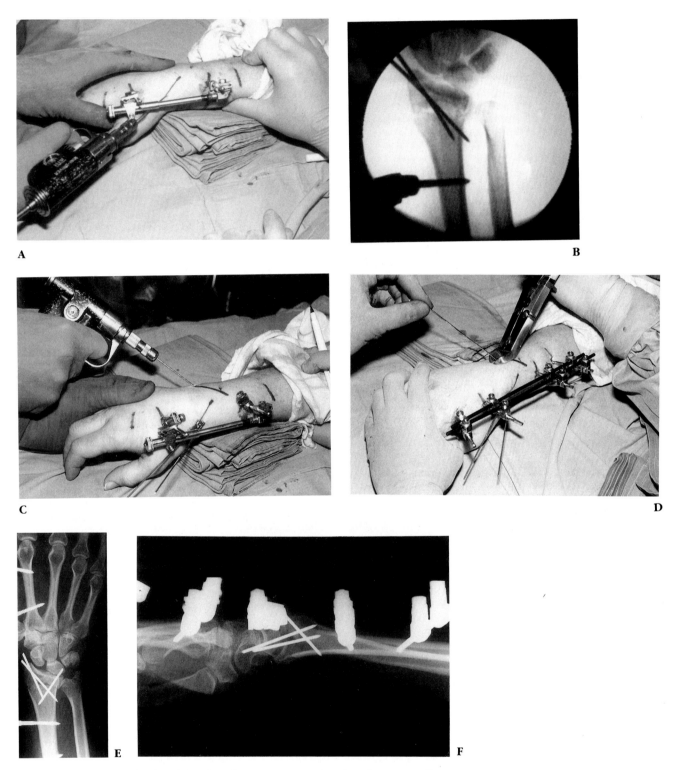

Figure 5.28. An unstable dorsal bending fracture associated with soft tissue swelling. The fracture was treated with a combination of the external skeletal fixation and percutaneous pins. A. Following application of the external fixation, two percutaneous pins were placed across the radial styloid. B. The radial styloid pins were confirmed using an image intensifier. C. An additional pin was placed into the dorsoulnar corner of the distal fragment and directed proximally from dorsal to palmarward. D. The pins were cut to lie just beneath the skin. E,F. Anteroposterior and lateral radiographs demonstrate the fracture anatomically reduced and the position of the percutaneous pins.

Figure 5.29. A 56-year-old woman presented with an unstable dorsal bending fracture which displaced following closed reduction and cast application. A,B. Anteroposterior and lateral radiographs of the displaced unstable bending fracture. C,D. Anteroposterior and lateral radiographs which show the fracture having displaced in the cast. E,F. The fracture was reduced and stabilized with two 0.062-inch smooth Kirschner wires placed into the radial styloid directed towards the opposite cortex. G,H. The fracture healed in a reduced position.

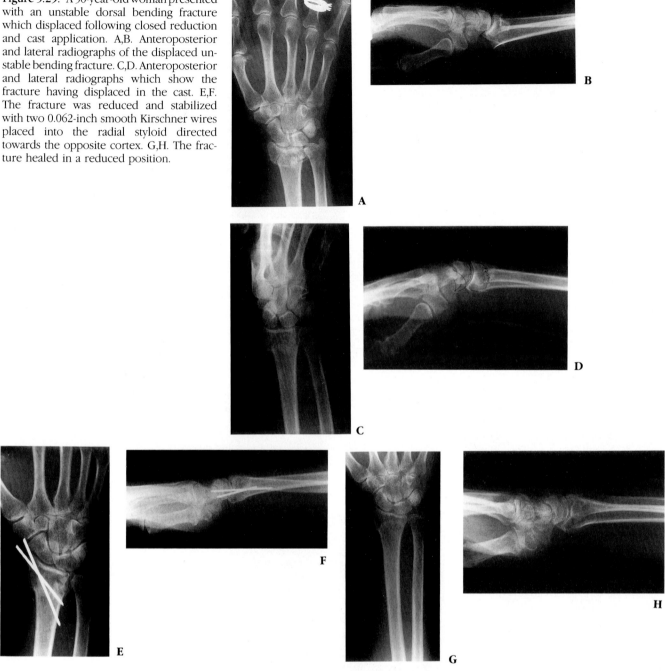

Although Kapandji suggested that plaster support be optional, it has been utilized by many who advocate this technique for approximately 4 to 6 weeks after pin insertion. The pins can be removed as well at the time of cast removal.

Percutaneous Kirschner wire

Indications	Unstable extraarticular dorsally displaced bending fractures
Advantages	Minimally invasive; relatively easy; limited equipment
Disadvantages	Requires additional cast or external fixation; pins may migrate; pin removal required

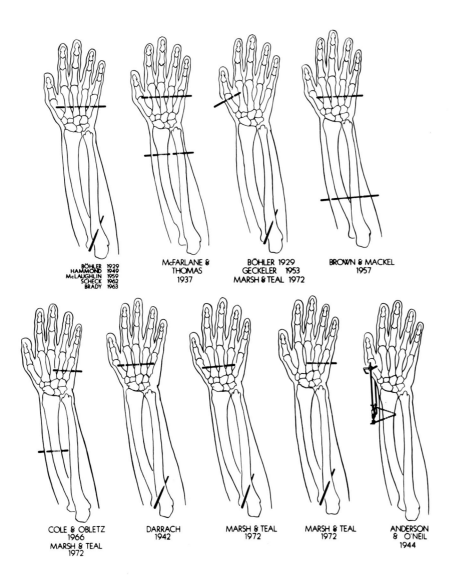

Figure 5.30. A variety of techniques have been described for the pins and plaster technique. Reprinted with permission from Green DP. Pins and plaster treatment of comminuted fractures of the distal end of the radius. *J Bone Joint Surg [Am]* 57A: 304–310, 1975.

Pins and Plaster

Since Böhler's initial description in 1929,[22] pins placed into the metacarpals and forearm bones and incorporated into a below-elbow cast have had a number of advocates. A variety of pin placements have been described in the literature (Fig. 5.30). The technique continues to draw favor in some circles due to its simplicity and relatively low cost.[165] By the same token, a number of studies have suggested that the technique is associated with a relatively high rate of complications.[30,35,225] These include pin loosening, pin tract infection, nerve palsies, iatrogenic fracture at the pin sites, and flattening of the transverse metacarpal arch.

In view of the fact that the authors' preferred means of controlling the unstable dorsal bending fractures is with percutaneous pin fixation and a below-elbow cast, the role of external pin fixation becomes important, primarily when associated soft tissue problems negate the use of a circular cast. In this setting, pins incorporated into a circular cast have fewer applications and have largely been supplanted by metal external fixateurs.

By the same token, pins and plaster techniques are of use and should be made familiar to anyone involved in the care of these more complex fractures.

We prefer to use a single pin, usually a smooth 3/32-inch Steinmann pin placed across the base of the second and third metacarpals. The thumb should be adducted and the first dorsal interosseous muscle pushed away from the second metacarpal prior to pin placement. Although others have advocated the use of the fourth and fifth metacarpals, we agree with Green[88] that this pin placement could have an adverse effect on the normal metacarpal arch as well as increasing the risk of iatrogenic fracture due to the narrow diameter of these metacarpals.[168] The pin can be bent as it exits the skin to afford greater purchase with the plaster as well as preventing interference with retropulsion of the thumb. Pring et al.[165] suggested placement of the distal pin into the thumb metacarpal held in palmar abduction to limit the potential for contracture of the first web as well as to help maintain a more direct line of distraction across the fracture site.

The proximal pin is placed into the radius between the muscles of the first and second dorsal extensor compartments, engaging both cortices of the radius. Again, either a smooth Steinmann pin is placed through a predrilled hole made with a smaller-diameter drill bit or, if available, a half pin with a manufactured threaded tip is used.

The pins are incorporated into a circular below-elbow plaster cast, with particular attention taken to trim the cast distally. The plaster is cut dorsally at the level of the metacarpophalangeal joints, while volarly the entire palm, including both thenar and hypothenar eminences, is left free (Fig. 5.31A–F).

If additional percutaneous pins are placed across the fracture site, the pins and plaster can be removed by 6 weeks, with the percutaneous Kirschner wires left in place an additional 2 weeks. If no percutaneous pins are used, it is preferable to leave the pins and plaster in place for 8 weeks, as the impacted dorsal metaphyseal bone may not support the distal fragment by 6 weeks, leading to a loss of reduction.[88]

Figure 5.31. An unstable and widely displaced fracture of the distal radius was reduced and immobilized in pins and plaster. A. The lateral radiograph reveals the displaced fracture. B,C. One smooth pin is placed across the second and third metacarpal and the more proximal pin is placed into the radius. The pins are bent for better holding with the plaster and to allow full extension of the thumb. D. The anteroposterior radiograph shows the placement of the metacarpal pin. The fracture is well reduced. E,F. The plaster is trimmed to permit full digital extension and flexion.

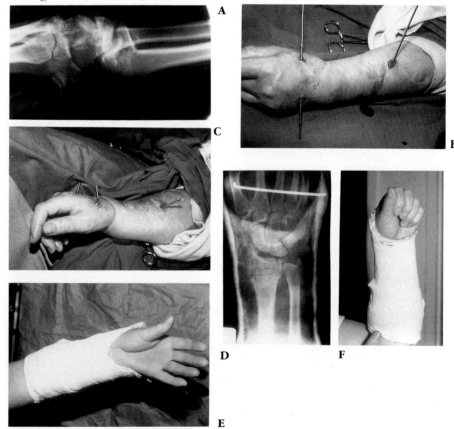

Pins and plaster

Indications	Unstable dorsal bending fractures
	Provide axial length and protect percutaneous pins
Advantages	Ease of application
	Low cost
	Good patient acceptance
Disadvantages	Circular plaster a problem with soft tissue swelling
	Cannot be adjusted
	Pin tract complications
	Iatrogenic nerve and skeletal injuries
	Indirect control over fracture

External Skeletal Fixation

External skeletal fixation has now become widely accepted in the management of complex fractures of the distal end of the radius. Improvements in pin and frame design as well as techniques of application have helped to decrease the recognized problems from pin-related complications.[7,8,38,58,67,77,101,112,134,135,151,190,191,219] Although the majority of unstable extraarticular dorsally displaced bending fractures can be effectively treated by percutaneous pins and a circular cast, the presence of soft tissue complications, associated neurologic deficits, or redisplacement following closed reduction and cast application represent defined indications for the application of external skeletal fixation.

Although it may be difficult to evaluate the literature on external fixation as it has been applied to a heterogenous group of fractures, the authors have widely applied techniques for external skeletal fixation of fractures and strongly support their use with specific complex bending fractures. At the same time, a number of specific issues remain regarding external fixation with not only bending fractures but with all fractures of the distal radius in general. These include specific indications, techniques of application, frame design, and avoidance of complications.

Indications

Although the application of external fixation for displaced unstable bending fractures has its primary indication when soft tissue swelling precludes plaster immobilization, the authors have found its utility to extend to patients of all ages, even those with underlying osteoporosis. This is in contrast to some studies which have suggested that it offers no advantage over plaster support for patients over 60 years of age.[100,122,123] Improvements in pin design and pin size, extending to larger 4-mm pins, as well as adjuvant use of percutaneous pins across the fracture, have provided stable skeletal fixation even in osteopenic bone. In addition, one must continue to bear in mind when evaluating much of the literature on the subject that multiple fracture types are included in most series, often presenting more complicated patterns than the extraarticular comminuted bending fracture. Nevertheless, most studies comparing external skeletal fixation to plaster cast immobilization have documented an improved ability to maintain fracture reduction with external skeletal fixation.[101,107,118,122,123,201,202]

In the case of a bending fracture that has redislocated, external fixation along with percutaneous pins should also be considered.[111,176,186]

Application

The application of external fixation demands the same attention to detail as one would expect with internal fixation. Regardless of the type of frame to be applied, the basic principles of application remain the same. An image intensifier is particularly useful not only for control of the fracture reduction but also for a more precise pin placement. Using the image intensifier, the location of pin placement with reference to both the fracture and the specific sites on the radius and metacarpals can be drawn on the skin (Fig. 5.32A and B) (see Chapter 4).

The authors' preference has been for a simpler type of external fixateur based on that designed by Roger Anderson for fractures of the distal radius.[10] The frame is based on the placement of individual pins, which are then connected together in a variety of designs offering extreme versatility. Two pins are placed into the second metacarpal and two into the distal third of the radius.

Placement of the pins in the distal third of the radius is generally at a locus about 10 to 12 cm proximal to the tip of the radial styloid. Seitz et al.,[189] in cadaver studies, identified this as a more optimal location as long as one takes

Figure 5.32. The application of external skeletal fixation for unstable bending fractures of the distal radius. A,B. Using the image intensifier, the precise location of the pin placement can be identified and marked onto the skin. C,D. Using a drill guide, the pins are individually placed into the metacarpals and the length confirmed on the image. E,F. The pin placement into the distal radius is also performed through a drill guide and confirmed on the image. G. The external frame is applied along with percutaneous pins.

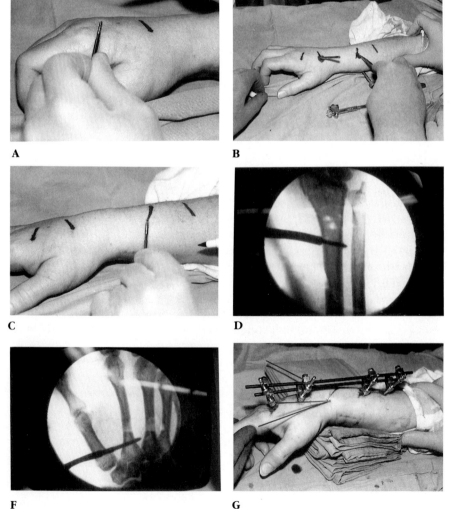

A

B

C

D

E

F

G

precautions regarding injury to the overlying tendons and radial sensory nerve. Through small incisions and use of dissecting scissors, the musculotendinous junctions of the brachioradialis and radial wrist extensors can be mobilized along with the radial nerve. A drill guide with a serrated end to hold onto the bone will ensure that the pin placement will not injure these soft tissue structures. In younger patients, initial holes should be drilled with a 2.0-mm drill bit into which are placed 2.5-mm Schanz pins. In older patients, we now prefer 4.0-mm Schanz pins that can be drilled directly into the bone through the drill guide. Using a more "open" technique of pin placement, Seitz and co-workers observed in 66 consecutive cases no tendon or nerve injury and only a 2 percent incidence of superficial pin infection without any case of deep bony infection.[190] This has been the authors' experience as well (Fig. 5.32C and D).

The distal two pins are placed into the second metacarpal. In a like manner to that described for the proximal pin placement, small incisions are used along with a protective drill guide to minimize the risk of injury to overlying tendons, first dorsal interosseous muscle, or branches of the radial sensory nerve. One pin is placed into the base of the metacarpal at the proximal flair of the bone, while the more distal pin is placed into the distal third of the bone, avoiding the sagittal fibers of the extensor mechanism over the meta-carpophalangeal joint. As the amount of cortical bone in the second metacarpal is limited, more thread purchase for each pin is gained by aiming the pins at approximately a 30-degree angle to the long axis of the metacarpal. The pins should be directed off the horizontal at approximately a 45-degree angle to avoid interference with retroposition of the thumb metacarpal (Fig. 5.32E and F).

Many have suggested that the frame be applied so that the hand and wrist are immobilized in a position similar to that with plaster support, i.e., some palmar flexion and ulnar deviation, however, we have not found this to be necessary. Furthermore, this position can be deleterious to maximizing functional recovery of digital function and strength of grip.[8] As we would attempt to support the fracture reduction with percutaneously placed Kirschner wires, the external frame would function effectively with the wrist in neutral or even 5 to 10 degrees of extension (Fig. 5.32F).

At the conclusion of the procedure, the skin should be without tension around the pins. Sterile gauze wraps are placed around each pin and pre-ferentially left in place for 3 to 6 days before removal and initiation of routine pin care. The latter consists of cleansing the pins daily with hydrogen peroxide and careful follow-up to release any areas of skin that become adherent to the pins. The patients, as a general rule, are permitted to shower by 10 to 14 days after application of the external fixation frame.

Frame Design

The vast majority of external fixation frames accomplish the intended goals of providing axial length and rotational control to maintain reduction of unstable dorsal bending fractures. In addition, most are lightweight, offer versatility in pin placement, and are relatively easy to apply.[77] In fact, there is little in the literature to suggest that one particular frame size, shape, or method of application offers demonstrable advantages over the other.[189] For this reason, we continue to have confidence in the basic pin-to-frame design, which is an adaptation of the original design of the Roger Anderson.[104]

Several variations of external fixation design and application may prove particularly useful with unstable extraarticular fractures that feature a large displaced distal fragment. As most designs are based upon maintenance of traction across the wrist, certain inherent problems have been noted. These include digital stiffness due to wrist positioning, intrinsic tightness,[7,115] or even delay in healing due to overdistraction.[118] Several authors have documented success by designing their frames to place pins into the distal fragment as well as the distal radial diaphysis, thereby avoiding traction across the wrist.[151]

Alternatively, there is increasing interest in the development of "dynamic" or mobile wrist external fixation frames which will maintain axial length and alignment while at the same time permitting wrist flexion and extension.[38,109,133] Enthusiasm for these has been tempered by the complexity of the operative protocol as well as the difficulty in controlling the more unstable fractures. Although some have attempted to correlate the duration and extent of distraction across the carpal ligaments with the development of long-term wrist stiffness,[115] these studies have not been well controlled and stratified to determine the specific effect of the external fixation as opposed to the nature of the injury. Furthermore, several investigators have confirmed the authors' own observations that upwards of 18 months to 2 years should be permitted to go by before determining final outcome.[47,58] More often than not, substantial wrist motion will be recovered over this duration of follow-up.

Finally, a surgical tactic has been established by Leung et al.[134,135] based on external fixation in conjunction with placement of autogenous cancellous bone in the metaphyseal defect that is always present following reduction of the comminuted unstable dorsal bending fractures.[134] In these authors' hands, this technique, albeit invasive, has yielded extraordinarily good results (Fig. 5.33A–H). While the vast majority of their cases involved intraarticular fractures, it does offer similar possibilities for these unstable extraarticular injuries. The fixateurs were left in place for only 3 weeks, following which a wrist brace was applied, permitting wrist motion from neutral to full flexion. At the end of 6 weeks, the brace was removed and full mobility encouraged. the brace was

Figure 5.33. An extremely dorsally displaced bending fracture in an active professional bowler. A,B. The preoperative anteroposterior and lateral radiographs demonstrate the extensive metaphyseal comminution and dorsal displacement. C,D. Following closed reduction and external fixation, autogenous iliac crest bone graft was placed in the metaphyseal defect. E,F. Anteroposterior and lateral radiographs at 6 weeks at the time of frame removal. G,H. An excellent radiographic and functional result at 1 year posttreatment.

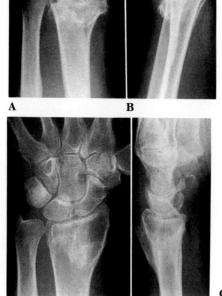
A   B

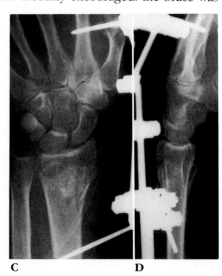
C   D

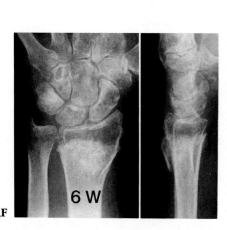
6 W
E,F

G,H

removed and full mobility encouraged. The authors reported on 100 consecutive cases, with the majority having excellent results. However, pin- or nerve-related complications occurred in 17 of these 100 cases.

Complications

As with many other aspects of the surgical experience with external skeletal fixation of fractures of the distal end of the radius, the identification and documentation of the incidence of complications in the literature vary widely. At times, one cannot be certain if some complications attributed to external fixation, e.g., wrist stiffness, loss of reduction, and soft tissue problems, are more accurately a reflection of the injury itself. As Sanders and co-workers have noted,[179] the complications may be more accurately categorized in three major groups: (1) problems attributable to the difficulty of reduction and maintenance of the fracture reduction, (2) pin-related problems, (3) problems inherent to the fracture regardless of the method of treatment.

In the first category, the dorsal unstable bending fractures are readily reduced, and the use of adjuvant percutaneous pins will offset the tendency for loss of reduction. With compression articular fractures, alternative techniques for maintaining the reduction will be addressed in Chapter 7.

Pin-related problems, so prevalent in the literature, can also be minimized by careful attention to detail as outlined above.

Finally, a number of the problems that have been attributed to the fracture, such as swelling, nerve compression, reflex sympathetic dystrophy, and digital stiffness, just to list a few, can also be minimized by early recognition and prompt attention (see Chapter 10).

Frame Removal

To some degree, problems associated with the use of external fixation can be minimized by early removal of the frame. The use of percutaneous pins or autogenous bone graft will permit the fixation frames to be removed by 3 to 4 weeks following their application. In a prior publication, one of the authors (JBJ) along with RJ McMurtry established a framework for timing of frame removal which has subsequently been modified.[148]

Fracture type and external fixation	Frame removal (weeks)
Extraarticular	
With percutaneous pins	4
With bone graft	3–4
With pins or bone graft	6

External skeletal fixation	
Indications	Unstable dorsal bending fracture
	Associated soft tissue complications
	When metaphyseal defect filled with autogenous graft
Advantages	Maintain length
	Allows soft tissue rehabilitation
Disadvantages	Indirect control over fracture fragments
	Pin-related complication
	More complicated
	Requires additional equipment

Operative Treatment

Operative exposure of displaced comminuted unstable dorsal bending fractures is not commonly required. Although the technique of open bone grafting and external skeletal fixation advocated by Leung et al. offers more direct control over the distal fragment without the need for internal fixation,[134] formal operative management of these fractures is reserved for certain situations including open fractures, fractures with associated soft tissue injuries, those associated with carpal ligament injury, or those seen beyond 3 weeks postinjury with unacceptable deformity.[66,113,114]

The surgical approach is extensile between either the second and the third, or the fourth and the fifth, dorsal extensor compartments (see Chapter 4). The crossing large dorsal veins and sensory nerve are identified and protected. The extensor retinaculum is opened between the second and third extensor compartments, with the fourth compartment elevated in a subperiosteal fashion. Once the fracture is identified, we prefer to apply a mini distractor with one pin in the distal fragment placed 5 to 10 degrees further dorsally angulated than the distal fragment itself. A second pin is placed perpendicular to the radial shaft proximal to the fracture (Fig. 5.34A–F).

If the fracture is beyond 2 weeks postinjury, the fracture line will be obscured by immature callus. Cautious removal will permit excellent exposure of the fracture lines. The distal fragment is now distracted until length and alignment is restored both visually and with radiographic control.

Figure 5.34. A dorsally displaced bending fracture seen at 3 weeks postfracture in an athletic college student. The fracture required operative exposure. Through a dorsal extensile exposure, the extensor retinaculum is exposed. A. The retinaculum is opened between the second and third extensor compartments. B. A mini distractor is applied with one pin in the distal fragment and distal part of the radial shaft. C. A dorsal T plate is applied once fracture reduction has been achieved. The postoperative radiographs reveal the anatomic reduction and plate application.

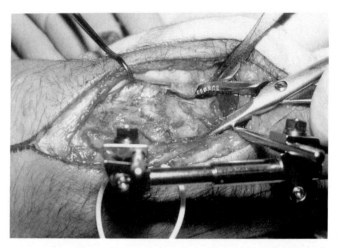

A

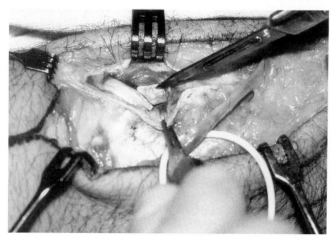

B

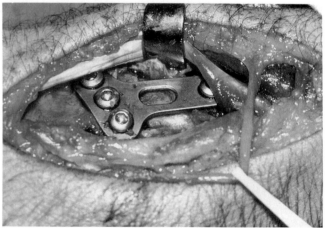

C

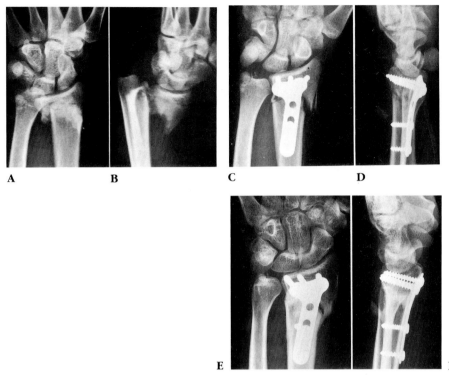

A B   C D

E   F

Figure 5.35. A high-energy displaced dorsal bending fracture which was grossly unstable in a 28-year-old laborer. A,B. Anteroposterior and lateral radiographs of the displaced fracture. C,D. An operative exposure and plate application provided anatomic reduction and stable internal fixation. The good quality of the patient's bone enabled screws to be placed into the distal fragment. E,F. Anatomic reduction was maintained though union and a full functional result was achieved.

A cancellous bone graft will be required to fill the defect that will have resulted once the fracture has been reduced. The bone graft can be obtained from the iliac crest using trephine biopsy needles. Definitive fixation is provided with an angled T plate. Our preference has been to avoid placing screws into the distal fragment unless the quality of the bone will assure excellent screw purchase (Fig. 5.35A–F).

Postoperatively, a thermoplastic splint worn for 2 to 3 weeks is ordinarily sufficient support unless screw purchase was insecure due to underlying osteoporosis. In the latter case, a short arm cast for 6 weeks is advisable.

Palmar Bending Fracture

Some confusion and even disagreement exists as to the proper identification and management of volarly displaced fractures of the distal radius. Although Goyrand's[86] and Smith's[197] original description suggested an extraarticular metaphyseal fracture, others later began to include intraarticular shearing fractures[34,212] under the overall grouping of Smith's fractures. What is clear is that not all of these are bending fractures, and, moreover, the bending-type volarly displaced fractures are not all to be viewed as mirror images of the dorsally displaced variant. The extent of overlying soft tissues, the rotational deformity, and the often oblique nature of the fracture line tend to make accurate closed reduction more difficult and, even further, maintenance of the reduction in a cast more unpredictable.

If one confines the discussion to only the extraarticular fractures, a treatment rationale can be established in a manner similar to that for the dorsally displaced bending fracture. For impacted fractures with little or no displacement, the immobilization technique described by Mills in 1957,[153] holding the wrist in slight extension, the forearm in full supination, and the elbow at 90 degrees of flexion, has proven effective. The cast is maintained for 6 weeks.

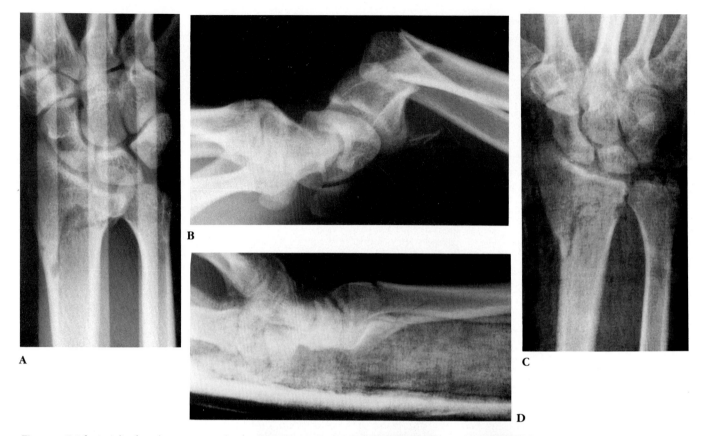

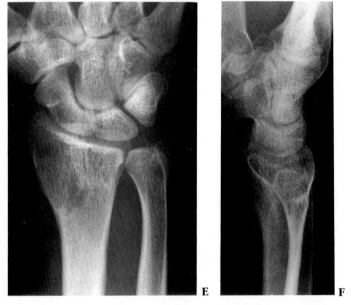

Figure 5.36. A displaced extraarticular palmar bending fracture in a 35-year-old laborer. A,B. Anteroposterior and lateral radiographs of the palmarly displaced extraarticular fracture. C,D. Following a closed manipulative reduction under axillary block anesthesia, an anatomic reduction was confirmed on x-ray. Initially a sugartong splint was applied with the forcarm in Supination and in 7 days converted to a long arm cast. E,F. At 1 year follow-up, excellent alignment and function was noted.

A displaced transverse bending pattern with only a limited zone of comminution is also one that can be managed by closed reduction and cast immobilization. By the same token, this fracture pattern will tend to include a rotational deformity. Therefore, reduction of the fractures will require disimpaction and manipulation of the distal fragment into extension, as well as supination of the hand and wrist. The type of immobilization will be that advocated by Mills (Fig. 5.36A–F).[153]

In contrast, the transverse volarly displaced bending fracture associated with metaphyseal comminution (Fernandez Type C or subgroups A3.2 or A3.3) and the oblique fracture pattern (Fernandez B) both tend to be more difficult to accurately reduce by manipulation and are definitely more difficult to maintain in a plaster support.[196] In these cases it is the authors' preference to perform an open reduction and plate fixation.

The surgical approach is extensile and is presented in detail in Chapters 4 and 6. As these are extraarticular fractures, the reduction can be effectively controlled by observing the reduction of the fracture lines without any need to visualize the articular surface. A volarly applied T plate which is contoured to the anatomy of the distal radius is preferred. By the same token, given that these fractures tend to require only a "buttress" type of plate support, other plate shapes or designs will also prove effective (Fig. 5.37A–F).[60,78]

The authors have compiled a series of 56 patients treated operatively for unstable palmarly displaced fractures of the distal radius.

Although the majority of these cases involved intraarticular shearing fractures, it was apparent from that experience that the operative treatment of these fractures can result in an excellent functional outcome with limited risks and complications. It is noteworthy in this series that almost 50 percent of the cases had displaced in a plaster cast following a closed manipulative reduction.

The Distal Radioulnar Joint

The significance of involvement of the distal radioulnar joint in extraarticular bending fractures is becoming increasingly apparent. As the anatomy and kinesiology of the distal radioulnar joint is complex,[20,69,160] injury to this articulation can lead to long-lasting symptoms and residual disability.[208] Reduction of overall grip strength,[40,177,217] restricted forearm rotation,[177] and residual pain[99] have all been noted in part of the wrist in association with a distal radius fracture.

Although late problems with the distal radioulnar joint are covered in detail in Chapter 10, assessment and management of involvement of the distal radioulnar joint at the time of treatment of the initial fracture may prove critical for assuring a functional outcome.

The relationship of the distal radioulnar joint in both the management and the outcome of extraarticular bending fractures was recognized relatively early by some investigators.[146,188] Scudder noted in 1939 that the integrity of the distal radioulnar joint, which in turn he attributed to a large degree to the triangular fibrocartilage, was crucial for successful management of these fractures.[188] He differentiated the fractures into two basic groups: those with an intact distal radioulnar joint and triangular fibrocartilage, and those with loss of integrity of support of the distal radioulnar joint. The latter were subdivided into those with rupture of the triangular fibrocartilage alone, with avulsion of the ulnar styloid at its base, or with severe comminution of the distal fragment of the radius with the distal radioulnar joint ligaments attached to a loose fragment of the distal radius. Physical examination at the time of fracture manipulation can identify hypermobility of the distal ulna, which would suggest loss of the intrinsic support of the distal radioulnar joint.

We have divided involvement of the distal radioulnar joint into three types (Fig. 5.9). In Type I, the joint is stable and congruous following reduction of the distal radius fracture. One may see an avulsion fracture of the ulnar styloid (Type IA) or a stable ulnar neck fracture (Type IB). No specific treatment apart from that directed at the distal radius fracture will be required.

Type II injuries represent subluxation or dislocation of the ulnar head in conjunction with the distal radius fracture. Type IIA injuries involve a substance tear of the triangular fibrocartilage complex with or without rupture of the

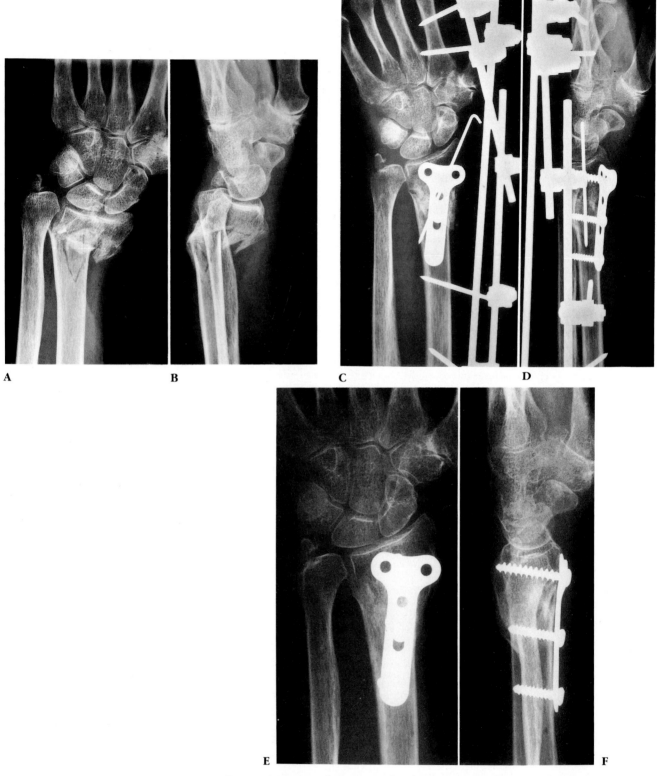

Figure 5.37. A multifragmented subgroup A3.3 comminuted palmarly displaced extraarticular fracture in an elderly woman with osteoporosis. The fracture was unstable and could not be held in a plaster cast. A,B. Anteroposterior and lateral radiographs reveal the complex fracture pattern of the palmarly displaced bending fracture. C,D. In view of the underlying osteoporosis, in addition to the palmar buttress plate and autogenous bone graft, an external skeletal fixateur was applied for 3 weeks. E,F. Follow-up at 1 year reveals an anatomic reduction. Excellent function was achieved.

dorsal and palmar capsular ligaments. Type IIB injuries involve an avulsion fracture at the base of the ulnar styloid.

With Type IIA problems, we recommend a closed reduction of the distal radioulnar joint and immobilization of the joint with the forearm in 45 degrees of supination for 4 to 6 weeks. Alternatively, for operative repair of the triangular fibrocartilage or with Type IIB fractures, internal fixation of the ulnar styloid is also a consideration. Following operative treatment, the forearm should also be immobilized in 30–40 degrees of supination for a period of 4 to 6 weeks to permit soft tissue healing.

The third type of distal radioulnar joint injuries consists of what the authors consider potentially unstable injuries. Type IIA injuries involve an intraarticular fracture of the sigmoid notch which would be part of the Type C distal radius fracture patterns or Type IIIB patterns involving an intraarticular fracture of the ulnar head. With these injuries, we favor a closed reduction and cast immobilization with the forearm in supination for 4 to 6 weeks and consider later reconstruction if posttraumatic arthrosis develops which is symptomatic.

Complications

The complications that have been identified with extraarticular bending fractures, which are related both to the fracture itself and to the treatment, are so substantial that the authors have decided to devote two entire chapters (Chapters 10 and 11) to these problems. The reader is encouraged to become thoroughly familiar with these problems, as all too many are avoidable!

Outcome

No fracture so frequently occurred and none, perhaps, was so little understood. Mr. Sully mentioned that recent case of an experienced surgeon, who had been proceeded against by his patient for damages, in consequence of some deformity having followed the treatment of a fracture of this kind.
                                        Royal Medical and Surgical Society, March 1847

Although the literature reflects attempts by some investigators to quantitate their results with objective as well as subjective evaluations,[45,81,89,120,136,180,184,191] it would seem accurate to suggest that many have felt that little would be gained by stringent evaluation criteria, given the fact that so many patients appeared to function relatively well. This attitude is perhaps best summarized by G.B. Smaill, who noted in 1965:

Objective results were not so satisfactory as the subjective but overall...no reason to depart from present methods of managing their injuries by manipulation and immobilization in plaster.[194]

One of the major difficulties that continues to exist in the literature is the lack of agreement on the optimal way to assess outcome. This may be due in part to the fact that some patients function relatively well in the presence of deformity following fractures of the distal radius. However, many do not do as well. Therefore, it is quite reasonable to strive for evaluation methods that combine the patient's perspectives with objective criteria.

One of the most widely applied evaluation systems is that developed by Gartland and Werley in 1951 (Table 5.1).[81] Although this method somewhat

Table 5.1. Point system used to evaluate end results of healed Colles' fracture.*

Result	Points
Residual deformity	
Prominent ulnar styloid	1
Residual dorsal tilt	2
Radial deviation of the hand	2–3
Point range	0–3
Subjective evaluation	
Excellent: No pain, disability, or limitation of motion	0
Good: Occasional pain, slight limitation of motion, no disability	2
Fair: Occasional pain, slight limitation of motion, feeling of weakness in wrist, no particular disability if careful, activities slightly restricted	4
Poor: Pain, limitation of motion, disability, activities more or less markedly restricted	6
Point range	0–6
Objective evaluation[†]	
Loss of dorsiflexion	5
Loss of ulnar deviation	3
Loss of supination	2
Loss of palmar flexion	1
Loss of radial deviation	1
Loss of circumduction	1
Pain in distal radioulnar joint	1
Point range	0–5
Complications	
Arthritic change	
Minimal	1
Minimal with pain	3
Moderate	2
Moderate with pain	4
Severe	3
Severe with pain	5
Nerve complications (median)	1–3
Poor finger function due to cast	1–2
Point range	0–5
End-result point range	0–2
Excellent	0–2
Good	3–8
Poor	9–20
Fair	21 and above

* Reprinted from Gartland JJ, Jr, Werley CC: Evaluation of healed Colles' fractures. *J Bone Joint Surg* 33A: 900, October 1951.
† The objective evaluation is based upon the following ranges of motion as being the minimum for normal function: dorsiflexion, 45 degrees; palmar flexion, 30 degrees; radial deviation, 15 degrees; ulnar deviation, 15 degrees; pronation, 50 degrees; and supination, 50 degrees.

arbitrarily assigns a numerical score to a host of parameters, they early on recognized the value of the patient's subjective impressions and symptoms. Lidström in 1959[136] established a less stringent evaluation method that was utilized as well by Frykman in 1967[76] in his exhaustive monograph on the distal radius fracture (Table 5.2). Scheck in 1962[184] presented an evaluation approach that placed emphasis on both the patient's symptoms and functional status and the presence of deformity (Table 5.3).

Table 5.2. Evaluation of function—subjective and objective.

Excellent	Unrestricted wrist function; no subjective complaints No visible deformity Limitation in volar and dorsal flexion not exceeding 15° No loss of strength
Good	Unrestricted wrist function; minor subjective complaints Deformity can be accepted if subjective complaints are not associated with deformity Movement limitation up to 20° and mild loss of strength
Fair	Less satisfactory wrist function when working with a tool or upon extreme movement. Function otherwise retained. Moderate loss of strength
Poor	Reduced work capacity and impaired general function Constant pain Significant loss of strength

From Frykman[76] and Lidström.[136]

Table 5.3. Evaluation of function.

Subjective	
Excellent	Fully satisfied with cosmetic result; no pain, weakness, or limitation of motion; no restriction in occupation or recreational activity
Good	Just noticeable difference in appearance or mild and occasional discomfort after exertion, or both; minor restriction in motion or strength or both; continuation of former occupation and recreational activities
Poor	Deformity, pain, weakness, and limitation of motion. Patient has not continued with former occupation or recreational activity
Visual	
Excellent	Normal appearance; no visible difference between the injured and uninjured wrists
Good	Just noticeable deformity because of some broadening of the wrist; slight radial drift of the hand, or slight prominence of the ulnar styloid process
Poor	Obvious deformity

From Scheck.[184]

Three more contemporary evaluation systems are that of Green and O'Brien,[89] as modified by Cooney et al.,[45] to apply to fractures of the distal radius (Table 5.4), the New York Orthopaedic Hospital Wrist Rating Scale (Table 5.5),[191] and that of de Bruijn (Table 5.6).[49]

Radiologic outcome has also been studied with an objective rating scale. Sarmiento modified Lidström's radiologic evaluation as to outcome based upon measuring dorsal angulation, shortening of the radius in relation to the distal ulna, and loss of the normal surface of the distal end of the radius (Table 5.7).[182,183] Knirk and Jupiter[120] further developed a radiologic grading for both articular congruity (Table 5.8) and radiologic evidence of arthritis (Table 5.9).

Table 5.4. Modified clinical scoring system of Green and O'Brien.

Category	Score (points)	Findings
Pain (25 points)	25	None
	20	Mild, occasional
	15	Moderate, tolerable
	0	Severe or intolerable
Functional status (25 points)	25	Returned to regular employment
	20	Restricted employment
	15	Able to work but unemployed
	0	Unable to work because of pain
Range of motion (25 points)		Percentage of normal
	25	100
	15	75–99
	10	50–74
	5	25–49
	0	0–24
		Dorsiflexion-palmar flexion arc (injured hand only)
	25	120° or more
	15	91–119°
	10	61–90°
	5	31–60°
	0	30° or less
Grip strength (25 points)		Percentage of normal
	25	100
	15	75–99
	10	50–74
	5	25–49
	0	0–24
Final result		
Excellent	90–100	
Good	80–89	
Fair	65–79	
Poor	<65	

Table 5.5. New York Orthopaedic Hospital wrist rating scale.

A. Objective
1. Motion (percentage of normal motion): 0–15 points.
   Dorsi/ulnar flexion + radioulnar deviation + supination/pronation (%)
   6.7%

2. Grip strength: 0–15 points
   Percentage of "normal"
   6.7%

3. Roentgenogram: 0–20 points
   a. Length
      Maintained — 7
      Loss of 0–2 mm — 5
      Loss of 2–3 mm — 3
      Loss of >5 mm — 0

   b. Articular surface
      Congruent — 7
      Incongruity of 0–1 mm — 5
      Incongruity of 1–2 mm — 3
      Incongruity of >2 mm — 0

   c. Joint space
      "Normal" — 4
      Decreased — 2
      Not apparent — 0

   d. Lateral alignment
      <20° dorsal tilt — 2
      >20° dorsal tilt — 0

B. Subjective
1. Pain: 0–20 points
   a. None — 20
   b. Only with heavy activities (e.g., contact sports, construction) — 16
   c. Occurs with moderate activity (e.g., swimming, heavy housework) — 12
   d. Frequent with light activity (desk work, washing dishes) — 8
   e. Present at all times but does not require analgesics — 4
   f. Present at all times requiring analgesics — 0

2. Function: 0–30 points
   a. Unlimited — 30
   b. Can no longer participate in heavy activity — 25
   c. Can no longer participate in moderate activity — 20
   d. Has difficulty with light activity — 15
   e. Uses injured hand only as a helper — 10
   f. Cannot use hand — 0

   Sum total (1–100)

Results: Excellent, 90–100; good, 70–89; fair, 55–69; poor <55.

Table 5.6. Scoring system of the final clinical assessment.

Complaints				Score
a. Pain while resting				10
b. Pain while moving				8
c. Pain during heavy work/excessive motion (if b = 0)				4
d. Numbness of paresthesia in the fingers				3
e. Restricted daily basic life activities				10
f. Pain while wringing out clothes (if b + c = 0)				3
g. Loss of power				3
h. Subjective judgment of the end result				5 or 10
i. Open question for any other complaints (if a + b + c = 0)				1, 2 or 3

Motion in the wrist region	0–40%	40–60%	60–80%	80–90%
Dorsal flexion	5	4	3	2
Volar flexion	5	4	3	2
Radial deviation	2	1	1	0
Ulnar deviation	2	1	1	0
Pronation	5	4	3	2
Supination	5	4	3	2

Motor functions of the hand	0–40%	40–60%	60–80%	80–90%
Grip power	8	5	3	2
Making a fist			8	
Finger extension			8	
Opposition			8	

	Abnormal	Impossible
Opening a door	5	8
Weight lifting	5	8
Picking up a pen	5	8
Crumpling a piece of paper	5	8
Lifting a cup and saucer	5	8

Signs and symptoms	
Swelling of hand/fingers	5
Abnormal color	2
Skin atrophy/hyperesthesia/hyperhidrosis	4
Ulnar compression pain	2

Cosmesis	
Cosmetic apperance	2, 3, or 5

From de Bruijn.[49]

Table 5.7. Criteria for anatomical results.

Result	Criteria
Excellent	No or insignificant deformity Dorsal angulation ≤0° Shortening <3 mm Loss of radial deviation <4°
Good	Slight deformity Dorsal angulation 1–10° Shortening 3–6 mm Loss of radial deviation 5–9°
Fair	Moderate deformity Dorsal angulation 11–14° Shortening 7–11 mm Loss of radial deviation 10–14°
Poor	Severe deformity Dorsal angulation >15° Shortening ≥12 mm Loss of radial deviation >15°

After Sarmiento et al.[183] modified from Lidström.[136]

Table 5.8. Articular congruity as measured according to the method of Knirk and Jupiter.

Grade	Step-off
0	0–1 mm
1	1–2 mm
2	2–3 mm
3	>3 mm

Table 5.9. Arthritis grading according to the method of Knirk and Jupiter.

Grade	Findings
0	None
1	Slight joint space narrowing
2	Marked joint space narrowing, osteophyte formation
3	Bone-on-bone, osteophyte formation, cyst formation

References

1. Abbaszadegan H, Adolphson P, Dalen N: Bone mineral loss after Colles' fracture: Plaster cast and external fixation equivalent. *Acta Orthop Scand* 62: 156–158, 1991.
2. Abbaszadegan H, Conradi P: Fixation not needed for undisplaced Colles' fracture. *Acta Orthop Scand* 60: 60–62, 1989.
3. Abbaszadegan H, Jonsson U: External fixation or plaster cast for severely displaced Colles' fracture? Prospective 1-year study of 46 patients. *Acta Orthop Scand* 61: 528–530, 1990.
4. Abbaszadegan H, Jonsson U: Regional anesthesia preferable for Colles' fracture. *Acta Orthop Scand* 61: 348–349, 1990.
5. Abbaszadegan H, Jonsson U, von Sivers K: Prediction of instability of Colles' fractures. *Acta Orthop Scand* 60: 646–650, 1989.
6. Abbaszadegan H, von Sivers K, Jonsson U: Late displacement of Colles' fractures. *Int Orthop* 12: 197–199, 1988.
7. Agee JM: Distal radius fracture: Multiplanar ligamentotaxis. *Hand Clin* 9: 577–586, 1993.
8. Agee JM: External fixation. *Orthop Clin North Am* 24: 265–274, 1993.
9. Amendola FH: The after-treatment of Colles' fracture. *JAMA* 112: 1803–1806, 1938.
10. Anderson R, O'Neil G: Comminuted fractures of the distal end of the radius. *Surg Gynecol Obstet* 78: 434–440, 1944.
11. Augustine RW: The Colles' fracture. *Missouri Med* 69: 421–426, 1972.
12. Bacorn RW, Kurtxke JF: Colles' fracture: A study of 2,000 cases from the New York State Workers' Compensation Board. *J Bone Joint Surg [Am]* 35A: 643, 1953.
13. Baltensperger A: Indikation, Technik und Ergebnisse der percutanen Spickung von distalen Radius Frakturen. *Hefte Unfallheilk* 48: 245–247, 1965.
14. Bartosh RA, Saldaña MJ: Intraarticular fractures of the distal radius. A cadaveric study to determine if ligamentotaxis restores palmar tilt. *J Hand Surg* 15A: 18–21, 1990.
15. Bate JT: Apparatus for use in reduction and fixation of fractures of the distal radius. *Clin Orthop Rel Res* 63: 190–195, 1969.
16. Baumgartl F, Kreme K, Schreiber H: Spezielle Chirurgie für die Praxis. Stuttgart: Georg Thieme Verlag, 1976.
17. Benjamin A: Injuries of the forearm. In: *Watson-Jones Fractures and Joint Injuries*, edited by Wilson JN, Edinburgh: Churchill-Livingstone, 1982, pp. 650–709.
18. Betts GW, Hodgkinson V, Densley GW, Karmat S: Original British trials on the functional bracing of Colles' fractures. *Nursing Times* 901–909, 1981.
19. Blichert-Toft M, Kælund JH: Colles' fracture treated with modified Böhler Technique. *Acta Orthop Scand* 42: 45–57, 1971.
20. Bowers WH: The distal radioulnar joint. In: *Operative Hand Surgery*, edited by Green DP, New York: Churchill-Livingstone, 1993.
21. Boyd LG, Horne JG: The outcome of fractures of the distal radius in young adults. *Injury* 19: 97–100, 1988.
22. Böhler J: Gelenknahe Frakturen des Unterarmes. *Chirurgie* 4: 198–203, 1969.
23. Böhler L: Die funktionelle Bewegungsbehandlung der "typischen radiusbrüche." *Münch Med Wochenschr* 20: 387, 1923.
24. Böhler L: *Treatment of Fractures*. New York: Grune and Stratton, 1929.
25. Bünger C, Solund K, Rasmussen P: Early results after Colles' fractures. Functional bracing in supination versus dorsal plaster immobilization. *Arch Orthop Trauma Surg* 103: 251–256, 1984.
26. Caldwell JA: Device for making traction on fingers. *JAMA* 96: 1226, 1931.
27. Callender GW: Fractures injuring joints—Fractures interfering with the movements at the wrist and with those of pronation and supination. *Saint Bartholomews Hospital Reports,*: 281–298, 1865.
28. Carothers RG, Berning DN: Colles' fracture. *Am J Surg* 80: 626–629, 1950.
29. Carothers RG, Boyd FJ: Thumb traction technic for reduction of Colles' fracture. *Arch Surg* 58: 848–852, 1949.
30. Carrozzella J, Stern PJ: Treatment of comminuted distal radius fractures with pins and plaster. *Hand Clin* 4 391–397, 1988.
31. Case RD: Haematoma block—a safe method of reducing Colles' fractures. *Injury* 16: 469–470, 1985.
32. Cassebaum WH: Colles' fractures. A study of end results. *JAMA* 143: 963–965, 1950.
33. Castaing J: Les fractures récentes de l'extrémité inférieure du radius chez l'adulte. *Rev Chir Orthop* 50: 581–696, 1964.
34. Cauchoix J, Duparc J, Potel M: Les fractures-luxations marginales antérieures du radius. *Rev Chir Orthop* 46: 233–245, 1960.

35. Chapman DR, Bennett JB, Bryan WJ, Tullos HS: Complications of distal radial fractures: Pins and plaster treatment. *J Hand Surg* 7: 509–512, 1982.

36. Charnley J: *The Closed Treatment of Common Fractures.* Baltimore: Williams & Wilkins, 1961, p. 142.

37. Clancey G: Percutaneous Kirschner wire fixation of Colles' fracture. *J Bone Joint Surg [Am]* 66A: 1008–1014, 1984.

38. Clyburn TA: Dynamic external fixation for comminuted intraarticular fractures of the distal end of the radius. *J Bone Joint Surg [Am]* 69A: 248–254, 1987.

39. Cole JM Obletz BE: Comminuted fractures of the distal end of the radius treated by skeletal transfixion in plaster cast: An end-result study of thirty-three cases. *J Bone Joint Surg [Am]* 48A: 931–45, 1966.

40. Coleman HM: Injuries of the articular disc at the wrist. *J Bone Joint Surg [Br]* 42B: 522–529, 1960.

41. Collert S, Isacson J: Management of redislocated Colles' fractures. *Clin Orthop Rel Res* 135: 183–186, 1978.

42. Colles A: On the fracture of the carpal extremity of the radius. *Edinburgh Med Surg J* 10: 182–186, 1814.

43. Conwell HE: Injuries to the wrist. *Clinical Symposia (CIBA)* 22: 2–30, 1970.

44. Cooney WP III: External fixation of distal radius fractures. *Clin Orthop Rel Res* 180: 44–49, 1983.

45. Cooney WP III, Bussey R, Dobyns JH, Linscheid RL: Difficult wrist fractures. Perilunate fracture-dislocations of the wrist. *Clin Orthop Rel Res* 214: 136–147, 1987.

46. Cooney WP III, Dobyns JH, Linscheid RL: Complications of Colles' fractures. *J Bone Joint Surg [Am]* 58A: 733, 1976.

47. Cooney WP III, Linscheid RL, Dobyns JH: External pin fixation for unstable Colles' fractures. *J Bone Joint Surg [Am]* 61A: 840–845, 1979.

48. D'Anca AF, Sternlieb SB, Byron TW, Feinstein PA: External fixation management of unstable Colles' fractures: An alternative method. *Orthopaedics* 7: 853–859, 1984.

49. de Bruijn HP: Functional treatment of Colles' fractures. *Acta Orthop Scand Suppl* 223: 1–95, 1987.

50. de Marbaux: Traitement des fractures du radius par la mobilisation immédiate sans réduction. *J Med Chir Pratique* 81: 882, 1911.

51. DePalma AF: Comminuted fractures of the distal end of the radius treated by ulnar pinning. *J Bone Joint Surg [Am]* 34A: 651–662, 1952.

52. Dias JJ, Wray CC, Jones JM: The radiological deformity of Colles' fractures. *Injury* 18: 304–308, 1987.

53. Dias JJ, Wray CC, Jones JM, Gregg PJ: The value of early mobilization in the treatment of Colles' fractures. *J Bone Joint Surg [Br]* 69B: 463–467, 1987.

54. Dinley RJ, Michelinakis E: Local anesthesia in the reduction of Colles' fractures. *Injury* 4: 345–346, 1973.

55. Docquier J, Soete P, Twahirwa J: L'embrochage intrafocal selon Kapandji dans la fracture Pouteau-Colles. *Acta Orthop Belg* 48: 794–810, 1982.

56. Dowling JJ, Sawyer B Jr: Comminuted Colles' fractures. Evaluation of a method of treatment. *J Bone Joint Surg [Am]* 43A: 657–668, 1961.

57. Dupuytren: *Injuries and Diseases of Bone.* London: 1847.

58. Edwards GS: Intraarticular fractures of the distal part of the radius. Treatment with the small AO external fixator. *J Bone Joint Surg [Am]* 73A 1241–1250, 1991.

59. Ekenstam FW, Hagert CG: The distal radioulnar joint: The influence of geometry and ligaments on simulated Colles' fracture. *Scand J Plastic Reconstr Surg* 19: 27–31, 1985.

60. Ellis J: Smith's and Barton's fractures—a method of treatment. *J Bone Joint Surg [Br]* 47B: 724–727, 1965.

61. Engkvist O, Lundborg G: Rupture of the extensor pollicis longus tendon after fracture of the lower end of the radius. A clinical and microangiographic study. *Hand* 11: 76–86, 1979.

62. Epinette JA, Lehut JM, Cavenaille M: Fracture de Pouteau-Colles: Double embrochage intrafocal en berceau selon Kapandji. *Ann Chir Main* 1: 71–83, 1982.

63. Fahey JH: Fractures and dislocations about the wrist. *Surg Clin North Am* 37: 19–40, 1957.

64. Fenyö G, Johansson O: Secondary displacement of reduced distal radius fractures. *Acta Orthop Scand* 45: 76–81, 1974.

64A. Ferre RL, Fernandez LL: Fracturas de la Muñeca. *Rev Med Ciencias Afines* 20: 27–32, 1940.

65. Fernandez DL: Smith Frakturen. *Z Unfallmed Berufskrankheiten* 3: 110–114, 1980.

66. Fernandez DL: Fractures of the distal radius. Operative treatment. *AAOS Instructional Course Lectures* 42: 73–88, 1993.

67. Fernandez DL, Jakob RP, Büchler U: External fixation of the wrist. Current indications and techniques. *Ann Chir Gyn* 72: 298–302, 1983.

68. Ferris BD, Thomas NP, Dewar ME: Brace treatment of Colles' fractures. *Acta Orthop Scand* 60: 63–65, 1989.

69. Fisk GR: The wrist: Review article. *J Bone Joint Surg [Br]* 66B: 396–407, 1984.

70. Fitzsimmons RA: Colles' fracture and Chauffeur's fracture. *Br Med J* 2: 357–360, 1938.

71. Ford LT, Key JA: Present day management of Colles' fracture. *J Iowa State Med Soc* 45:324–327, 1955.

72. Forgon M, Mammel E: The external fixator in the management of unstable Colles' fractures. *Int Orthop* 5: 9, 1981.

73. Fournier P, Bardy A, Roche G: Approche d'une définition du cal vicieux du poignet. *Int Orthop* 4: 299–305, 1981.

74. Friberg S, Lundström B: Radiographic measurements of the radio-carpal joint in normal adults. *Acta Radiol Diag* 17: 249–256, 1976.

75. Fritsche K: Konservative oder operative Therapie der typischen Radiusfraktur. *Z Chir* 103: 435–438, 1978.

76. Frykman GK: Fracture of the distal radius including sequelae—Shoulder hand finger syndrome. Disturbance in the distal radioulnar joint and impairment of nerve function. A clinical and experimental study. *Acta Orthop Scand* Suppl 108: 1–155, 1967.

77. Frykman GK, Tooma GS: Comparison of 11 external fixators for treatment of unstable wrist fractures. *J Hand Surg* 14: 247–254, 1989.

78. Fuller DJ: The Ellis plate operation for Smith's fractures. *J Bone Joint Surg [Br]* 55B: 173–178, 1973.

79. Futami T, Yamamoto M: Chinese external fixation treatment for fractures of the distal end of the radius. *J Hand Surg* 14A: 1028–1032, 1989.

80. Garner RW, Grimes DW: Percutaneous pinning of displaced fractures of the distal radius. *Orthop Rev* 6: 87–91, 1977.

81. Gartland JJ, Werley CW: Evaluation of healed Colles' fractures. *J Bone Joint Surg [Am]* 33A: 895–907, 1951.

82. Geckeler EO: Treatment of comminuted Colles' fractures. *J Int Coll Surg* 20: 596–601, 1953.

83. Gelberman RH, Szabo RM, Mortensen WW: Carpal tunnel pressures and wrist position in patients with Colles' fractures. *J Trauma* 24: 747–749, 1984.

84. Ghormley RK, Mroz RJ: Fractures of the wrist: A review of 176 cases. *Surg Gynecol Obstet* 55: 377–381, 1932.

85. Golden GN: Treatment and prognosis of Colles' fracture. *Lancet* 1: 511–514, 1963.

86. Goyrand G: Memoirs sur les fractures de l'extrémité inférieure du radius qui simulent les luxations du poignet. *Gaz Med* 3: 664–667, 1832.

87. Greatting MD, Bishop AT: Intrafocal (Kapandji) pinning of unstable fracture of the distal radius. *Orthop Clin North Am* 24: 301–307, 1993.

88. Green DP: Pins and plaster treatment of comminuted fractures of the distal end of the radius. *J Bone Joint Surg [Am]* 57A: 304–310, 1975.

89. Green DP, O'Brien ET: Open reduction of carpal dislocation. Indications and operative techniques. *J Hand Surg* 3: 250–265, 1978.

90. Gupta A: The treatment of Colles' fracture: Immobilization with the wrist dorsiflexed. *J Bone Joint Surg [Br]* 73B: 312–315, 1991.

91. Hammond G: Comminuted Colles' fractures. *Am J Surg* 78: 617–624, 1949.

92. Hawkins LD, Storey SD, Wells GG: Intravenous lidocaine anesthesia for upper extremity fractures and dislocations. *J Bone Joint Surg [Am]* 52A: 1647–1649, 1970.

93. Heath ML: Deaths after intravenous regional anaesthesia. *Br Med J* 285: 913, 1982.

94. Heffington CA, Thompson RC: The use of interscaline block anesthesia for manipulative reduction of fractures and dislocations. *J Bone Joint Surg [Am]* 55A 83–86, 1973.

95. Helal B, Chen SC, Iwegbu G: Rupture of the extensor pollicis longus tendon in undisplaced Colles' type of fracture. *Hand* 14: 41–47, 1982.

96. Heppenstall RB: *Fracture Treatment and Healing*. Philadelphia: WB Saunders, 1980.

97. Hinding E: Fractures of the distal end of the forearm. *Acta Orthop Scand* 43: 357–365, 1972.

98. Hiraswa Y, Katsumi Y, Akiyoshi T: Clinical and microangiographic studies on rupture of the extensor pollicis longus tendon after distal radius fracture. *J Hand Surg* 15B: 51–57, 1990.

99. Hollingsworth R, Morris J: The importance of the ulnar side of the wrist in fractures of the distal end of the radius. *Injury* 7: 263–266, 1976.

100. Horne JG, Devane P, Purdie G: A prospective randomized trial of external fixation

and plaster cast immobilization in the treatment of distal radius fractures. *J Orthop Trauma* 4: 30–34, 1990.

101. Howard PW, Stewart HD, Hind RE, Burke PD: Externa fixation of plaster for severely displaced comminuted Colles' fractures? A prospective study of anatomical functional results. *J Bone Joint Surg [Br]* 71B: 68–73, 1989.

102. Hudson OC, Rusnack TJ: Comminuted fractures of the lower end of the radius. *Am J Surg* 95: 74–80, 1958.

103. Jahss SA: Fractures of the metacarpals: A new method of reduction and immobilization. *J Bone Joint Surg [Am]* 20: 178, 1938.

104. Jakob RP, Fernandez DL, The treatment of wrist fractures with the small AO external fixation device. In: *Current Concepts of External Fixation of Fractures*, edited by Uhthoff HK. Berlin: Springer-Verlag, 1982, pp. 307–314.

105. Jenkins NH: The unstable Colles' fracture. *J Hand Surg* 14B: 149–154, 1989.

106. Jenkins NH Jones DG, Johnson SR, Mintowt-Czyz WT: External fixation of Colles' fractures: An anatomical study. *J Bone Joint Surg [Br]* 69B: 207–211, 1987.

107. Jenkins NH, Jones DG, Mintow CW: External fixation and recovery of function following fractures of the distal radius in young adults. *Injury* 19: 235–238, 1988.

108. Jenkins NH, Mackie IG: Late rupture of the extensor pollicis longus tendon: The case against attrition. *J Hand Surg* 13B: 448–449, 1988.

109. Jones KG: A modification of the use of extraskeletal immobilization for comminuted fractures of the distal radius. *Clin Orthop Rel Res* 123: 83–86, 1977.

110. Jones R: *Injuries of the Joints*. London: Henry Frowde and Hodder & Stoughton, 1915.

111. Jonsson U: External fixation for redislocated Colles' fractures. *Acta Orthop Scand* 54: 878–883, 1983.

112. Jupiter JB: External skeletal fixation of the upper extremity. *AAOS Instructional Course Lectures* 39: 209–218, 1990.

113. Jupiter JB: Current concepts review. Fractures of the distal end of the radius. *J Bone Joint Surg [Am]* 73A: 461–469, 1991.

114. Jupiter JB: Operative treatment of fractures of the distal radius. In: *Treatment of Wrist Disorders*, edited by Gelberman R. New York: Raven Press, 1994.

115. Kaempffe FA, Wheeler DR, Peimer CA: Severe fractures of the distal radius: Effects of amount and duration of external fixator dislocation on outcome. *J Hand Surg* 18A: 33–41, 1993.

116. Kapandji A: L'ostéosythèse par double embrochage intrafocal. Traitement fonctionnel des fractures non articulaires de l'extrémité inférieure du radius. *Ann. Chir* 30: 903–908, 1976.

117. Kapandji A: L'embrochage intrafocal des fractures de l'extrémité inférieure du radius: Dix ans après. *Ann Chir Main* 6: 57, 1987 (Abstract).

118. Kaukonen JP, Karaharju EO, Luthje P, Porras M: External fixation of Colles' fracture. *Acta Orthop Scand* 60: 54–56, 1989.

119. Kaukonen JP, Karaharju EO, Porras M: Functional recovery after fractures of the distal forearm: Analysis of radiographic and other factors affecting the outcome. *Ann Chir Gyn* 77: 27–31, 1988.

120. Knirk JL, Jupiter JB: Intraarticular fractures of the distal end of the radius in young adults. *J Bone Joint Surg [Am]* 68A: 647–659, 1986.

121. Kongsholm J, Olerud C: Plaster cast versus external fixation for unstable intraarticular Colles' fractures. *J Bone Joint Surg [Am]* 68A: 647–659, 1986.

122. Kongsholm J, Olerud C: Comminuted Colles' fractures treated with external fixation. *Arch Orthop Trauma Surg* 106: 220–225, 1987.

123. Kongsholm J, Olerud C: Plaster cast versus external fixation for unstable intra-articular Colles' fractures. *Clin Orthop Rel Res* 241: 57–65, 1989.

124. Kozin SH, Wood MB: Early soft tissue complications after distal radius fractures. *AAOS Instructional Course Lectures*, Chapter 6: 89–98, 1993.

125. Kwasny O, Fuchs M, Hertz H: Skeletal transfixation in treatment of comminuted fractures of the distal end of the radius. *J Trauma* 30: 1278–1284, 1990.

126. Kwasny O, Hertz H, Schabus R: Percutaneous drill wire fixation for treating distal radius fractures at dislocation risk [German]. *Arch Traumatol* 20: 97, 1990.

127. LaFontaine M, Hardy D, Delince PH: Stability assessment of distal radius fractures. *Injury* 20: 208–210, 1989.

128. Lambrinudi C: Injuries to the wrist. *Guy's Hosp Gaz* 52: 107, 1938.

129. Latta LL, Sarmiento A, Tarr RR: The rationale of functional bracing of fractures. *Clin Orthop Rel Res* 140: 28–36, 1980.

130. Ledingham WM, Wytch R, Göring CC: On immediate functional bracing of Colles' fracture. *Injury* 22: 197–201, 1991.

131. Ledoux A: La consolidation en position vicieuse des fractures de l'extrémité inférieure du radius. *Acta Chir Belg* 7: 477–502, 1969.

132. Ledoux A, Ravis A, van der Ghinst M: Pinning of fractures of the inferior extremity of the radius [French] *Rev Chir Orthop* 59: 427–438, 1973.

133. Lennox JD, Page BJ, Mandell RM: Use of the Clyburn external fixator in fractures of the distal radius. *J Trauma* 29: 326–331, 1989.

134. Leung KS, Shen WY, Leung PC: Ligamentotaxis and bone grafting for comminuted fractures of the distal radius. *J Bone Joint Surg [Br]* 71B: 838–842, 1989.

135. Leung KS, Shen WY, Tsang HK, Chiu KH, Leung PC, Hung LK: An effective treatment of comminuted fracture of the distal radius. *J Hand Surg* 15A: 11–17, 1990.

136. Lidström A: Fractures of the distal end of the radius. A clinical and statistical study of end results. *Acta Orthop Scand* 30 (Suppl 41): 1–118, 1959.

137. Liles R, Frierson JN, Wolf CL, Frnka T: Reduction of Colles' fracture by weight traction under local anesthesia. *Southern Med J* 62: 45–48, 1962.

138. Lippman RK: Laxity of the radioulnar joint following Colles' fracture. *Arch Surg* 35: 772–782, 1937.

139. Lucas-Championnière J: Traitement des fractures du radius et du péroné par le massage. Traitement des fractures pararticulaires simples et compliquées de plaie sans immobilisation, mobilisation et massage. *Bull Mem Soc Chir Paris* 12: 560, 1886.

140. Lynch AL, Lipscomb PR: The carpal tunnel syndrome and Colles' fractures. *JAMA* 185: 363–366, 1963.

141. MacAusland WR Jr: Colles' fractures. *Am J Surg* 36: 320, 1937.

142. Mah E, Atkinson R: Percutaneous Kirschner wire stabilization following closed reduction of Colles' fractures. *J Hand Surg* 17B: 55–61, 1992.

143. Mandell BB: Assessment of results of treatment of 100 cases of Colles' fracture. *South Afr Med J* 39: 171–174, 1965.

144. Mannerfelt L, Oetker R, Ostlund B: Rupture of the extensor pollicis longus tendon after Colles' fracture and by rheumatoid arthritis. *J Hand Surg* 153: 49–50, 1990.

145. Mason ML: Colles' Fracture: Survey of end results. *Br J Surg* 40: 340–346, 1953.

146. Mayer JH: Colles' fractures. *Br J Surg* 27: 629–642, 1940.

147. McAuliffe TB, Hilliar KM, Coates CJ, Grange WJ: Early mobilization of Colles' fractures. A prospective trial. *J Bone Joint Surg [Br]* 69B: 727–729, 1987.

148. McMurtry RY, and Jupiter JB, Fractures of the distal radius. In: *Skeletal Trauma*, edited by Browner, BD, Jupiter JB, Levine AM Trafton PG, Philadelphia: WB, Saunders, 1992, pp. 1063–1094.

149. McQueen M, Caspers J: Colles' fracture: Does the anatomic result affect the final function? *J Bone Joint Surg [Br]* 70B: 649, 1988.

150. McQueen M, MacLaren A, Chalmers J: The value of remanipulation of Colles' fractures. *J Bone Joint Surg [Br]* 68B: 232–233, 1986.

151. Melendez EM, Mehne DK, Posner PC: Treatment of unstable Colles' fractures with a new radius minifixator. *J Hand Surg* 14A: 807–811, 1989.

152. Milch H: Torsional malalignment in transverse fractures of the lower end of the radius. *Surgery* 55: 396–406, 1964.

153. Mills TJ: Smith's fracture and anterior marginal fracture of the radius. *Br Med J* 2: 603–605, 1957.

154. Mohanti RC, Kar N: Study of triangular fibrocartilage of the wrist joint in Colles' fracture. *Injury* 11: 321–324, 1980.

155. Mortier JP, Kuhlmann JN, Richet C, Baux S: Brochage horizontal cubito-radial dans les fractures de l'extremité inférieure du radius comportent un fragment postero-interne. *Rev Chir Orthop* 72: 567–571, 1986.

156. Müller ME, Nazarian S, Koch P, Schatzker J: *The Comperhensive Classification of Fractures of Long Bones.*. Berlin, Springer-Verlag, 1990.

157. Nakata RY, Chand Y, Matiko JD, Frykman GKm, Wood VE: External fixators for wrist fractures: A biomechanical and clinical study. *J Hand Surg* 10A: 845–851, 1985.

158. Nonnemacher J, Neumeier K: Intrafokale Verdrantung bei Handgelenkfrakturen. *Hand Chir* 19: 67, 1987.

159. Older TM, Stabler EV, Cassebaum WH: Colles' fracture: Evaluation of selection of therapy. *J Trauma* 5: 469–476, 1965.

160. Palmer AK, Werner FW: The triangular fibrocartilage complex of the wrist: Anatomy and function. *J Hand Surg* 6: 153–162, 1981.

161. Patterson SD, Richards RS: Distal radius fractures. *Curr Opin Orthop* 4: 20–28, 1993.

162. Petersen F: Zur Behandlung des Typischen Radiusbrüchen. *Arch Klin Chir* 84: 708–715, 1894.

163. Pool C: Colles' fracture. A prospective study of treatment. *J Bone Joint Surg [Br]* 55B: 540, 1973.

164. Porter M, Stockley I: Fractures of the distal radius. Intermediate and end results in relation to radiograph parameters. *Clin Orthop Rel Res* 220: 241–251, 1987.

165. Pring DJ, Barber L, Williams DJ: Bipolar fixation of fractures of the distal end of the radius. A comparative study. *Injury* 19: 145–148, 1988.

166. Pyrgos NM, Argyropoulos EI, Pyrgos VN: The use of intravenous regional anesthesia for the reduction of Colles' fractures. *Resuscitation* 5: 59–63, 1976.

167. Quinton DN: Local anesthetic toxicity of haematoma blocks in manipulation of Colles' fracture. *Injury* 19: 239–240, 1988.

168. Raskin KB, Melone CP, Jr: Unstable articular fractures of the distal radius: Comparative techniques of ligamentotaxis. *Orthop Clin North Am* 24: 275–286, 1993.

169. Ravis A, Ledoux A, Thiebant A, van der Ghinst M: Bipolar fixation of fractures of the distal end of the radius. *Int Orthop* 3: 89–93, 1979.

170. Rayhack J: The history and evolution of percutaneous pinning of displaced distal radius fractures. *Orthop Clin North Am* 24: 287–300, 1993.

171. Richter D: Behandlungsergebnisse bei typischen radiusfrakturen nach Einführung von "Gruppenturnen." *Deutsche Gesundsheitswesen* 21: 1983–1986, 1966.

172. Riis J, Fruensgård S: Treatment of unstable Colles' fractures by external fixation. *J Hand Surg* 14B: 145–148, 1989.

173. Rogers SC: An analysis of Colles' fracture. *Br Med J* 1: 807–809, 1944.

174. Rosen E: Fractura extremitatis distalis radii. *Ugesk Laeger* 109: 603, 1947.

175. Rosetsky A: Colles' fractures treated by plaster and polyurethane braces: A controlled clinical study. *J Trauma* 22: 910–913, 1982.

176. Roumen RM, Hesp WL, Bruggink E: Unstable Colles' fractures in elderly patients: A randomized trial of external fixation for redisplacement. *J. Bone Joint Surg [Br]* 73B: 307–311, 1991.

177. Roysam GS: The distal radioulnar joint in Colles' fractures. *J Bone Joint Surg [Br]* 75B: 58–60, 1993.

178. Ruiz GR: Percutaneous pinning of comminuted Colles' fractures. *Clin Orthop Rel Res* 108: 174–180, 1975.

179. Sanders RA, Keppel FL, Waldrop JI: External fixation of distal radius fractures. Results and complications. *J Hand Surg* 11A: 385–390, 1991.

180. Sarmiento A: The brachioradialis as a deforming force in Colles' fractures. *Clin Orthop Rel Res* 38: 86–92, 1965.

181. Sarmiento A, Latta LL: *Closed Functional Treatment of Fractures*. Berlin, Heidelberg, New York: Springer-Verlag, 1981.

182. Sarmiento A, Pratt GW, Berry NC, Sinclair WF: Colles' fracture: Functional bracing in supination. *J Bone Joint Surg [Am]* 57A: 311–317, 1975.

183. Sarmiento A, Zagorski JB, Sinclair WF: Functional bracing of Colles' fracture: A prospective study of immobilization in supination vs. pronation. *Clin Orthop Rel Res* 146: 175–183, 1980.

184. Scheck M: Long-term follow-up of treatment of comminuted fractures of the distal end of the radius by transfixation with Kirschner wires and cast. *J Bone Joint Surg [Am]* 44A: 337–351, 1962.

185. Schmalholz A: Closed reduction of axial compression in Colles' fracture is hardly possible. *Acta Orthop Scand* 60: 57–59, 1989.

186. Schmalholz A: External skeletal fixation versus cement fixation in the treatment of redislocated Colles' fracture. *Clin Orthop Rel Res* 254: 236–241, 1990.

187. Schuind F, Donkerwolcke M, Rusguin C, Burny F: External fixation of fractures of the distal radius: A study of 225 cases. *J Hand Surg* 14A: 404–407, 1989.

188. Scudder CL, *Treatment of Fractures*. Philadelphia: WB Saunders, 1939, pp. 716–748.

189. Seitz WH Jr, Froimson AI, Brooks DB: Biomechanical analysis of pin placement and pin size for external fixation of distal radius fractures. *Clin Orthop Rel Res* 251: 207–212, 1990.

190. Seitz WH Jr, Froimson AI, Leb R, Shapiro JD: Augmented external fixation of unstable distal radius fracture. *J Hand Surg* 16A: 1010–1016, 1991.

191. Seitz WH Jr, Putnam MD, Dick HM: Limited open surgical approach for external fixation of distal radius fractures. *J Hand Surg* 15A: 288–293, 1990.

192. Shang TY, Gu YW, Dieng FH: Treatment of forearm bone fractures by an integrated method of Chinese and Western medicine. *Clin Orthop Rel Res* 215: 56–64, 1987.

193. Sirbu AB, Colloff B: Colles' fracture. A study of end results with conservative management. *World J Surg* 59: 635–643, 1951.

194. Smaill GB: Long-term followup of Colles' fracture. *J Bone Joint Surg [Br]* 47B: 80–85, 1965.

195. Smith FM: Late rupture of extensor pollicis longus tendon following Colles' fracture. *J Bone Joint Surg [Am]* 28A: 49–59, 1946.

196. Smith RJ, Floyd WE III: Smith's and Barton's Fractures. In: *Fractures of the Hand and Wrist*, edited by Barton NJ London: Churchill Livingstone, 1988, pp. 252–266.

197. Smith RW: *A Treatise on Fracture in the Vicinity of Joints and on Certain Forms of*

Accidental and Congenital Dislocations. Dublin: Hodges and Smith, 1847.

198. Solgård S: Classification of distal radius fractures. *Acta Orthop Scand* 56: 249–252, 1984.

199. Solgård S: Early displacement of distal radius fractures. *Acta Orthop Scand* 57: 229–231, 1986.

200. Solgård S: Function after distal radius fractures. *Acta Orthop Scand* 59: 39–42, 1988.

201. Solgård S: External fixation or a cast for Colles' fracture. *Acta Orthop Scand* 60: 387–391, 1989.

202. Solgård S, Bünger C, Solund K: Displaced distal radius fractures. A comparative study of early results following external fixation, functional bracing in supination, or dorsal plaster immobilization. *Arch Orthop Trauma Surg* 109: 34–38, 1989.

203. Solgård S, Petersen VS: Epidemiology of distal radius fractures. *Acta Orthop Scand* 56: 391–393, 1985.

204. Spira E, Weigl K: The comminuted fracture of the distal end of the radius. *Recon Surg Traumat* 11: 128–138, 1969.

205. Stein A, Katz S: Stabilization of comminuted fractures of the distal inch of the radius: Percutaneous pinning. *Clin Orthop Rel Res* 108: 174–181, 1975.

206. Stewart HD, Innes AR, Burke PD: Functional cast bracing for Colles' fractures. *J Bone Joint Surg* [Br], 66B: 749–753, 1984.

207. Stewart HD, Innes AR, Burke PD: The hand complications of Colles' fractures. *J Hand Surg* 10B: 103–106, 1985.

208. Stewart HD, Innes AR, Burke PD: Factors influencing the outcome of Colles' fracture: An anatomical and functional study. *Injury* 16: 289–295, 1985.

209. Strong JM: Treatment of Colles' fracture. *Surg Gynecol Obstet* 121: 107–112, 1955.

210. Szabo RM: Comminuted distal radius fractures. *Orthop Clin of North Am* 23: 1–6, 1992.

211. Taylor GW, Parsons CL: The role of the discus articularis in Colles' fracture. *J Bone Joint Surg [Am]* 20: 149–152, 1938.

212. Thomas FB: Reduction of Smith's fracture. *J Bone Joint Surg [Br]* 39B: 463–470, 1957.

213. Thorn BJ: Colles' fracture in the over 60 age group. *J Bone Joint Surg [Br]* 66B: 613, 1984.

214. Trevor D: Rupture of the extensor pollicis longus tendon after Colles' fracture. *J Bone Joint Surg [Br]* 32B: 370–375, 1950.

215. Van der Linden W, Ericson R: Colles' fracture. How should its displacement be measured and how should it be immobilized? *J Bone Joint Surg [Am]* 63A: 1285–1288, 1981.

216. Vaughn PA, Lui SM, Harrington IJ, Maistrelli GL: Treatment of unstable fractures of the distal radius by external fixation. *J Bone Joint Surg [Br]* 67B: 385–389, 1985.

217. Villar RN, March D: Three years after Colles' fracture. A prospective review. *J Bone Joint Surg [Am]* 69B: 635–638, 1987.

218. Wadsworth TG: Colles' fracture. *Br Med J* 301: 192–194, 1990.

219. Wagner HE, Jakob RP: Operative Behandlung der distalen Radiusfrakturen mit Fixateur externe. *Unfallchirurgie* 88: 473–480, 1985.

220. Wahlström O: Treatment of Colles' fracture. *Acta Orthop Scand.*, 53: 225–228, 1982.

221. Wardrope J, Flowers M, Wilson DH: Comparison of anesthetic techniques in the reduction of Colles' fractures. *Arch Emerg Med* 2: 67–72, 1985.

222. Warwick D, Prothew D, Field J, Bannister GC: Radiological measurement of radial shortening in Colles' fracture. *J Hand Surg* 18B: 50–52, 1993.

223. Watson-Jones R: *Fractures and Joint Injuries* 6th ed. Edinburgh: Churchill-Livingstone, 1982.

224. Weber ER: A rational approach for the recognition and treatment of Colles' fracture. *Hand Clin* 3: 13–21, 1987.

225. Weber SC, Szabo RM: Severely comminuted distal radius fractures as an unsolved problem: Complications associated with external fixation and pins and plaster techniques. *J Hand Surg* 11A: 157–165, 1986.

226. Wiklund T, Müllern-Aspegren J: "Typisk Radiusfraktur." *Nord Med* 56: 1411, 1956.

227. Willenegger H, Guggenbuhl A: Zur operativen Behandlung bestimmter Fálle von distalen Radius Frakturen. *Helv Chir Acta* 26: 81–89, 1959.

228. Wilson PD: *Management of Fractures and Dislocations.* Philadelphia: WB Saunders, 1929.

229. Woolson ST, Dev P, Fellingham LL, Vassiliadis A: Three dimensional imaging of the ankle joint from computerized tomography. *Foot Ankle* 6: 2–6, 1985.

Chapter Six

Articular Marginal Shearing Fractures

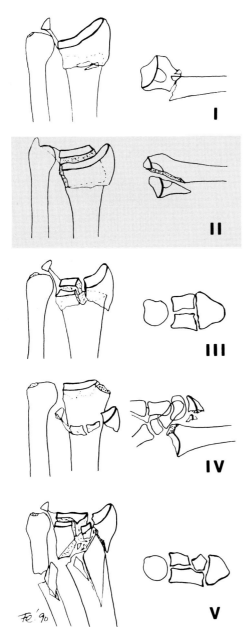

The accidents which are to be the principal subject of my remarks, usually pass either for sprains or dislocations of the wrist...This accident must not be confounded with those which are also of frequent occurrence, namely fractures of the radius and ulna, just above, and not involving the joint. The fragment may be, and usually is, quite small and is broken from the end of the radius on the dorsal side and through the cartilagenous face of it, and necessarily into the joint.

John Rhea Barton, 1838

A Practical, Treatment Oriented Classification of Fractures of the Distal Radius and Associated Distal Radioulnar Joint Lesions.
Diego L. Fernandez, M.D. PD

FRACTURE TYPES (ADULTS) BASED ON THE MECHANISM OF INJURY		CHILDREN FRACTURE EQUIVALENT	STABILITY/INSTABILITY: high risk of secondary displacement after initial adequate reduction	DISPLACEMENT PATTERN	NUMBER OF FRAGMENTS	ASSOCIATED LESIONS carpal ligament, fractures, median, ulnar nerve, tendons, ipsilat., fx upper extremity, compartment syndrome	RECOMMENDED TREATMENT
TYPE I BENDING FRACTURE OF THE METAPHYSIS		DISTAL FOREARM FRACTURE SALTER II	STABLE UNSTABLE	NON-DISPLACED DORSALLY (Colles-Pouteau) VOLARLY (Smith) PROXIMAL COMBINED	ALWAYS 2 MAIN FRAGMENTS + VARYING DEGREE OF METAPHYSEAL COMMINUTION (instability)	UNCOMMON	CONSERVATIVE (stable fxs) PERCUTANEOUS PINNING (extra- or intrafocal) EXTERNAL FIXATION (exceptionally BONE GRAFT)
TYPE II SHEARING FRACTURE OF THE JOINT SURFACE		SALTER IV	UNSTABLE	DORSAL RADIAL VOLAR PROXIMAL COMBINED	TWO-PART THREE-PART COMMINUTED	LESS UNCOMMON	OPEN REDUCTION SCREW/PLATE FIXATION
TYPE III COMPRESSION FRACTURE OF THE JOINT SURFACE		SALTER III, IV, V	STABLE UNSTABLE	NON-DISPLACED DORSAL RADIAL VOLAR PROXIMAL COMBINED	TWO-PART THREE-PART FOUR-PART COMMINUTED	COMMON	CONSERVATIVE CLOSED, LIMITED, ARTHROSCOPIC ASSISTED, OR EXTENSILE OPEN REDUCTION PERCUTANEOUS PINS COMBINED EXTERNAL AND INTERNAL FIXATION BONE GRAFT
TYPE IV AVULSION FRACTURES, RADIO CARPAL FRACTURE DISLOCATION		VERY RARE	UNSTABLE	DORSAL RADIAL VOLAR PROXIMAL COMBINED	TWO-PART (radial styloid ulnar styloid) THREE-PART (volar, dorsal margin) COMMINUTED	FREQUENT	CLOSED OR OPEN REDUCTION PIN OR SCREW FIXATION TENSION WIRING
TYPE V COMBINED FRACTURES (I - II - III - IV) HIGH-VELOCITY INJURY		VERY RARE	UNSTABLE	DORSAL RADIAL VOLAR PROXIMAL COMBINED	COMMINUTED and/or BONE LOSS (frequently intraarticular, open, seldom extraarticular)	ALWAYS PRESENT	COMBINED METHOD

Fracture of the distal radius: associated distal radioulnar joint (DRUJ) lesions.

	Patho-anatomy of the lesion	Degree of joint surface involvement	Prognosis	Recommended treatment
Type 1 **Stable** (following reduction of the radius the DRUJ is congruous and stable)	A Avulsion fracture tip ulnar styloid B Stable fracture ulnar neck	None	Good	A+B Functional aftertreatment Encourage early pronation-supination exercises Note: Extraarticular <u>unstable</u> fractures of the ulna at the metaphyseal level or distal shaft require stable plate fixation
Type II **Unstable** (subluxation or dislocation of the ulnar head present)	A Substance tear of TFCC and/or palmar and dorsal capsular ligaments B Avulsion fracture base of the ulnar styloid	None	• Chronic instability • Painful limitation of supination if left unreduced • Possible late arthritic changes	A <u>Closed treatment</u> Reduce subluxation, sugar tong splint in 45° of supination four to six weeks A+B <u>Operative treatment</u> Repair TFCC or fix ulnar styloid with tension band wiring Immobilize wrist and elbow in supination (cast) or transfix ulna/radius with k-wire and forearm cast
Type III **Potentially unstable** (subluxation possible)	A Intraarticular fracture of the sigmoid notch B Intraarticular fracture of the ulnar head	Present	• Dorsal subluxation possible together with dorsally displaced die punch or dorso-ulnar fragment • Risk of early degenerative changes and severe limitation of forearm rotation if left unreduced	A Anatomic reduction of palmar and dorsal sigmoid notch fragments. If residual subluxation tendency present immobilize as in type II injury B Functional aftertreatment to enhance remodelling of ulnar head If DRUJ remains painful: partial ulnar resection, darrach or sauvé-kapandji procedure at a later date

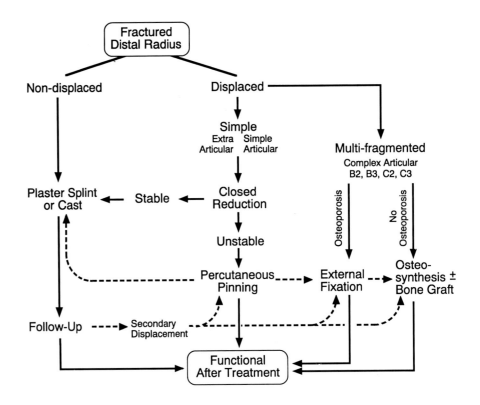

Articular Marginal Shearing Fracture

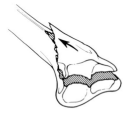

The basic feature common to all the "shearing" fractures is that a portion of the metaphyseal and epiphyseal area of the distal radius remains intact and in continuity with the unaffected area of the articular surface. This feature offers a more favorable prognosis in the management of these injuries, given the fact that in most instances the displaced articular fragment(s) can be anatomically reduced back onto the intact remaining articular surface. Although the obliquity of the fracture line makes these fractures inherently unstable, the reduction of the fracture can usually be solidly fixed to the intact column of the distal radius. As these fractures may be found in younger adults with more substantial cancellous bone, the holding power of the internal fixation is more likely to be sound (Fig. 6).

Incidence

Barton considered the injury that still bears his name to be commonplace, but this is, in fact, not the case. Although the literature has more than amply described the marginal shearing fracture,[1–20,22–26,29–35] only a few reports have specifically addressed the relative frequency of these injuries as they are compared to all types of distal radius fractures.

From those few reports that have reviewed relative incidence, it is quite evident that the marginal shearing fractures are exceptionally uncommon, representing less than 5 percent of all distal radius fractures in these studies (Table 6.1). By the same token, with expanding knowledge of the specific

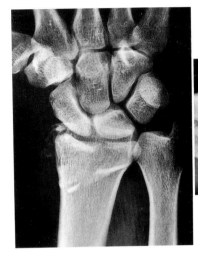 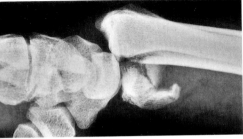

Figure 6.1. An oblique shearing fracture of the distal radius will more likely be found in younger adults with more substantial cancellous bone facilitating stable internal fixation.

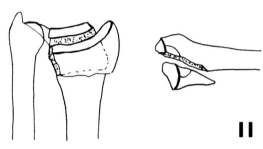

II

Table 6.1. Relative frequency of shearing fractures.

Author(s)	No. distal radius fractures	No. shearing fractures	%	Dorsal	Volar	Styloid
Böhler (1943)	448	7	1.5	7	10	
King (1975)	1252	17	1.3	7	10	
Thompson and Grant (1977)*	662	15	2.3	5	10	
Bengner and Johnell (1985)	1914	35	1.8			35
Pattee and Thompson (1988)†	1788	21	1.2	8	12	

* Radial styloid fracture in 13 cases (4 separate fragments).
† One patient lost to follow-up.

fracture patterns as well as computer-generated fracture documentation, it is possible that these data may change.[12]

Mechanism

As with the vast majority of distal radius fractures, the mechanism of the shearing marginal fracture has been attributed to an axial load onto the end of the radius.[1,6,10,15,16,19,23,26,29,31,35] King postulated that in certain positions, upon impact, a portion of the intrinsic ligamentous support of the lunate is injured sufficiently to permit it to migrate along with the sheared articular fragment of the end of the radius.[19] In contrast to a true radiocarpal dislocation (Type IV), he postulated that the extrinsic radiocarpal ligaments arising from the radius and inserting onto the capitate remain intact.

In the contemporary, high-speed, mechanized world, the volar and dorsal marginal fractures are becoming more often seen in association with a high-velocity impact. Thompson and Grant suggested that compressive forces occurring with the wrist locked in palmar flexion, such as when holding the handlebars of a motorcycle, or with the wrist fixed in extension at impact, as when holding an automobile steering wheel, will lead to anterior and dorsal shearing fractures, respectively.[32] This association with higher-impact injury has also been observed by de Oliveira[8] as well as Fellmann.[12] It is not surprising that in association with high-velocity trauma, a younger age population is involved, often with associated ipsilateral trauma or even polytrauma. Pattee and Thompson noted a 15 percent incidence of associated carpal injuries.[24]

Fractures of the radial styloid, known as "chauffeur" or "backfire" fractures due to early observations of their association with cranking automobile engines,[9] are now recognized as potentially complex radiocarpal injuries.[21] In a study of 14 such cases, Helm and Tonkin observed seven to be due to a motorcycle accident and six to a fall from a height.[18] Nine patients had associated skeletal injuries, including four ipsilateral scaphoid fractures.

Nonoperative Treatment: Technique

Anterior and Dorsal Shearing

Closed manipulative reduction of the marginal shearing fracture was described by Barton, who also recognized their inherent instability.[2] He noted that the displacement was easily reduced using longitudinal traction. However, once released, redisplacement would inevitably occur. For this reason he recommended that splints be applied while traction was maintained. By the same token, Barton appeared cognizant of the potential difficulty with residual wrist stiffness if the splints were continued for a prolonged period of time. He recommended the use of a dorsal and palmar splint to be changed every 4 to 5 days to encourage wrist mobilization. This approach, parenthetically, is still in use by traditional physicians in China and elsewhere in the world.

In the century that followed Barton's early descriptions, the approach to the marginal fractures paralleled that of all distal radius fractures, i.e., fixed periods of immobilization in splints or plaster casts. Wrist extension was recommended for anterior marginal fractures, although the possibility of redisplacement was well recognized.[1] To offset this problem, Böhler suggested adding adhesive plaster traction with a metacarpal wire incorporated into a cast.[5]

Thomas in 1957 recommended that anteriorly displaced distal radius fractures (both extra- and intraarticular) be treated by a closed reduction using longitudinal traction, followed by the application of an above-elbow plaster cast with the forearm in supination and wrist in slight palmar flexion. This approach was followed by subsequent authors, all emphasizing the importance of forearm supination.[1,7,10,15,23]

King developed a rationale for the position of immobilization based upon his impression of the mechanism of these fractures.[19,20] He suggested the anterior marginal fracture be immobilized with the wrist in volar flexion, which would place the dorsal radiocarpal ligaments in tension and help hold the lunate in position. The opposite would be the case with a posterior marginal shear fracture. He recommended casting for 6 weeks, with frequent control radiographs, given the tendency of this type of fracture to redisplace.

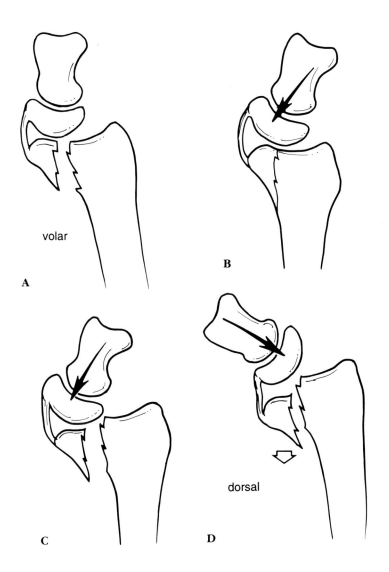

volar

A

B

C

dorsal

D

Figure 6.2. As suggested by Smith and Floyd, the closed reduction and immobilization of anterior marginal shear fractures is a paradox, as the position in which the fracture is reduced is that which tends to displace the articular reduction. A. The anterior marginal fracture with attached radiocarpal ligament to the lunate. B. Traction and wrist extension pulls the marginal articular fracture into position. C. Compression forces through the carpus will tend to redisplace the fracture. D. Placing the wrist in palmar flexion will prove unsuccessful as the tension on the volar radiocarpal ligaments is released.

Smith and Floyd, by contrast, found this approach paradoxical, as the wrist position that would effectively reduce this fracture would also be the position that would lead to fragment displacement (Fig. 6.2). They felt that these fractures were inherently unstable and recommended operative intervention.

Radial Styloid

Closed treatment of isolated radial styloid fractures has traditionally involved a reduction by traction and ulnar deviation of the hand and wrist, followed by immobilization of the limb in an above-elbow support with the forearm in supination.

Nonoperative Treatment: Results

Little is known regarding the outcome of Barton's cases. The facts that he never confirmed his clinical impression of the injury pattern with an autopsy specimen and that he suggested these to be primarily dorsal injuries would also raise some questions as to any observations on outcome.

What can be gleaned from later studies of closed treatment is that redisplacement is commonplace. Coincident with that is a direct correlation with functional disability, such as pain or loss of motion and loss of the articular realignment.[15,19,24,29,32,35] Woodyard, using Thomas's classification and techniques of immobilization, treated 13 marginal shearing fractures.[35] The results in this group were not as satisfactory as those with the extraarticular bending fractures. The results of the 13 patients were eight good, one fair, and one poor, with four cases of radiocarpal arthritis. He noted that loss of motion and pain were both related to residual loss of articular reduction.

Pattee and Thomson treated 18 of their 20 cases with a closed reduction and cast, using the approach recommended by King.[19,24] Reduction was maintained in only eight fractures, while 10 required alternative methods, including external fixation in three and open reduction and internal fixation in seven. The outcome of the patients who did not have operative reduction (eight with cast and three with external fixation) revealed six excellent and five good, with a relatively short follow-up. Of note, however, is that fact that 65 percent of the cases in their series had evidence of radiographic arthritis at the radiocarpal joint.

Thomson and Grant also observed less favorable results in those marginal shear fractures treated nonoperatively.[32]

Shearing Fractures: Cuneiform (Group B1)

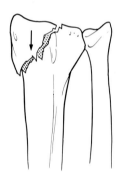

Fractures of the radial styloid are usually associated with a fall on the outstretched hand, with the wrist forced into extension and slight radial deviation. In this position, the scaphoid directly transmits the force of impact onto the radial styloid, which can fracture in an oblique pattern. At the beginning of this century, the fracture was noted in association with the backfire of the starting handles of cars, resulting in the name "chauffeur's fracture."[16] Avulsion fractures of the styloid can also be seen in association with combinations of perilunar dislocations of the carpus. The so-called greater arc injuries include radial styloid fractures associated with various combinations of trans-scaphoid, trans-capitate, or trans-triquetral injuries (Fig. 6.3). Mayfield and co-workers described the effects of forced hyperextension, ulnar deviation, and intercarpal

Figure 6.3. Schematic illustration of the possible volar intracapsular ligament injuries associated with a large styloid fracture. RC = radial collateral ligament. RSC = radioscaphocapitate ligament. RLT = radiolunatocapitate ligament. RSL = radioscapholunate ligament. (Reprinted with permission from Siegel D, Gelberman R. Radial styloidectomy: An anatomical study. *J Hand Surg* 16A: 43, 1991.)

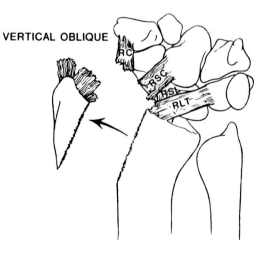

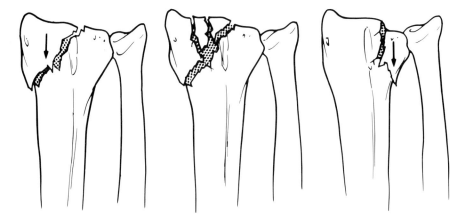

Figure 6.4. (left) A vertical shearing radial styloid fracture (subgroup B1.1).

Figure 6.5. (middle) A multifragmented shearing radial styloid fracture (subgroup B1.2).

Figure 6.6. (right) A unique vertical shearing fracture involving the lunate facet of the distal radius (subgroup B1.3). This unusual pattern differs from the impact-type "die-punch" fracture.

supination of the wrist and demonstrated that avulsion fractures of the body of the radial styloid are the result of a tensile load on the radiocapitate ligament.[17] Anatomic studies have also confirmed the fact that the smaller avulsion styloid fractures will be found attached to the radial collateral ligaments, whereas the larger styloid fractures are likely to have both radial collateral and radiocapitate ligaments attached.[18,19] Thus, in addition to restoring the articular congruity and radial buttress, the anatomic restoration of displaced styloid fractures helps to restore the length, alignment, and integrity of the supporting volar capsular ligaments of the wrist. Shearing fractures involving the radial styloid may be a single-fragment subgroup B1.1 (Fig. 6.4) or subgroup B1.2 (Fig. 6.5). A third cuneiform-type shearing fracture has been determined to involve a vertical shear fracture of the lunate facet subgroup B1.3 of the distal radius (Fig. 6.6).[27]

Preoperative Planning

The possible association of an intracapsular or interosseous ligament injury must be kept in mind and the patient so informed. Accurate x-rays both preoperatively and following reduction of the fracture are essential to carefully evaluate the radiographic relationships of the carpal bones to each other and to the radius. Should questions arise regarding the possibility of associated ligament injury, the adjuvant use of an arthroscope may be most helpful, particularly in defining the condition of the scapholunate interosseous ligament (Fig. 6.7).

Management

Nondisplaced radial styloid fractures can be treated by immobilization in an above-elbow cast with the forearm in supination and the wrist in slight ulnar deviation. For displaced fractures, closed reduction should be attempted with longitudinal traction and ulnar deviation of the hand and wrist. Given the inherent instability of these fractures, however, our preference is to place two oblique Kirschner wires or cannulated screws percutaneously, even when an anatomic reduction can be achieved.

Figure 6.7. A fracture of the radial styloid may be part of a greater arc intercarpal ligament injury. The increased space between the scaphoid and lunate was recognized only after the styloid fracture had united.

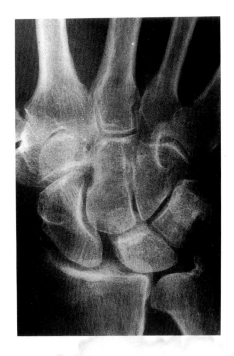

Surgical Tactic

Preferably under image intensification, the reduction of the styloid is controlled in several projections. Additionally, careful evaluation must be extended towards the radiographic alignment of the carpal bones. The radial styloid lies anterior to the mid-axis of the distal radius. Therefore, percutaneous Kirschner wires or the guide wires to cannulated screws should be placed into the

Figure 6.8. (left) The placement of any implant for styloid fractures should be in a proximal dorsoulnar direction. The surgeon should be cognizant of the fact that the radial styloid lies anterior to the mid-axis of the distal radius.

Figure 6.9. (right) The surgical tactics of a percutaneous cannulated screw into the radial styloid.

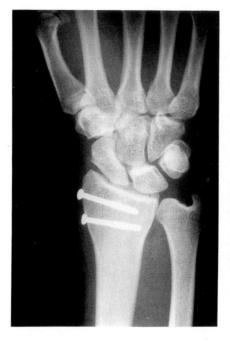
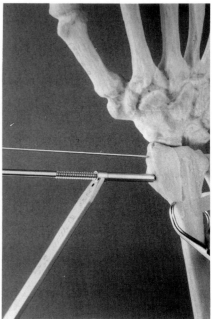

Figure 6.10. The dorsal approach to the radial styloid fracture. Particular care should be taken to avoid injury to the radial artery and the superficial radial nerve. The radius is approached through the first and second extensor compartment.

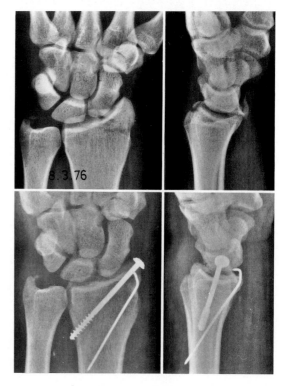

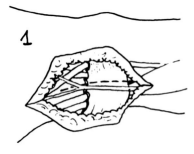

Figure 6.11. A displaced radial styloid was approached dorsally and reduced anatomically. Stable fixation was achieved with a screw and Kirschner wire. Note on the lateral radiograph both implants extend from a radial palmar to a dorsal ulnar direction.

styloid aiming proximally, ulnarward, and somewhat dorsally to gain purchase into the proximal dorsoulnar cortex (Fig. 6.8). Given the proximity of the branches of the radial sensory nerve, drill guides are mandatory when placing screws percutaneously into the radial styloid (Fig. 6.9).

The reduction and internal fixation are protected with a long arm cast for 6 weeks.

If a closed reduction cannot be obtained or if there is evidence of either associated trans-styloid greater arc injuries or a comminuted styloid fracture (subgroup B1.2), open reduction and internal fixation are advised. A dorsoradial, longitudinal incision is created, with particular care to identify and protect the superficial radial nerve, the radial artery, and the extensor pollicis longus tendon in the anatomic snuff box (Figs. 6.10 and 6.11). Comminuted fractures will require a dorsal capsulotomy of the wrist to assure the accuracy of the anatomic reduction (Fig. 6.12).

The ulnar wedge subgroup B1.3 fracture is most unusual, but it can be treacherous due to the instability of these fractures by virtue of an almost vertical fracture plane (Fig. 6.13). These fractures are difficult to reduce by closed methods, as they tend to be impacted in their displaced position. With longitudinal traction, the fracture may be successfully elevated, using a pointed awl, through a small incision under image intensification (Fig. 6.14A–E). A limited open reduction may be necessary through a dorsal incision just ulna to

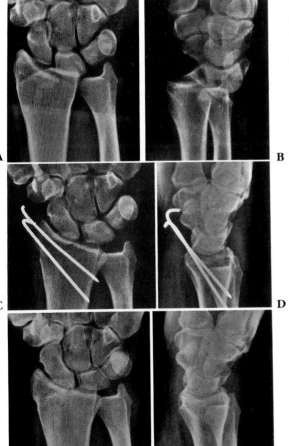

Figure 6.12. A complex comminuted radial styloid fracture with dorsal displacement of the carpus. A,B. Anterior and posterior x-rays of the fracture in a 28-year-old laborer. C,D. Anatomic reduction and stable internal fixation were accomplished through a dorsal surgical approach. A dorsal capsulotomy was made both to assure anatomic restoration and to evaluate the scapholunate interosseous ligament. E,F. Follow-up at 1 year reveals an anatomic restoration without evidence of intercarpal instability.

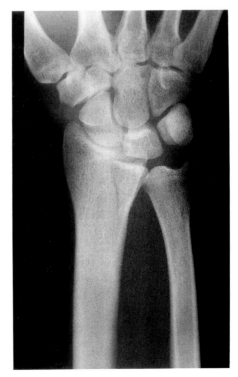

Figure 6.13. A vertical shear medial cuneiform fracture of the lunate facet. This fracture is extremely unstable when elevated.

170   6. Articular Marginal Shearing Fractures

Figure 6.14. Under image intensification, the shearing lunate facet fracture can at times be elevated using a pointed awl applied through a small dorsal incision. A,B. AP and lateral radiograph of a complex shearing fracture. C. The Iunate facet is elevated with a pointed awl. D,E. Both shearing fractures are stabilized.

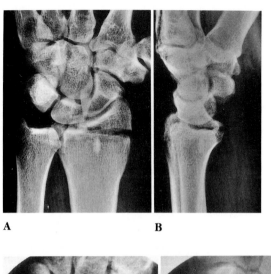

A   B

C   D   E

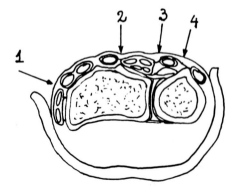

Figure 6.15. The dorsal surgical approach to the impacted, displaced medial cuneiform shear fracture.

the extensor digitorum communis tendons (Fig. 6.15). The fragment can be elevated under direct vision and held with percutaneously placed Kirschner wires passed in an ulnar direction across the distal radius (Fig. 6.16). Care must be taken to avoid transfixing the distal radioulnar joint. In these instances, external skeletal fixation is advisable to maintain axial length and protect the percutaneous Kirschner wires.

Styloid shearing fractures

Pitfalls	Pearls
Failure to appreciate ligamentous injury	Consider dorsal arthrotomy or intraoperative arthroscopy
Failure to recognize articular comminution	Lateral and anterior tomography may be of help
Inadequate internal fixation	Appreciate the anterior position of the styloid. Aim the screws of Kirschner wires in a dorsal, proximal, and ulna direction
Failure to appreciate associated carpal injuries	Traction views may reveal either carpal fractures or ligamentous injury

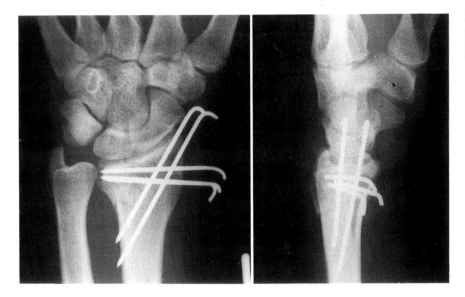

Figure 6.16. The fragment can be held by percutaneously placed Kirschner wires passed in an ulnar direction with care taken to avoid entering the sigmoid notch.

Shearing Fracture: Dorsal (Group B2)

Despite the fact that the fracture likely described by Barton involved the dorsal aspect of the radiocarpal joint, an isolated dorsal marginal fracture (subgroup B2.1) is extremely uncommon (Fig. 6.17). In contrast, the combined lesion of a radial styloid and dorsal marginal fracture (subgroup B2.2) is considerably more common (Fig. 6.18). Yet because of similar appearance on the lateral x-ray, this fracture can well be misdiagnosed as a Colles' fracture. Careful assessment of the x-ray will reveal an intact volar and ulna aspect of the articular surface.

Dorsal marginal fractures may also be found in association with massively displaced dorsal radiocarpal dislocations (subgroup B2.3), which are discussed in more detail in Chapter 8 (Fig. 6.19).

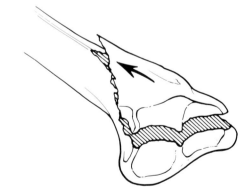

Figure 6.17. A dorsal marginal shearing fracture (subgroup B2.1) is uncommon.

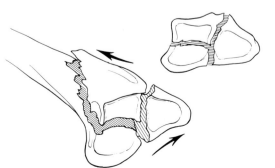

Figure 6.18. A combination of a dorsal marginal fracture with a radial styloid fracture (subgroup B2.2) is the more common dorsal shearing fracture pattern.

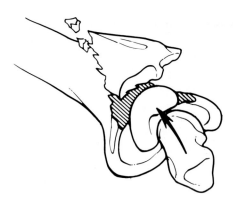

Preoperative Planning

As the dorsal marginal shearing fractures are less common than anterior marginal fractures, preoperative planning is enhanced by the lateral and anteroposterior tomogram. These may particularly help define the radial styloid involvement more clearly.

Nonoperative

By virtue of the relatively subcutaneous nature of the dorsal cortex of the distal radius, there is a definite place for an attempt at closed manipulative reduction of dorsal marginal subgroup B2.1 and subgroup B2.2 fractures. By the same token, the shearing mechanism and obliquity of the fracture line would suggest that the results with cast immobilization will be unpredictable. For this reason, percutaneous pins and external skeletal fixation are needed to maintain the reduction. The fixateur is left in place for a minimum of 6 weeks, while the percutaneous pins should remain at least 2 weeks after removal of the external fixateur (Fig. 6.20).

Operative

The goal in the management of these fractures is to restore both the normal radiocarpal relationships and the articular surface to within 1 to 2 mm of congruency. In many instances, this will require open reduction and internal fixation.

Surgical Tactic

These fractures are approached through a dorsal longitudinal incision. The extensor retinaculum is opened between the second and fourth extensor compartments, taking care to elevate and mobilize the extensor pollicis longus tendon (Fig. 6.21). The initial procedure, particularly with an subgroup B2.2 fracture involving both the radial styloid fragment and a shearing marginal fracture, is to restore the radial styloid fragment and provisionally fix the styloid with a smooth Kirschner wire. The dorsal lip fracture is next reduced

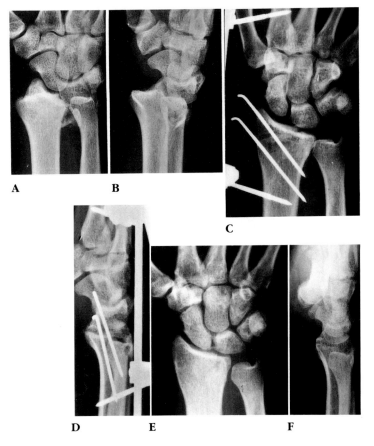

A   B

C

D   E   F

Figure 6.20. A 27-year-old laborer fell off a scaffold, sustaining a dorsal shearing fracture involving the radial styloid as well as the dorsal articular rim of the distal radius. A,B. Anteroposterior and lateral x-rays of the initial fracture. C,D. Closed manipulative reduction combined with longitudinal traction gained an anatomic reduction. Percutaneous Kirschner wires placed through the radial styloid held the fracture. An external fixateur provided axial length. E,F. At 1 year follow-up, the anteroposterior and lateral x-rays reveal an anatomic reduction has been maintained. Excellent clinical function was restored.

against the scaphoid and lunate, correcting the dorsal subluxation of the carpus (Fig. 6.22A–G).

The intraarticular congruity is checked either with an image intensifier or by direct vision through a dorsal longitudinal capsular incision.

At times following reduction and proximal fixation with Kirschner wires, a defect will be noted in the metaphyseal bone that will require cancellous bone graft to help support the distal anatomy. Depending upon the size of the dorsal rim fracture, either a small T or L plate or even a larger plate may be required for stable fixation and to prevent recurrence of the deformity.

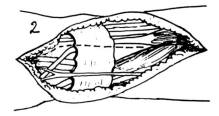

Figure 6.21. The surgical approach to the dorsal marginal fracture is through a longitudinal incision creating an interval between the second and fourth dorsal extensor compartments.

Dorsal shearing marginal fractures

Pitfalls	Pearls
Failure to recognize the fracture as a marginal shearing fracture	Lateral tomography or axial computed tomography will accurately define the fracture
Failure to appreciate the subgroup B2.2 with a radial styloid component	A more extensile dorsal surgical approach is preferred for the complex fracture patterns
Lack of definitive implant for dorsal surface of the distal radius	Have available small and mini implants as well as external fixation.

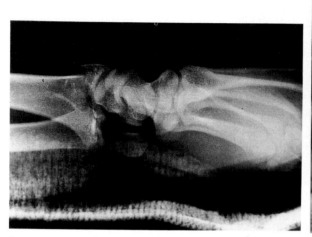

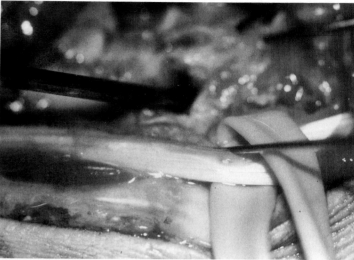

A

B

Figure 6.22. A 22-year-old male was injured in a high-speed motor vehicle accident, sustaining a dorsal marginal fracture as well as polytrauma. A. Lateral x-ray showing a dorsal marginal fracture with radiocarpal subluxation. B. Open reduction was performed through a dorsal longitudinal approach. C. Following reduction and provisional fixation with Kirschner wires, a defect in the metaphysis was filled with autogenous iliac crest bone graft. (*Figure continues on facing page.*)

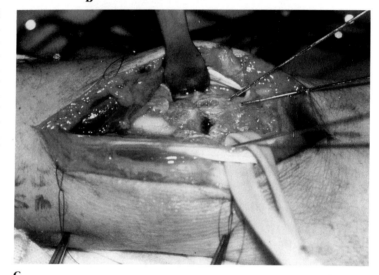

C

Shearing Fracture: Anterior (Group B3)

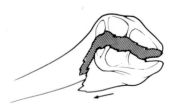

:Due in large part to the obliquity of the fracture line and loss of palmar support of the carpus, these fractures tend to be intrinsically unstable. Shortening and palmar displacement of the fragment(s) are always associated with a volar subluxation of the carpus.

With increased experience in the operative management of these fractures has come an awareness that these fractures may have distinct anatomic features that prove important in their management. The fracture may be a single fragment involving only the most radial aspect of the palmar articular surface (subgroup B3.1) (Fig. 6.23) and sparing the sigmoid notch or it may extend ulnarward to also include the ulnar notch (subgroup B3.2) (Fig. 6.24). Depending upon the quality of the bone as well as the severity of the impact, variable amounts of articular or metaphyseal comminution of the fracture fragment may be present (subgroup B3.3) (Fig. 6.25).

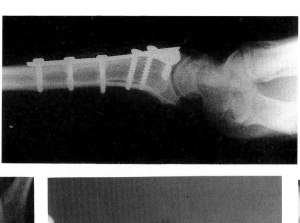

D,E. The fracture was stabilized with a cloverleaf plate with the projecting tip cut off. F,G. Excellent function resulted.

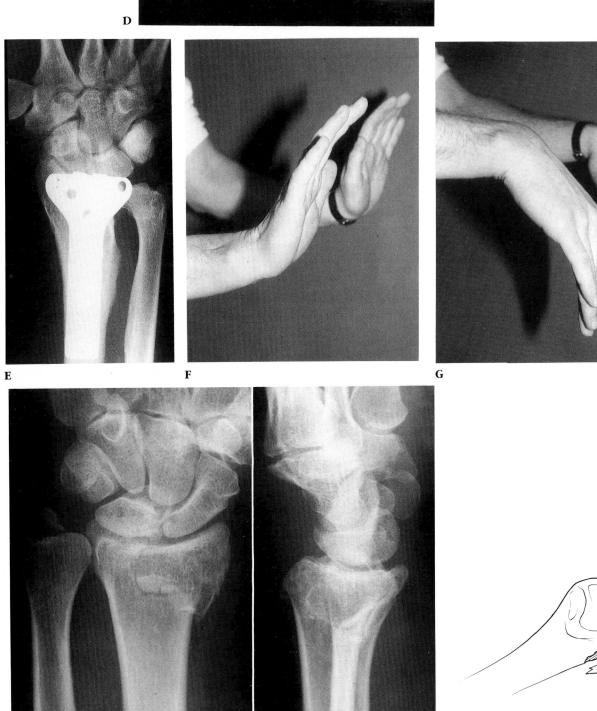

E   F   G

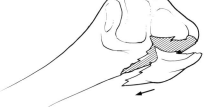

Figure 6.23. Anterior marginal fracture involving only the most radial aspect of the volar articular surface (subgroup B3.1).

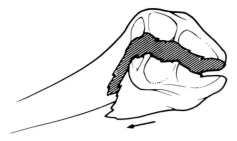

Figure 6.24. Anterior marginal fracture involving the sigmoid notch (subgroup B3.2).

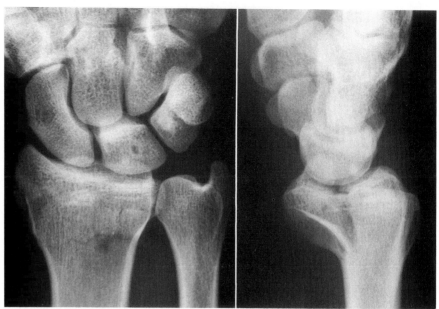

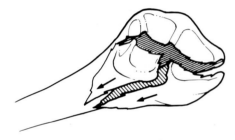

Figure 6.25. Multifragmented anterior marginal shearing fracture (subgroup B3.3).

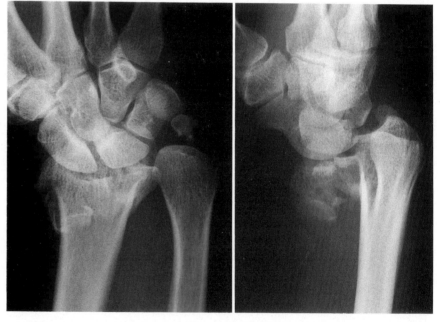

Fractures associated with a higher energy of impact or more extensive displacement may also be associated with an avulsion of the ulnar styloid or tear of the triangular fibrocartilage (Fig. 6.26A–F).

Preoperative Planning

A careful assessment of the surrounding soft tissues and neurologic status is mandatory, as these fractures may be associated with high-energy trauma. Median nerve compression or a forearm compartment syndrome may be coexistent and mandate a more expeditious operative intervention.

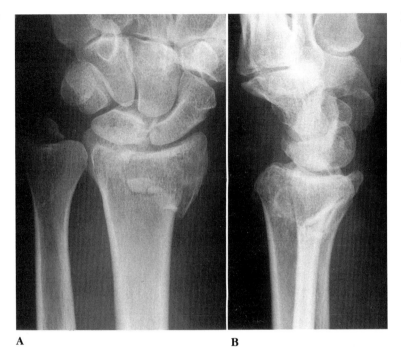

A   B

Figure 6.26. An anterior marginal fracture not involving the sigmoid notch in an anesthesiologist (subgroup B3.1). A,B. Anteroposterior and lateral x-rays show the intraarticular fracture. An ulnar styloid fracture is evident. C,D. The fracture was anatomically reduced and supported with an anterior buttress plate. The styloid was also anatomically reduced and internally fixed. E,F. Radiographs at two years after treatment. Full function returned.

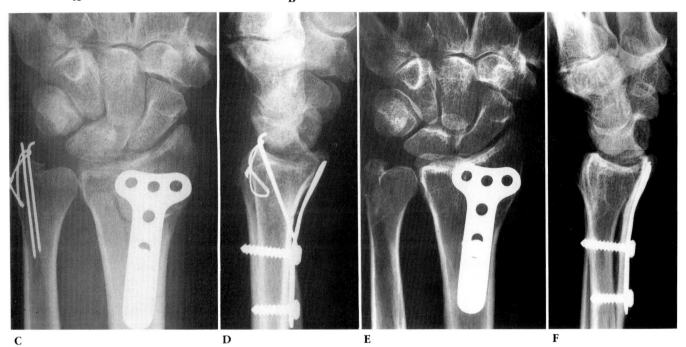

C   D   E   F

When the standard x-rays suggest the possibility of comminution, lateral tomography of the wrist is especially helpful to identify the presence and location of small impacted articular fragments (Fig. 6.27A–C). The presence of these will have a considerable influence on the surgical tactic.

The majority of these fractures are best treated operatively, as functional results have been shown to correlate directly with an anatomic restoration of this unstable fracture. Cast immobilization is reserved for nondisplaced fractures, particularly those not involving the sigmoid notch, or for displaced fractures in patients considered medically unfit or who refuse surgery. Closed reduction is performed with longitudinal traction applied to the extended

Figure 6.27. A 30-year-old sky diver sustained a high-energy impact on his dominant hand. A,B. Anteroposterior and lateral x-rays reveal an anterior marginal shear fracture. C. The lateral tomogram suggested the presence of an impacted articular fragment involving the lunate facet of the distal radius. D. The fracture was anatomically secured and stabilized with a volar buttress plate as well as an additional 2.7-mm lag screw. E,F. Follow-up at 1 year shows anatomic restoration to be maintained. A nearly full functional result was present.

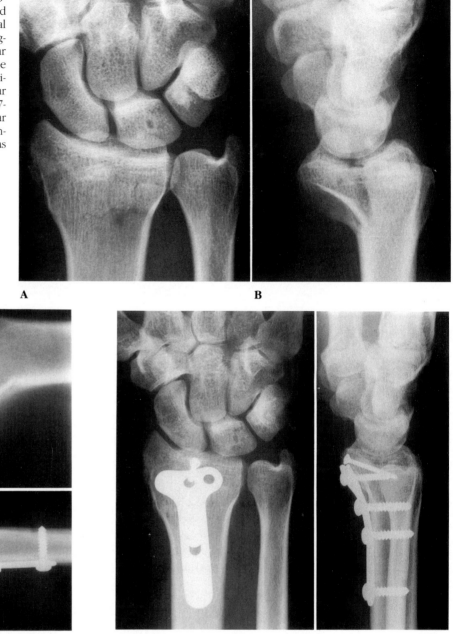

C   A   B

D   E   F

hand and wrist in order to utilize the intact volar radiocarpal ligaments. The reduction is maintained, immobilizing the arm with the forearm in maximal supination and the wrist in neutral or slight palmar flexion in an above-elbow cast.[8,9,10] Careful and frequent radiographic control is necessary over the next 2 weeks due to the intrinsic instability of the fracture. The above-elbow cast is maintained for 6 weeks in view of the complexity of this fracture.

Operative Management

Operative reduction and stable internal fixation more reliably assure the anatomic reduction of the joint and realignment of the radiocarpal articulation. In addition, the buttress effect of a plate supporting the reduced fracture fragment will help maintain the articular reduction by virtue of the fact that it directly compresses the anterior fragment against the intact dorsal column of the radius.

For most subgroup B3.1 and subgroup B3.2 fractures, we prefer an anterior surgical approach along the radial border of the distal forearm (Fig. 6.28) (see Chapter 4). The fracture can be exposed through the interval between the flexor carpi radialis tendon and the radial artery and the accompanying venae comitantes along with radial detachment of the pronator quadratus muscle (Fig. 6.29). When the fracture is associated with symptoms of acute median nerve compression, a second incision can be made in the palm in line with the ring finger to release the transverse carpal ligament. This is preferable to extending the radial incision across the volar wrist crease onto the palm, as this would place the palmar cutaneous nerve in jeopardy of injury. An alternative approach is a more ulnar-based incision extending from the mid-palmar crease across onto the distal forearm (Fig. 6.30). (see Chapter 4).

Once the fracture is exposed, the hematoma is gently cleansed away with a dental pic and irrigation. When dealing with a subgroup B3.1 or subgroup B3.2 fracture without evidence of intraarticular comminution, the fracture can be reduced by realigning the metaphyseal fracture lines. This is facilitated by hyperextending the wrist over a rolled towel with the forearm in maximal supination (Fig. 6.31A–J). It is imperative *not* to open the volar wrist capsule to visualize the articular surface, as this can lead to injury to the volar radiocarpal ligaments and postoperative instability.

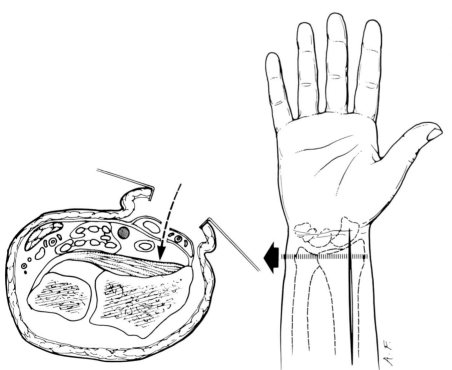

Figure 6.28. An anterior surgical approach will be satisfactory for most volar marginal shearing fractures. The interval between the radial artery and the flexior carpi radialis is used to gain access to the distal radius.

Figure 6.29. The longitudinal approach to the volar marginal shearing fracture. A. The interval between the radial artery and the flexor carpi radialis. B. The pronator quadratus is identified. C. The pronator quadratus is elevated from its radial insertion. D. Full exposure is gained to the distal radius fracture.

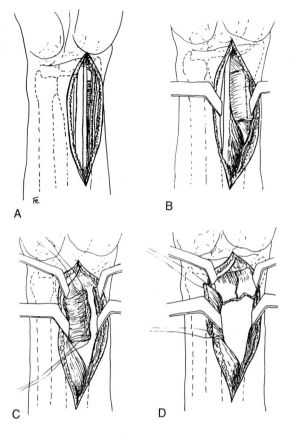

Figure 6.30. An alternative incision is more ulnar based and can be used to release the carpal tunnel (A) as well as approach those fractures which extend into the sigmoid notch (B).

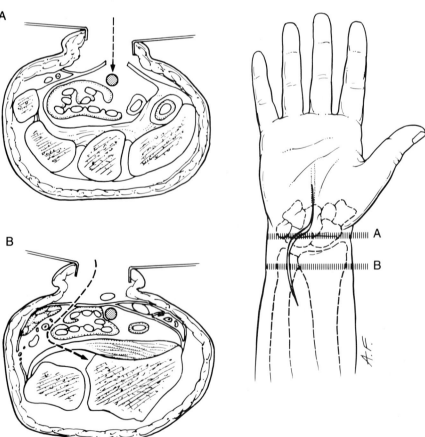

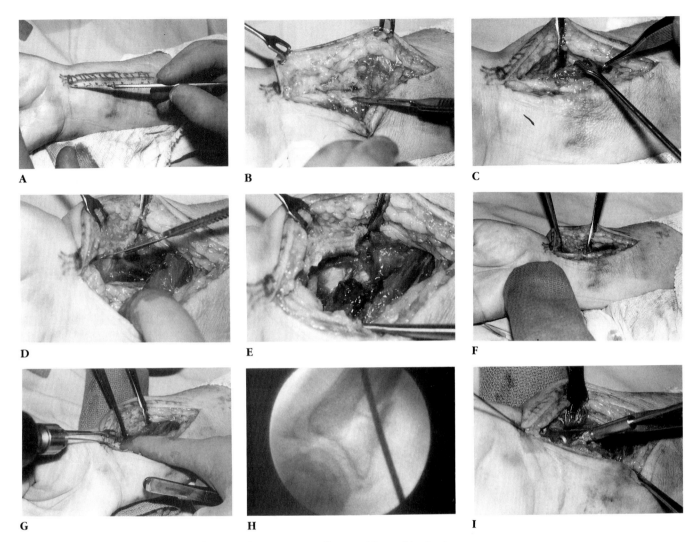

A   B   C

D   E   F

G   H   I

Figure 6.31. A complex anterior shearing fracture in a 62-year-old psychiatrist is approached along the radial border of the distal forearm. A. The incision parallels the radial artery. B. The flexor carpi radialis tendon is identified. C. An interval is created between the radial artery and the flexor carpi radialis and flexor pollicis longus. D. The pronator quadratus is incised along its radial border. E. The pronator is elevated in an ulnar direction exposing the fracture. F. A rolled towel is prepared which will help in fracture reduction. G. With the wrist extended over the rolled towel, the reduced fracture is provisionally fixed with Kirschner wire. H. The reduction is confirmed on the image intensifier. I. A small buttress plate is readily placed onto the anterior cortex of the distal radius.

Should the preoperative or intraoperative x-rays suggest the presence of a displaced articular fragment, it is preferable to reduce this under direct vision by pulling apart the anterior shearing fragment(s), exposing the fracture surface. This will permit elevation and reduction of the articular piece without additional injury to the volar capsular ligaments.

It is not surprising to identify small areas of metaphyseal comminution with these fractures, which also adds to the inherent instability of the fracture (Fig. 6.27).

Provisional fixation of the fracture with 0.45-inch smooth Kirschner wires facilitates the ease of applying the buttress plate. One must take heed that the point of entry of the Kirschner wires does not interfere with the placement of the plate. The wires should be put in obliquely from a distal to proximal

Figure 6.32. Provisional fixation with smooth Kirschner wires. Whenever possible, the wires are placed from a distal to a proximal direction to avoid the placement of the definitive implant.

Figure 6.33. If the provisional Kirschner wires interfere with positioning of the plate, they can be driven out of the dorsal cortex of the radius and the skin to be flush with the volar cortex.

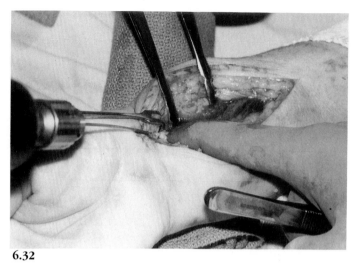

6.32

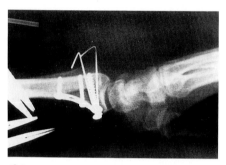

6.33

direction (Fig. 6.32). An alternative approach is to pass the wires out through the dorsal cortex and dermis until the end is flush with the anterior cortex. The wires can be readily removed once the plate has been applied (Fig. 6.33).

Definitive fixation for the single-fragment subgroup B3.1 or subgroup B3.2 fractures is achieved with a 3.5-mm T plate applied to the anterior cortex. The plate should be prebent in such a way that there is still a small space between the mid-portion of the plate and an area just proximal to the fracture site. The most proximal screw is applied first and tightened securely. The introduction of the second screw just distal to the first screw will firmly compress the plate against the radial shaft. This in turn will compress the articular fracture fragment against the intact distal radius, enhancing its buttress effect (Fig. 6.34). The reduction and placement of the plate must be confirmed using

Figure 6.34. The anterior buttress T plate is pre-bent so that it sits slightly off the radial cortex. After the most proximal screw (No. 1) is placed, tightening the second screw (No. 2) will push the plate up against the anterior fracture fragment, enhancing its buttressing effect. This is illustrated in the clinical example of an anterior shearing fracture in a 28-year-old lawyer. Additional stability is achieved by screws placed distally through the fracture fragment into the dorsal cortex.

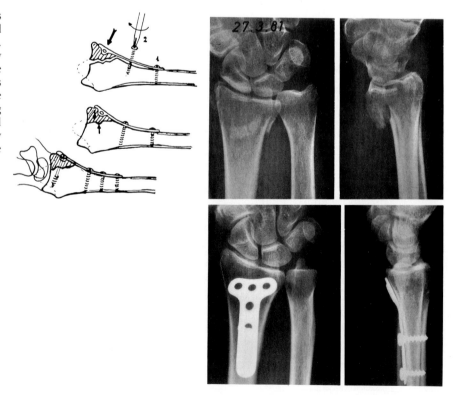

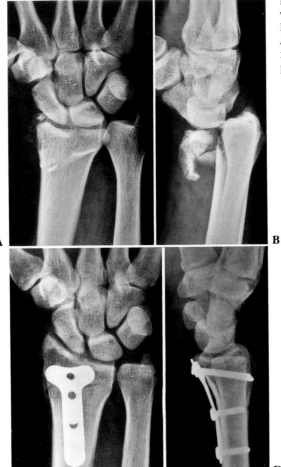

Figure 6.35. An anterior marginal fracture with two major articular fragments subgroup B3.3). Note the metaphyseal comminution. A,B. The preoperative anterior and posterior x-rays. C,D. Stable fixation with a screw placed distally into each fracture fragment.

either the image intensifier or biplanar x-rays. If the articular congruity is not satisfactory, the more distal screw is removed and the volar fragment is gently pushed into place with either a periosteal elevator or a sharp pointed awl, and the screw is replaced. For most subgroup B3.1 or subgroup B3.2 fractures which involve a single shearing fracture fragment, stability can be achieved by the buttressing effect of the plate alone without the need for additional screw fixation through the distal part of the plate (Fig. 6.26).

Additional stability may be desirable when more than one fragment is identified (subgroup B3.3). In such instances, screws can be placed into the distal radius either through the plate (Figs. 6.34 and 6.35) or separately into the fracture fragments.

When faced with more comminution, particularly that extending out into the radial styloid resulting in instability of the individual fragments, the surgeon should be prepared to use a combination of fixation methods. The styloid can be held in a reduced position by Kirschner wires placed percutaneously (Fig. 6.36), by a screw (Fig. 6.37), or by both (Fig. 6.38).

Wound closure is achieved by replacing the pronator quadratus back in its original position and closing the skin over a suction drain. A bulky dressing and a volar splint are applied. We prefer to leave the splint in place for 14 days, at which time the sutures are removed. At that point, a removable splint is worn for another few weeks, with the patient permitted to use the involved

Figure 6.36. A complex shearing fracture with displacement of the radial styloid. A,B. Initial anteroposterior and lateral x-rays C,D. The anterior shearing fracture was supported by a buttress plate while percutaneous Kirschner wires secured the styloid fragment. E,F. At 2-year follow-up, excellent function resulted with maintenance of an anatomic result.

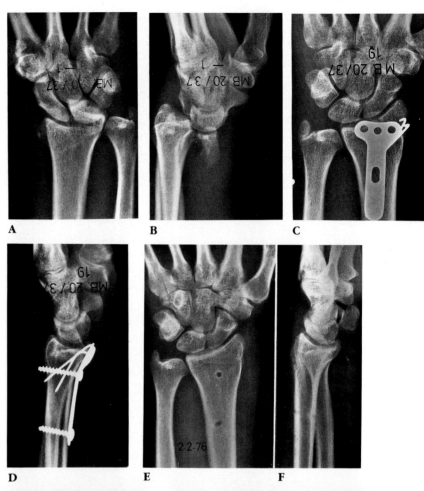

Figure 6.37. A complex marginal fracture secured with a buttress plate and a cannulated screw holding the radial styloid fragment.

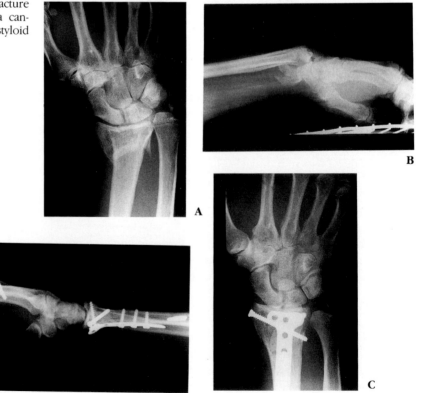

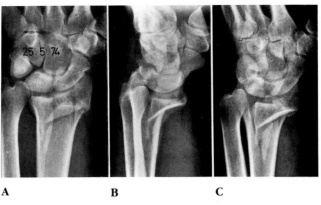

A　　　　　　　B　　　　　　　C

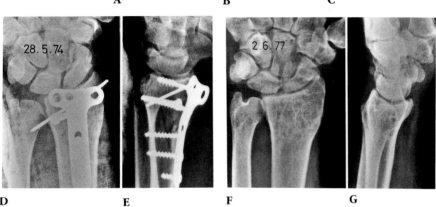

D　　　　　　　　E　　　　　　F　　　　　　　　G

Figure 6.38. A complex marginal fracture with metaphyseal comminution. A–C. Initial x-rays reveal the complex fracture pattern. D,E. Articular restoration was maintained by a combination of fixation modalities. F,G. Follow-up at 3 years revealed excellent function and no evidence of arthrosis on x-ray.

hand for activities of daily living. Manual work and sport are forbidden until fracture healing is assured, usually by 2 months postinjury.

Anterior marginal shearing fractures

Pitfalls	Pearls
Failure to recognize a split or comminuted shearing fracture (Fig. 6.39)	Tomography can help in preoperative planning
The buttress plate's inability to secure the entire fracture fragment	Consider Kirschner wires or a cannulated screw through the radial styloid
Elevation of an impacted articular fragment	Avoid opening the volar capsule. Elevate the fragment from within the fracture. Support with autogenous bone graft

Articular Shearing Fractures: Complications

Untoward outcomes following articular marginal shearing fractures can be divided into those occurring as a direct result of the injury and those assocated with difficulties of treatment.

Fracture Complications

Radial styloid fractures present two distinct foci of injury: disruption of the articular surface of the scaphoid facet at the end of the radius, and "greater arc" injuries involving a portion of the radiocarpal and intercarpal ligamentous

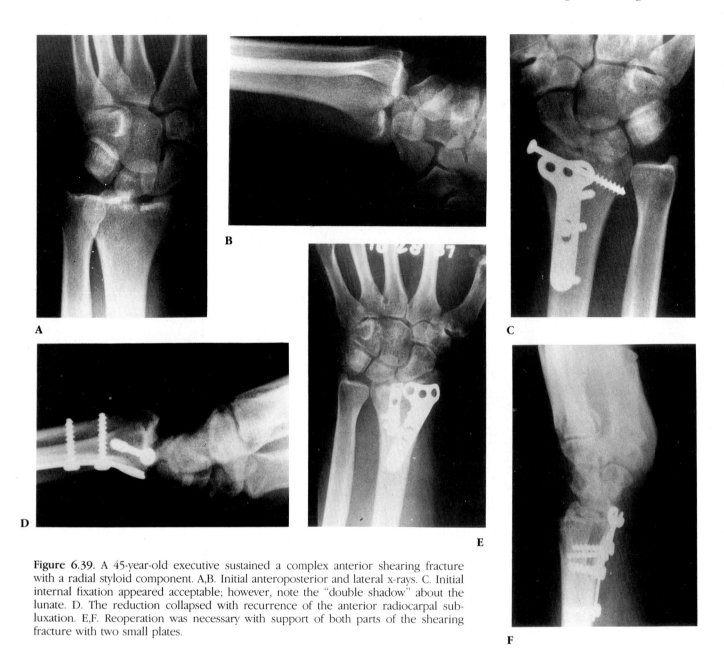

Figure 6.39. A 45-year-old executive sustained a complex anterior shearing fracture with a radial styloid component. A,B. Initial anteroposterior and lateral x-rays. C. Initial internal fixation appeared acceptable; however, note the "double shadow" about the lunate. D. The reduction collapsed with recurrence of the anterior radiocarpal subluxation. E,F. Reoperation was necessary with support of both parts of the shearing fracture with two small plates.

complex.[21,28] Failure to recognize this association can result in long-term disabilities, including radiocarpal arthrosis, loss of grip strength, and loss of radiocarpal mobility.[18]

In a similar light, the articular marginal shearing fractures, unless properly reduced and allowed to heal in an anatomic position, will result in the later development of arthrosis, loss of wrist strength, loss of wrist mobility, and at times disruption of the normal distal radioulnar joint mobility.[15,20,23,24,32]

Complications Associated with Treatment

Inadequate reduction, loss of internal fixation, stiffness, and overlying soft tissue problems have all been identified with the surgical management of these unstable shearing fractures.

A particular source of problems consists of the fracture patterns that represent combinations of styloid and marginal shearing fractures involving the remainder of the distal radius (subgroup B2.2 or subgroup B3.3). In these cases, failure to recognize the extent of the injury because of lack of appropriate preoperative x-rays or of intraoperative surgical exposure, or unstable internal fixation may lead to persistent articular incongruity and result in disability.

The surgical problems that may arise are well illustrated in this case report:

A forty-five-year-old executive sustained a complex anterior shearing fracture while skiing at high speed. On the day of injury, he underwent an open reduction and internal fixation of the fracture through an anterior surgical approach (Fig. 6.39A and B).

His initial fracture reduction was deemed adequate at the time of surgery, and early postoperative radiographs suggested an adequate articular reduction (Fig. 6.39C). By the same token, a careful scrutiny of the x-rays would suggest that the lunate facet of the distal radius had not been anatomically reduced.

When he was seen at 7 weeks postsurgery, it was quite apparent that anterior subluxation of the lunate had recurred, best seen on the lateral x-ray (Fig. 6.39D). Therefore, at 8 weeks postinjury he underwent a repeat surgical procedure. The fracture callus was taken down and the articular marginal fracture was re-reduced and securely supported now with two small plates (Fig. 6.39E and F). An excellent functional result was noted at a follow-up of 6 years.

References

1. Aufranc OE, Jones WN, Turner RH: Anterior marginal articular fracture of the distal radius. *JAMA* 196: 108–111, 1966.
2. Barton JR: Views and treatment of an important injury of the wrist. *Medical Examiner and Record of Medical Science*, p. 367, 1838.
3. Bassett RL, Ray MJ: Carpal instability associated with radial styloid fractures. *Orthopaedics* 7: 1356–1361, 1984.
4. Bengner U, Johnell O: Increasing incidence of forearm fractures. *Acta Orthop Scand* 56: 158–160, 1985.
5. Böhler L: *Treatment of Fractures* Bristol: John Wright & Sons, Ltd., 1943.
6. Cauchoix J, Duparc J, Potel M: Les fractures-luxations marginales antérieures du radius. *Rev Chir Orthop* 46: 233–235, 1960.
7. Charnley J: *The Closed Treatment of Common Fractures* Baltimore: Williams & Wilkins, 1963, p. 142.
8. DeOliveira JC: Barton's fracture. *J Bone Joint Surg* 55A: 586–594, 1973.
9. Edwards HC: The mechanism and treatment of backfire fracture. *J Bone Joint Surg [Am]* 8: 701–717, 1926.
10. Ellis J: Smith's and Barton's fractures—a method of treatment. *J Bone Joint Surg [Am]* 47B: 724–727, 1965.
11. Emmett JE, Breck LW: A review and analysis of 11,000 fractures seen in a private practice of orthopaedic surgery. *J Bone Joint Surg [Am]* 40A: 1169, 1958.
12. Fellman T: *Smith-Frakturen*. Doctoral Thesis, University of Bern, 1991.
13. Fernandez DL: Smith Frakturen. *Hefte Unfallheilk* 148: 91–95, 1980.
14. Fernandez DL, Maeder G: Die Behandlung der Smith-Frakturen. *Arch Orthop Unfallchir* 88: 153–161, 1977.
15. Flandreau RH, Sweeney RM, O'Sullivan WD: Clinical experience with a series of Smith fractures. *Arch Surg* 84: 288–291, 1962.
16. Fuller DJ: The Ellis plate operation for Smith's fractures. *J Bone Joint Surg [Am]* 55B: 173–178, 1973.
17. Hamilton FH: *A Practical Treatise on Fractures and Dislocations* Philadelphia: Blanchard & Lea, 1860.
18. Helm RH, Tonkin MA: The chauffeur's fracture: Simple or complex? *J Hand Surg* 17B: 156–159, 1992.
19. King RE: Barton's fracture-dislocation of the wrist. In: *Current Practice in Orthopaedic Surgery*, edited by Ahstran JP Jr. St. Louis: C.V. Mosby, 1975, pp. 133–144.

20. King RE, Lovell W: Barton's enigma. *J Bone Joint Surg* 41A: 762–728, 1959.
21. Mayfield JK, Johnson RP, Kilcoyne RF: Carpal dislocations: Pathomechanics and progressive perilunar instability. *J Hand Surg* 5: 226–241, 1980.
22. McMurtry RY, Jupiter JB: Fractures of the distal radius. In: *Skeletal Trauma*, edited by Browner B, Jupiter J, Levine A, Trafton P. Philadelphia: WB Saunders, 1991, pp. 1063–1094.
23. Mills TJ: Smith's fracture and anterior marginal fracture of the radius. *Brit Med J* 2: 603–605, 1957.
24. Pattee GA, Thompson GH: Anterior and posterior marginal fracture-dislocation of the distal radius. *Clin Orthop Rel Res* 231: 183–195, 1988.
25. Pleeves L: Colles' and Smith's fractures. *J Bone Joint Surg* 44B: 227, 1962.
26. Roberts JB: A clinical, pathological, and experimental study of fracture of the lower end of the radius with displacement of the carpal fragment toward the flexor or anterior surface of the wrist. *Am. J. Med. Sci* 113: 10–80, 1897.
27. Saito H, Shibata M: Classification of fractures at the distal end of the radius with reference to treatment of comminuted fractures. In: *Current Concepts in Hand Surgery*, edited by Boswick JA Jr. Philadelphia: Lea & Febiger, 1983, pp. 129–145.
28. Siegel DB: Gelberman RH: Radial styloidectomy: An anatomical study with special reference to radiocarpal intrascapular ligamentous morphology. *J Hand Surg* 16A: 40–44, 1991.
29. Smith RJ, Floyd WE: III: Smith's and Barton's fractures. In: *Fractures of the Hand and Wrist*, edited by Barton NJ. London: Churchill Livingstone, 1988, pp. 252–266.
30. Smith RW: *A Treatise on Fracture in the Vicinity of Joints and on Certain Forms of Accidental and Congenital Dislocations*. Dublin: Hodges and Smith, 1847, pp. 162–163.
31. Thomas FB: Reduction of Smith's fracture. *J Bone Joint Surg* 39B: 463–470, 1957.
32. Thompson GH, Grant TT: Barton's fractures—reverse Barton's fractures. Confusing eponyms. *Clin Orthop Rel Res* 122: 210–221, 1977.
33. Wagner HE, Jakob RP: Operative Behandlung der distalen Radiusfrakturen mit Fixateur externe. *Unfallchirurgie* 88: 473–480, 1985.
34. Weiss H, Wilde CD, Berns H: Vergleichende Behandlungsergebnisse zwischen operativ und konservativ versorgten besonderen Frakturformen am Radius loco typico. *Hefte Unfallheilk* 132: 418, 1977.
35. Woodyard JE: A review of Smith's fractures. *J Bone Joint Surg* 51B: 324–329, 1969.

Chapter Seven

Compression Fractures of the Articular Surface

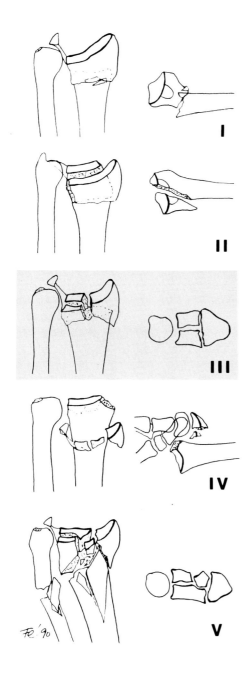

It is conceivable that in the case of a sudden and violent fall, the force of which is sustained by the hand, the rounded articular surface of the carpal mass, before the movement of backward flexion is completed, may be driven up against the concave articular surface of the radius with such force as to split it or perforate it.

L.S. Pilcher, M.D. 1917

A Practical, Treatment Oriented Classification of Fractures of the Distal Radius and Associated Distal Radioulnar Joint Lesions.
Diego L. Fernandez, M.D. PD

FRACTURE TYPES (ADULTS) BASED ON THE MECHANISM OF INJURY	CHILDREN FRACTURE EQUIVALENT	STABILITY/INSTABILITY: high risk of secondary displacement after initial adequate reduction	DISPLACEMENT PATTERN	NUMBER OF FRAGMENTS	ASSOCIATED LESIONS carpal ligament, fractures, median, ulnar nerve, tendons, ipsilat., fx upper extremity, compartment syndrome	RECOMMENDED TREATMENT
TYPE I BENDING FRACTURE OF THE METAPHYSIS	DISTAL FOREARM FRACTURE SALTER II	STABLE UNSTABLE	NON-DISPLACED DORSALLY (Colles-Pouteau) VOLARLY (Smith) PROXIMAL COMBINED	ALWAYS 2 MAIN FRAGMENTS + VARYING DEGREE OF METAPHYSEAL COMMINUTION (instability)	UNCOMMON	CONSERVATIVE (stable fxs) PERCUTANEOUS PINNING (extra- or intrafocal) EXTERNAL FIXATION (exceptionally BONE GRAFT)
TYPE II SHEARING FRACTURE OF THE JOINT SURFACE	SALTER IV	UNSTABLE	DORSAL RADIAL VOLAR PROXIMAL COMBINED	TWO-PART THREE-PART COMMINUTED	LESS UNCOMMON	OPEN REDUCTION SCREW-/PLATE FIXATION
TYPE III COMPRESSION FRACTURE OF THE JOINT SURFACE	SALTER III, IV, V	STABLE UNSTABLE	NON-DISPLACED DORSAL RADIAL VOLAR PROXIMAL COMBINED	TWO-PART THREE-PART FOUR-PART COMMINUTED	COMMON	CONSERVATIVE CLOSED, LIMITED, ARTHROSCOPIC ASSISTED, OR EXTENSILE OPEN REDUCTION PERCUTANEOUS PINS COMBINED EXTERNAL AND INTERNAL FIXATION BONE GRAFT
TYPE IV AVULSION FRACTURES, RADIO CARPAL FRACTURE DISLOCATION	VERY RARE	UNSTABLE	DORSAL RADIAL VOLAR PROXIMAL COMBINED	TWO-PART (radial styloid ulnar styloid) THREE-PART (volar, dorsal margin) COMMINUTED	FREQUENT	CLOSED OR OPEN REDUCTION PIN OR SCREW FIXATION TENSION WIRING
TYPE V COMBINED FRACTURES (I - II - III - IV) HIGH-VELOCITY INJURY	VERY RARE	UNSTABLE	DORSAL RADIAL VOLAR PROXIMAL COMBINED	COMMINUTED and/or BONE LOSS (frequently intraarticular, open, seldom extraarticular)	ALWAYS PRESENT	COMBINED METHOD

Fracture of the distal radius: associated distal radioulnar joint (DRUJ) lesions.

	Patho-anatomy of the lesion	Degree of joint surface involvement	Prognosis	Recommended treatment
Type I Stable (following reduction of the radius the DRUJ is congruous and stable)	A Avulsion fracture tip ulnar styloid B Stable fracture ulnar neck	None	Good	A+B Functional aftertreatment Encourage early pronation-supination exercises Note: Extraarticular unstable fractures of the ulna at the metaphyseal level or distal shaft require stable plate fixation
Type II Unstable (subluxation or dislocation of the ulnar head present)	A Substance tear of TFCC and/or palmar and dorsal capsular ligaments B Avulsion fracture base of the ulnar styloid	None	• Chronic instability • Painful limitation of supination if left unreduced • Possible late arthritic changes	A Closed treatment Reduce subluxation, sugar tong splint in 45° of supination four to six weeks A+B Operative treatment Repair TFCC or fix ulnar styloid with tension band wiring Immobilize wrist and elbow in supination (cast) or transfix ulna/radius with k-wire and forearm cast
Type III Potentially unstable (subluxation possible)	A Intraarticular fracture of the sigmoid notch B Intraarticular fracture of the ulnar head	Present	• Dorsal subluxation possible together with dorsally displaced die punch or dorso-ulnar fragment • Risk of early degenerative changes and severe limitation of forearm rotation if left unreduced	A Anatomic reduction of palmar and dorsal sigmoid notch fragments. If residual subluxation tendency present immobilize as in type II injury B Functional aftertreatment to enhance remodelling of ulnar head If DRUJ remains painful: partial ulnar resection, darrach or sauvé-kapandji procedure at a later date

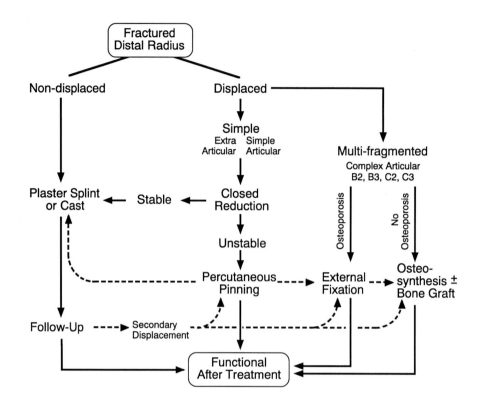

Compression Fractures of the Articular Surface

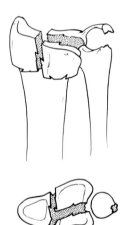

Compression fractures of the distal radius are those injuries whose major feature is an impaction of the subchondral and metaphyseal cancellous bone in concert with disruption of the distal radius articular surface (Fig. 7.1). In some instances, restoration of the articular disruption is readily achieved by applying longitudinal tension on the radiocarpal ligaments,[3] while in other instances, the disimpaction of the cartilage-bearing fragments may require operative reduction with replacement of the metaphyseal bony defect with a bone graft.

Historical Perspective

Much of the efforts of early investigators centered on refining the original descriptions of Petit,[37] Pouteau,[40] and Colles,[10] who primarily described bending-type fractures (see Chapter 1). Given the fact that for most of the nineteenth century, recognition of fracture patterns was made on post-mortem specimens, it is of interest to observe descriptions of compression-type fractures dating back as early as 1842, when Voillemier described such an injury in a patient who died 4 hours following a fall from a three-story height.[49] Callendar in 1865 reported on similar patterns in specimens housed in the museums of the London Hospital as well as St. Bartholomew's Hospital,[5] while across the Atlantic, Cotton in 1904 identified many of the contemporary sub-classifications of impaction injuries which he found in specimens at the Massachusetts General Hospital (Fig. 7.2).[13] With the invention of x-ray came a wider recognition of the varying patterns of distal radius fractures. Morton[35] and Pilcher,[38] among others, described such impaction-type injuries during radiographic evaluations of distal radius fractures.

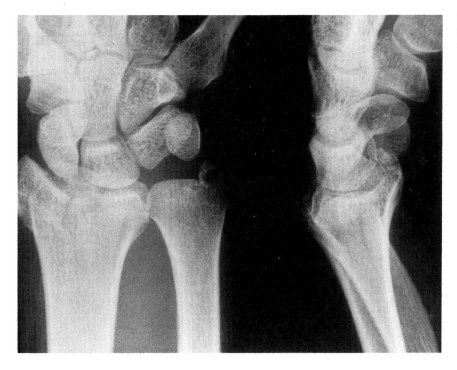

Figure 7.1. A compression fracture of the articular surface in a 41-year-old secretary who fell while doing in-line rollerblading.

Stevens in 1920 postulated that the lunate acted as the driving force in impaction injuries of the articular surface.[46] He described situations in which the lunate impacted the posteromedial aspect of the articular surface when the injury occurred with the forearm held in full pronation.

Scheck in 1962 coined the term "die-punch" injury for this lunate impaction against the posteromedial aspect of the radius.[43] He hypothesized that in some cases both compression and bending forces were exerted in the direction of the longitudinal axis of the radius (Fig. 7.3). This pattern was observed in 75 percent of the 24 fractures in his series, and he also suggested that these injuries had been commonly described in several prior reports such as that by Rogers in 1944[42] and Gartland and Werley in 1951.[21]

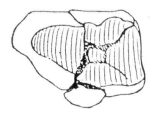

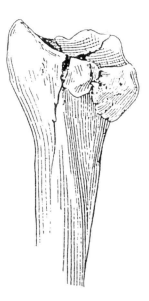

Figure 7.2. An autopsy specimen found in the Warren Museum at the Harvard Medical School described by Cotton in 1900 reveals an articular compression pattern quite similar to a subgroup C3.1. (Reprinted with permission from Cotton FJ. Fractures of the lower end of the radius. *Ann Surg* 32: 194, 1900.)

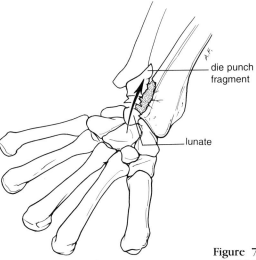

die punch fragment

lunate

compressive force

Figure 7.3. Scheck coined the term "die-punch" injury to describe the mechanism of the lunate impacting the articular surface of the radius.

Figure 7.4. The nature of the impaction injury to the distal radius will be influenced by a number of factors, including the position of the hand upon impact.

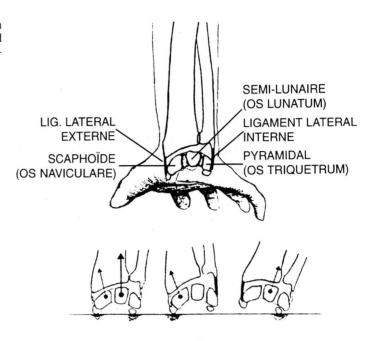

Castaing in 1964 presented a series of injuries representing patterns of compression-type injuries involving both the articular and the metaphyseal regions of the radius (see Chapter 2).[6] Mortier and colleagues[33,34] also stressed the importance of the lunate impaction into the posteromedial aspect of the articular surface of the distal radius (Fig. 7.4).

In several important publications, Melone expanded on the lunate impaction concept.[30,31] He identified four basic components to the impaction injury:

1. The radial shaft
2. The radial styloid
3. The posteromedial part of the lunate facet of the distal radius
4. The palmar medial part of the lunate facet

Melone felt that if the mechanism of injury was primarily that of compression, the medial aspect of the radius was most affected. He called this the "medial complex" to describe the lunate facet fracture fragments and their ligamentous attachment with the proximal row of carpal bones as well as the ulnar styloid. The fact that the lunate would be the focus of the direct compression helped to explain why the dorsomedial aspect of the distal radius was involved much more commonly than its palmar counterpart. This was suggested to be the case, as the injury most often occurred with the hand flat on the ground, thus driving the lunate into the dorsal aspect of the distal radius. However, with higher-velocity impaction injuries, wider separation of the lunate facet could be observed, which at times would result in the palmar-medial facet fragment being displaced and rotated as much as 180 degrees (Fig. 7.5).

The fracture patterns depicted by Castaing were expanded to form the basis of the current Comprehensive Classification of Fractures classifications (see Chapter 2).[17] The major grouping, Type C, includes those fractures involving a complete articular injury. The various subgroups are classified according to the orientation of the articular fracture line. In general terms, fractures oriented in the sagittal plane are more easily reduced than those in the frontal plane.

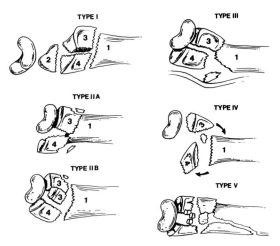

Figure 7.5. Melone divides the lunate impaction injury into four major components: (1) radial shaft; (2) radial styloid; (3) posteromedial part of the lunate facet; (4) anteromedial part of the lunate facet. Subgroups were later added to identify unique characteristics of these injuries. (Reprinted with permission. WB Saunders, Philadelphia. *Orthopaedic Clinics of North America*, 24: 1993.)

C1: Complete articular fractures of the radius, articular simple, metaphysis simple (Fig. 7.6).
C1.1: Posteromedial articular fracture line.
C1.2: Sagitall articular fracture line.
C1.3: Frontal articular fracture line.
C2: Complete articular fracture of the radius, articular simple, metaphyseal multifragmentary (Fig. 7.7).
C2.1: Sagitall articular fracture line.
C2.2: Frontal articular fracture line.
C2.3: Extending into diaphysis.

C   COMPLEX ARTICULAR: Fracture affects the joint surfaces (radio-ulnar and/or radio-carpal) and the metaphyseal area

C1 Complete articular fracture, of the radius, articular simple, metaphyseal simple

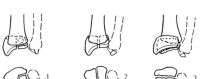

1 postero-medial articular fragment
2 sagittal articular fracture line
3 frontal articular fracture line

C2 Complete articular fracture, of the radius, articular simple, metaphyseal multifragmentary

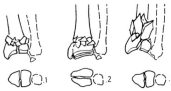

1 sagittal articular fracture line
2 frontal articular fracture line
3 extending into the diaphysis

Figure 7.6. Group C1 fractures involve a "simple" (two-fragment) intraarticular component and no metaphyseal. A. C1.1: Posteromedial articular fragment. B. C1.2: Sagittal articular fracture line. C. C1.3: Frontal articular fracture line.

Figure 7.7. Group C2 fractures involve a simple (two fragments) intraarticular component and metaphyseal multifragmented. A. C2.1: Sagittal articular fracture line. B. C2.2: Frontal articular fracture line. C. C2.3: Extending into the diaphysis.

C3: Complete articular fracture of the radius, multifragmentary.
C3.1: Metaphyseal simple.
C3.2: Metaphyseal multifragmentary.
C3.3: Extending into diaphysis.

Figure 7.8. Group C3 fractures are complex, involving multifragmentation of the articular surface. A. C3.1: Metaphyseal simple. B. C3.2: Metaphyseal multifragmentary. C. C3.3: Extending into diaphysis.

C3 Complete articular fracture, of the radius, multifragmentary

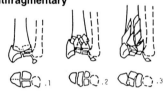

1 metaphyseal simple
2 metaphyseal multifragmentary
3 extending into the diaphysis

Goals of Treatment

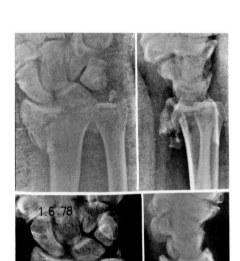

Figure 7.9. A compression articular fracture in a 29-year-old policewoman. Failure to maintain an anatomic reduction led to symptomatic arthrosis at a 4-year follow-up. Note the Scapholunate dissociation.

Displaced compression-type fractures make up a distinct group of distal radius injuries which have an inherent tendency to shorten, along with collapse of the subchondral support of the articular fracture components. At times the result of a high-energy impact, these fractures tend to be less amenable to closed manipulative reduction and are inherently unstable when immobilized in plaster.

Several studies have addressed the outcome of displaced intraarticular distal radius fractures, identifying a distinct association with posttraumatic arthrosis and residual articular incongruity.[4,27,28,48] Knirk and Jupiter retrospectively studied the outcome of 43 intraarticular fractures in 40 young adults who had a mean age of 27.6 years at the time of injury. At a mean follow-up of 6.7 years, 26 percent were rated excellent, 35 percent good, 33 percent fair, and 6 percent poor. Radiographic findings of posttraumatic arthrosis were evident in 28 (65 percent) of cases and, moreover, in 91 percent of fractures that healed with a visible incongruity of the articular surface (Fig. 7.9). This was in sharp contrast to the 11 percent incidence of radiographic arthrosis in 19 fractions that healed with a congruous radiocarpal joint. In this retrospective series, the "die-punch" compression fracture pattern was anatomically reduced in only 49 percent of cases and was responsible for a residual radiocarpal incongruity in 75 percent of the articular malalignment seen at late follow-up. If the articular step-off of the "die-punch" impaction fracture was 2 mm or greater, 100 percent of these cases went on to radiographic arthrosis, and 66 percent of these were symptomatic at follow-up.

Based upon the results of this study as well as other investigations,[4,28,48] it has become generally accepted that one should strive to achieve and maintain an anatomic or near-anatomic reduction of compression fractures of the articular surface.

Preoperative Planning

When embarking on the treatment of a compression fracture of the articular surface, the surgeon should take heed to carefully define the fracture pattern, the presence or absence of associated soft tissue or ligamentous injury, and the patient's functional requirements.

In addition to standard anteroposterior and lateral radiographs both before and after longitudinal traction, important information can be obtained with oblique x-rays taken with the forearm either partially pronated (to highlight the radial styloid) or partially supinated (to show the dorsomedial region of the distal radius). Trispiral tomography or computed tomography will be of particular benefit in accurately assessing three- and four-part articular fractures for both the number of fragments and their displacement (Fig. 7.10).

When faced with soft tissue swelling or signs and symptoms of associated

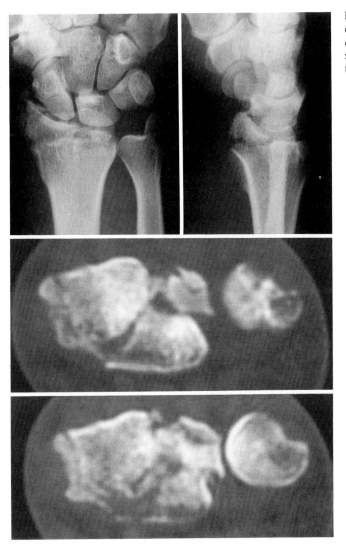

Figure 7.10. A complex compression articular fracture in a young sportsman. The computed tomogram demonstrates the dorsoulnar impaction and involvement of both the lunate and scaphoid facets.

neurologic dysfunction, we have generally found that early intervention is beneficial. The neurologic deficit should be documented by light touch and two-point discrimination prior to embarking on an operative procedure. Carpal tunnel pressure monitoring can also be useful (see Chapter 11). If dense sensory loss, demonstrable motor weakness, or an elevated carpal tunnel pressure measurement exists, release of the median nerve both in the carpal canal and in the distal forearm is recommended. If, however, demonstrable improvement occurs with longitudinal traction reducing the fracture deformity, the surgeon may elect to follow the patient's clinical signs and symptoms following definitive fracture care.

Treatment

In contradistinction to extraarticular bending fractures, which will often respond to conservative treatment (see Chapter 5), displaced or impacted compression fractures of the articular surface more often than not will require manipulative reduction and internal and/or external fixation to prevent redisplacement.[7–9,12,14–16,20,22,24,25,29,39,41,43,47,51]

In contrast to the shearing articular fractures (Chapter 6), treatment of articular compression fractures includes not only the restoration of the articular congruity but also correction of the metaphyseal angulation and maintenance of radial length with respect to the distal ulna.

Treatment approaches are based upon the recognition that compression fractures of the distal radius involve one or more fundamental components, including the radial styloid, the radial shaft, and the lunate facet, which can be split coronally into two units.[29]

Although the treatment of each fracture must be tailored to meet the specific features of the injury, some general concepts can be extended. If the fracture has a simple intraarticular component (two-part fracture) and no metaphyseal comminution, it will generally respond to closed manipulative reduction and percutaneous pinning. A percutaneous reduction may also be necessary in some instances of impaction of a dorsomedial articular fragment (Fig. 7.11A–F).

When the simple articular fracture is associated with comminution of the radial metaphysis (subgroup C3.2), external fixation and autogenous bone graft is the most effective method to prevent radial shortening. Unless there is a displaced anterior fragment, a dorsal surgical approach is preferred. The most commonly used approach is between the third and fourth extensor compartments. The fourth compartment is elevated subperiosteally to preserve its overall integrity. Through a transverse incision of the dorsal wrist capsule, the displaced and often impacted articular fragments can be well visualized and are elevated and reduced against the scaphoid and lunate. Following fixation of the bony fragments with Kirschner wires introduced transversely from the radial styloid towards the sigmoid notch, thus supporting the fragments with their meager subchondral bone, the metaphyseal defects are filled with compacted autogenous cancellous bone graft.

The possibility of associated soft tissue injury should be borne in mind. Through the dorsal capsulotomy, the scapholunate interosseous ligament should be inspected and probed, as associated scapholunate diastasis has been noted to occur in the presence of some articular compression injuries (Fig. 7.12A and B).[36] Similarly, once the radial articular fracture and metaphyseal defects have been reduced and securely held with Kirschner wires, the stability of the distal radioulnar joint must be assessed.

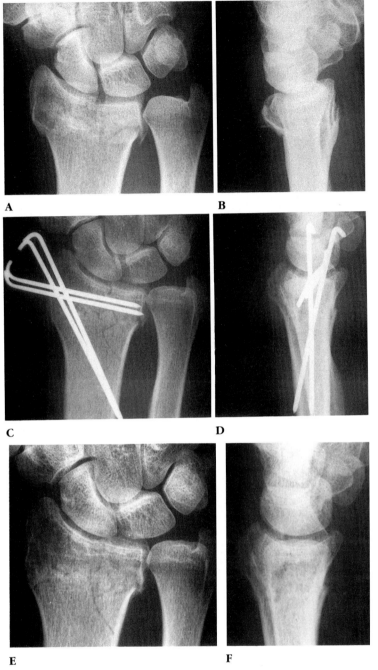

A   B

C   D

E   F

Figure 7.11. Manipulative reduction is often successful when one combines longitudinal traction, palmar flexion, and ulnar deviation. This is illustrated in this compression fracture in a 56-year-old woman. A,B. Antero-posterior and lateral x-rays of a two-part compression fracture. C,D. Following longitudinal traction and closed manipulation of the fracture, the anatomic reduction was secured with smooth Kirschner wires. E,F. The fracture healed with an anatomic restoration of the intra- and extraarticular fractures.

As a general rule, we tend to avoid the use of plates on the dorsal surface of the distal radius, preferring instead the use of Kirschner wires, autogenous bone graft, and external skeletal fixation. The major reason for this is the fact that current plate designs have a tendency to lead to irritation of the overlying extensor tendons, requiring a second surgical procedure for their removal.

For many three- and four-part articular fractures with an increasing amount of metaphyseal comminution, longitudinal traction and external fixation alone may not be adequate to reduce impacted small cartilage-bearing fragments or displaced and rotated volar lunate facet fractures. In these instances there will be a greater need for open reduction together with autogenous bone grafting. These injuries, as well, may be associated with soft tissue trauma, distal radioulnar joint instability, or carpal ligament disruption (Table 7.1).

Figure 7.12. Scapholunate diastasis may accompany compression fractures of the distal end of the radius. The "axial" scaphoid shift sign may identify this injury. A. The proximal carpal row contour shows a uniform radiographic arc. This is a sign of intercarpal stability, as the nondisrupted Shenton-Menard arc is for a stable hip. B. When traction is applied to the wrist with a scapholunate ligament tear, the scaphoid shifts distally, disrupting the "carpal Shenton's arc."

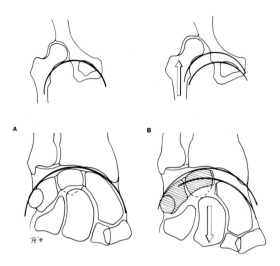

Table 7.1. Articular compression fractures: *general guidelines.*

Fracture type	Treatment
Two-part articular. Metaphysis not multifragmented	Closed reduction Percutaneous K-wire Cast
Two-part articular. Metaphysis multifragmented	Closed ± percutaneous reduction External fixation ± Autogenous bone graft
Three- or four-part articular. Metaphysis multifragmented	External fixation Open reduction Autogenous bone graft

Articular Two-Part (C1)

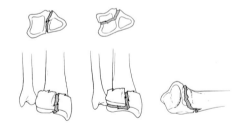

These "simple" compression fractures involve no more than two articular fragments without multifragmentation of the underlying metaphyseal bone. These would be considered under the group of C1 fractures (Fig. 7.6). Although these fractures can often be reduced by closed means—either with longitudinal traction or with manipulation—they have long been recognized to be extremely unstable when immobilized in plaster casts alone. It is for this reason that percutaneous pinning has assumed a central role in the management of these fractures.[2,7,18,22,41,43,44,50]

These fractures should be treated in the operating room with adequate anesthesia to permit a careful and controlled procedure. The involved limb as well as the iliac crest are prepped and draped in the event that autogenous bone graft will be required. With the image intensifier in position, a closed manipulative reduction is performed using longitudinal traction, palmar flexion of the wrist, and ulnar deviation of the hand and wrist. Alternatively, longitudinal traction may be more effectively gained using sterile finger traps or a small distractor (Fig. 7.13A and B). The latter devices are useful in freeing up the surgeon's hands for fragment manipulation and pinning.

When a radial styloid fragment is displaced, manipulation and fixation of this fragment should be addressed as the initial step. Reduction is likely to be successful through traction in ulnar deviation of the hand and wrist. The

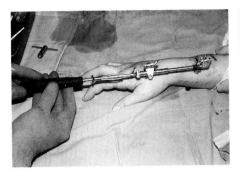 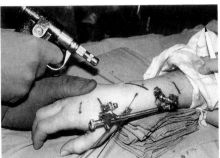

Figure 7.13. The use of a distractor applied to the second metacarpal and radius will provide longitudinal traction while allowing for the surgeon to simultaneously manipulate and percutaneously pin the articular fragments.

fragment is secured with one or two 0.62-inch smooth Kirschner wires driven obliquely from the volar radial tip of the styloid into the dorsal cortex of the radial shaft along its ulnar border (Fig. 7.14A–H). It is imperative that the Kirschner wires obtain a secure purchase in the cortex and the position of the reduction as well as of the Kirschner pins be confirmed using the image intensifier (Fig. 7.15).

When faced with a "die-punch" component to the lunate facet (subgroups C1.2 or C2.1) which can be anatomically reduced through the traction maneuvers, it is recommended that this fragment also be stabilized with the placement of percutaneous 0.62-inch smooth Kirschner wires directed transversely from the radial styloid aiming toward the sigmoid notch (Figs. 7.15 and 7.16). The wire is directed to lie just beneath the subchondral bone, in effect to "buttress" the reduced lunate facet fragment. Care is taken to avoid allowing the wire to penetrate into the distal radioulnar joint.

In the event that satisfactory reduction of the "die-punch" cannot be achieved by closed manipulative techniques, the fragment can be manipulated into position using a pointed awl or small elevator applied through a small (1–2 cm) incision. Intraoperative fluoroscopy is necessary both to guide the placement of the awl and to confirm the adequacy of the reduction (Fig. 7.17). When an impacted fragment is elevated, it is often useful to place autogenous bone graft into the deficit in the metaphyseal bone. As only small amounts of graft will be required, obtaining the bone graft from the iliac crest can be easily achieved using trephine biopsy needles, which will minimize the morbidity associated with using the iliac crest as a donor site (Fig. 7.18).

The two-part articular compression fracture may involve a sagittal split of the two main fragments (subgroup C1.3). In these instances, interfragmentary compression is possible using a large pointed bone reduction clamp (Fig. 7.14A–H). One point of the clamp is placed through a dorsomedial incision into the lunate facet fragment, while the other point grabs the radial styloid percutaneously. The fragments are gently compressed together, followed by the placement of transverse Kirschner wires (Fig. 7.19).

One can leave the Kirschner wires either outside the skin or cut sharply just beneath the skin. The advantage of the latter is primarily with regard to the possibility of pin tract inflammation, although the pins beneath the skin may tend to irritate adjacent sensory nerves or even the extensor tendons.

With the group C1 fractures, if the articular reduction can be achieved by closed means or with limited surgical exposure, and there is little soft tissue injury following application of the Kirschner wires, the fractures can be supported with an above-elbow plaster for 2 to 3 weeks, followed by a short-arm plaster for an additional 3 weeks. The pins are left in place a total of 8 weeks,

Figure 7.14. A three-part articular compression fracture is approached with following tactics: A. Following longitudinal traction, the styloid fragment is secured with smooth Kirschner wires. B,C,D. A displaced lunate impaction fragment can be elevated through a small dorsal incision using a pointed awl to push up the fragment. *(Figure continues on facing page.)*

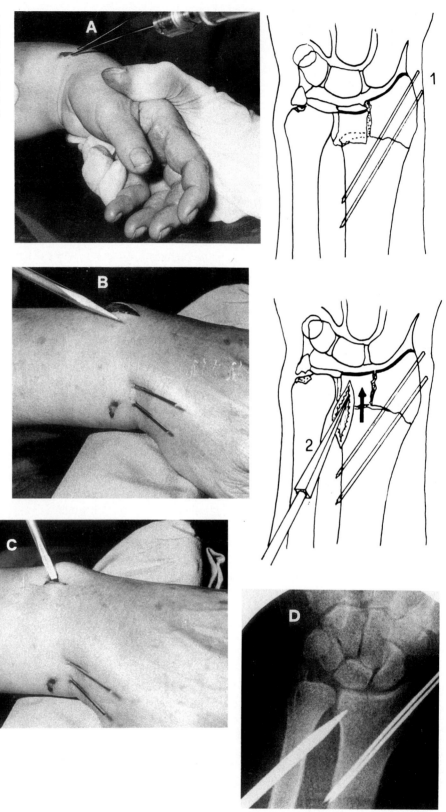

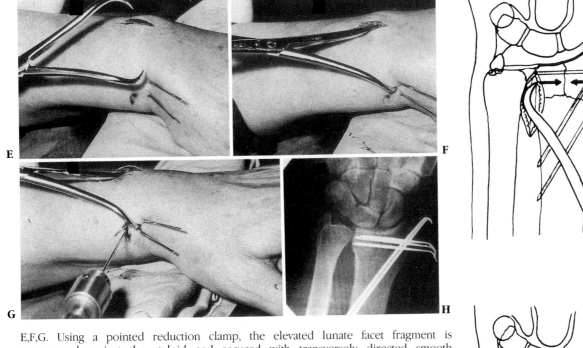

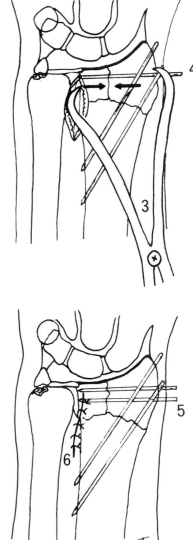

E,F,G. Using a pointed reduction clamp, the elevated lunate facet fragment is compressed against the styloid and secured with transversely directed smooth Kirschner wires. H. Secure fixation is achieved and the small wound closed with sutures.

Figure 7.15. Confirmation of the reduction of the articular fragments and position of the Kirschner wires is best accomplished with the image intensifier.

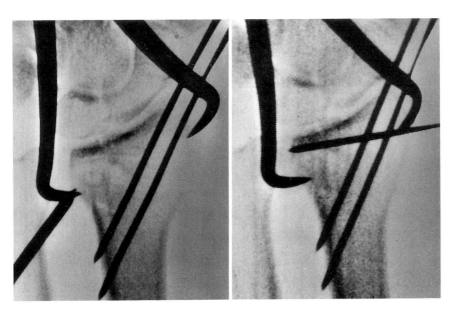

Figure 7.16. A two-part articular fracture in a 50-year-old woman was reduced with longitudinal traction and fragment manipulation. A,B. Initial anteroposterior lateral radiographs. C,D. Following reduction and pinning of the fragments, external skeletal fixation was applied because of massive soft tissue swelling. E,F. At 2 year follow-up, excellent alignment and function was present.

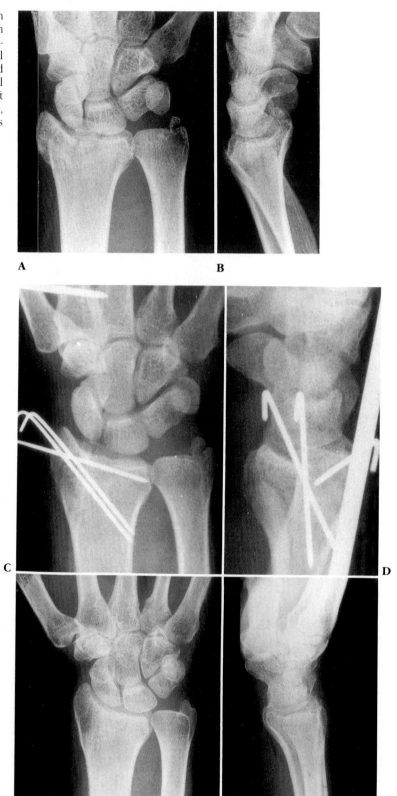

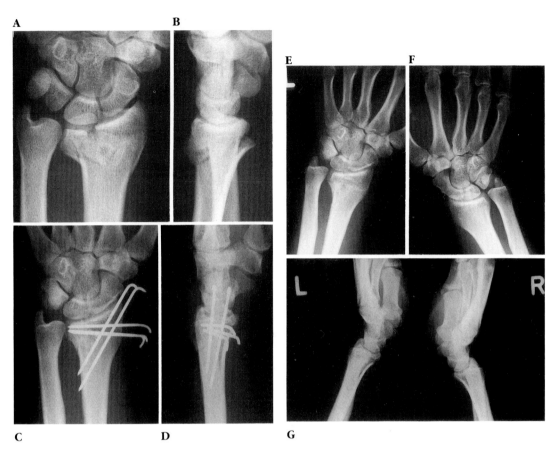

Figure 7.17. A two-part articular fracture with a displaced dorsomedial "die-punch" fragment in the left radius of a 45-year-old attorney. A,B. Anteroposterior and lateral x-rays of the displaced articular compression fracture. C,D. Stable fixation was achieved with smooth Kirschner wires following anatomic repositioning of the "die-punch" fragment. E–G. At 5-year follow-up, excellent function and a near-anatomic alignment can be seen when compared to the uninjured right radius.

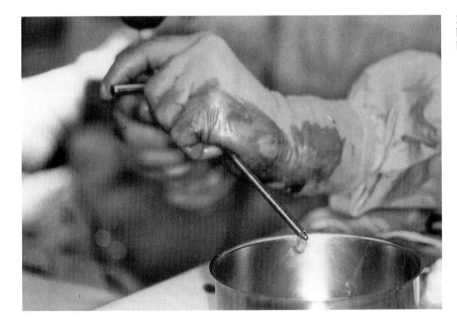

Figure 7.18. Ample autogenous iliac crest bone graft can be obtained using trephine biopsy needles.

Figure 7.19. A two-part articular fracture associated with metaphyseal comminution in a 65-year-old woman. A,B. Anteroposterior and lateral x-rays of the fracture revealing two major articular fragments and underlying metaphyseal comminution. C,D. Following longitudinal traction and application of an external fixateur, the styloid fragment was pinned and the lunate facet reduced using a pointed awl under image intensifier control. E,F. A 2.5-mm Schanz pin was used to buttress the lunate facet given the lack of metaphyseal support. Autogenous bone graft was also used. Note the axial scaphoid shift sign in this case.

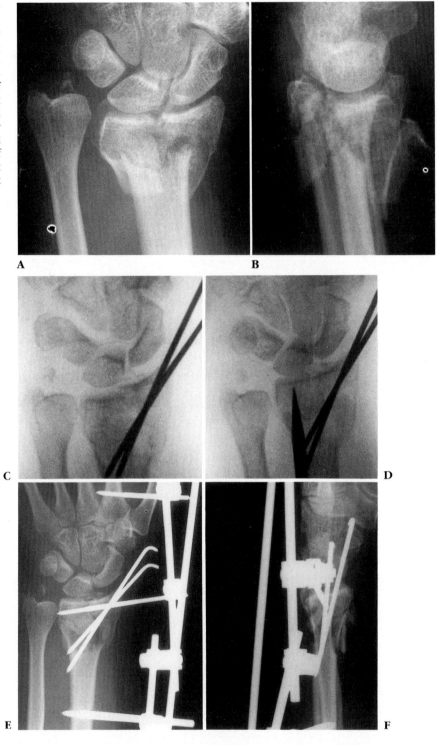

at which time they can be removed either in the clinic or using regional anesthesia.

In the event of soft tissue swelling and impaction of the articular fragments requiring elevation and bone grafting, as a general rule we prefer the use of external skeletal fixation. The external fixation can be left in place a minimum of 4 weeks and preferably 6 weeks—again with the internal pins left in place a total of 8 weeks.

Two-Part Articular Fractures with Metaphyseal Comminution (C2)

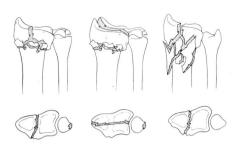

When the metaphyseal support of the articular fragments is further compromised by multifragmentation, there is a greater need for both external skeletal fixation and autogenous bone graft.[11,18,19,22,29] The bone graft supports the articular fragments, enhances the rapidity of healing, and permits earlier removal of the external fixation. Without this early support, it was not uncommon to see settling of the articular reduction as late as 8 to 12 weeks following fracture (Fig. 7.20). As described above, for the most part bone graft can be obtained using trephine core biopsy needles, and compact cancellous bone graft can be placed through very limited skin incisions.

On occasion, a fracture line in the frontal plane may require fixation with interfragmentary screws from the dorsal to the ulnar cortex (Fig. 7.21).

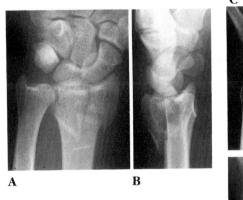

A   B

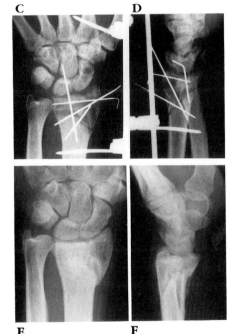

C   D

E   F

Figure 7.20. An articular compression fracture was reduced and held in external fixation. No bone graft was used, and the fracture settled following removal of the Kirschner wires and external fixation. A,B. Initial anteroposterior and lateral x-rays of the compression fracture with a suggestion of some metaphyseal multifragmentation. C,D. Excellent reduction was achieved. An external fixation device was left in place for 6 weeks and Kirschner wires for 8 weeks. E,F. Note the loss of radial length and ulnar inclination following removal of the fixation.

Complex Compression Articular Fractures (C3)

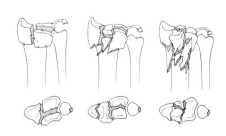

When the fracture pattern now involves the splitting of the lunate facet, reduction by closed or even percutaneous means becomes less predictable. The volar part of the so-called medial complex fracture has a tendency to rotate as longitudinal traction is applied. In these instances, open reduction through an anterior approach will be necessary.[1,19,22,23,26,30,32,45]

As with the two-part articular compression fractures, in most cases longitudinal traction will be helpful to restore axial length and realign the radial styloid fragments. External fixation will be extremely useful at this juncture to provide continuous traction during the operative intervention.

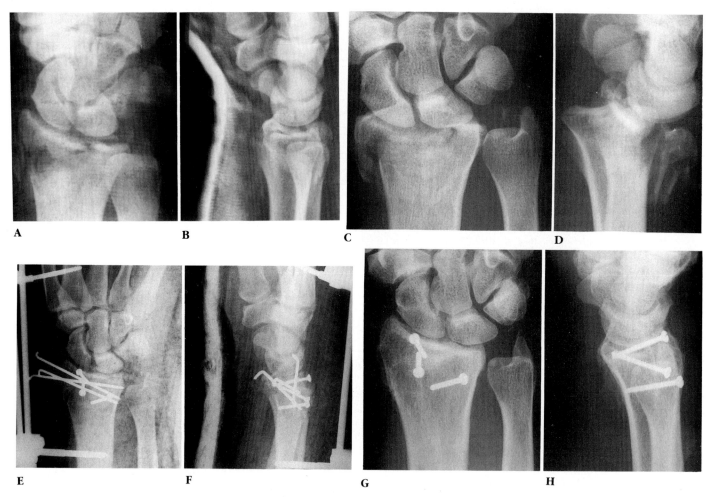

Figure 7.21. A more complex articular compression fracture with a major fracture line involving the styloid and lunate facet in the frontal plane. A,B. Initial anteroposterior and lateral x-rays of the displaced articular fracture. C,D. Following longitudinal traction in the emergency ward and a provisional splint, the fracture may be more readily appreciated. E,F. In the operating room, external fixation was applied. The styloid was secured using Kirschner wires and the frontal plane fracture was compressed with 2.7-mm screws. Autogenous bone graft was also placed in the metaphyseal defect. G,H. At 2-year following, the joint alignment is well maintained.

Figure 7.22. An extensile volar approach is recommended when exposing a displaced anterior articular fragment. The transverse retinacular ligament is opened, permitting added mobility to the flexor tendons and median nerve, which can be retracted radialward. The pronator quadratus need only be split part way.

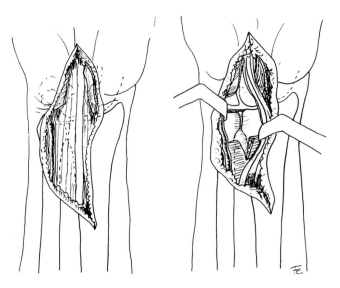

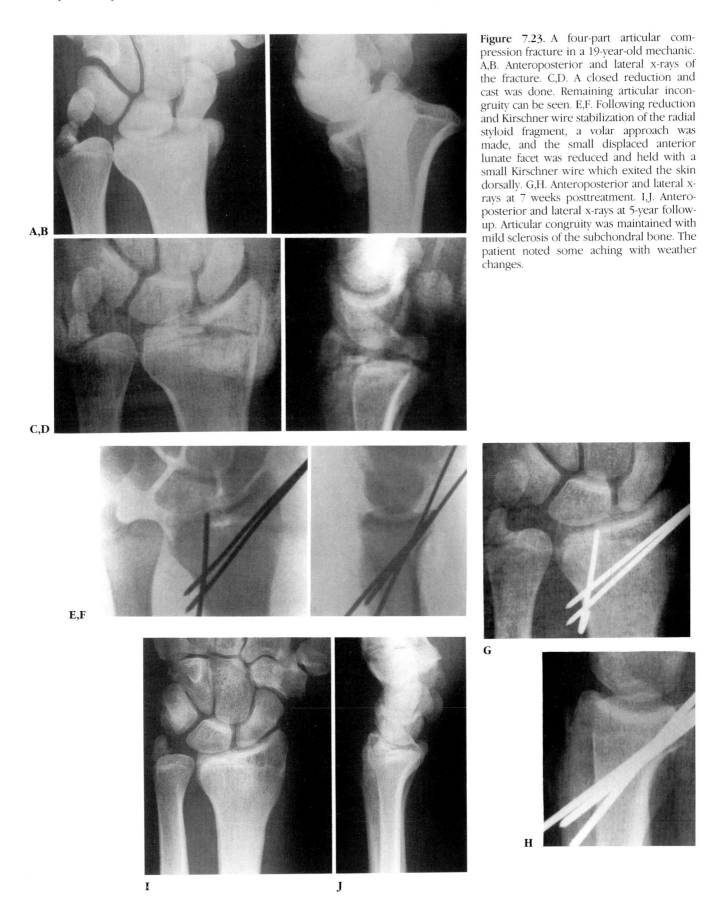

Figure 7.23. A four-part articular compression fracture in a 19-year-old mechanic. A,B. Anteroposterior and lateral x-rays of the fracture. C,D. A closed reduction and cast was done. Remaining articular incongruity can be seen. E,F. Following reduction and Kirschner wire stabilization of the radial styloid fragment, a volar approach was made, and the small displaced anterior lunate facet was reduced and held with a small Kirschner wire which exited the skin dorsally. G,H. Anteroposterior and lateral x-rays at 7 weeks posttreatment. I,J. Anteroposterior and lateral x-rays at 5-year follow-up. Articular congruity was maintained with mild sclerosis of the subchondral bone. The patient noted some aching with weather changes.

A,B

C,D

E,F

G

H

I   J

The radial styloid is stabilized with percutaneous pins, as previously described. Open reduction of the displaced volar fragment is recommended through an extensile approach (Fig. 7.22) (see Chapter 4).

The transverse retinacular ligament is opened and the interval between the ulnar artery and ulnar nerve developed. The distal border of the pronator quadratus is partially incised and elevated from the displaced volar-ulnar fragment. Reduction of the fragment is performed without additional soft tissue dissection, taking particular care to avoid disturbing the soft tissue attachments to this fragment, which include those of the triangular fibrocartilage complex as well as volar intracapsular ligaments. If the fragment is small, fixation is carried out with a single Kirschner wire introduced obliquely from the volar surface of the fragment across the metaphysis and retrieved through the dorsal skin of the forearm (Fig. 7.23). For most fragments, however, a small, 2.7-mm L or T plate is preferred to buttress the bony fragments (Figs. 7.24 and 7.25).

When this four-part articular pattern is associated with metaphyseal comminution, subgroup C3.2 external fixation and autogenous bone graft is the most effective method to prevent radial shortening (Fig. 7.26). As a general rule, we prefer this approach rather than plate fixation if the comminution extends primarily to the dorsal aspect of the distal radius, as plates in this region can prove problematic with the overlying tendons.

One should always be cautious in respecting the presence of soft tissue injury when dealing with these fractures.

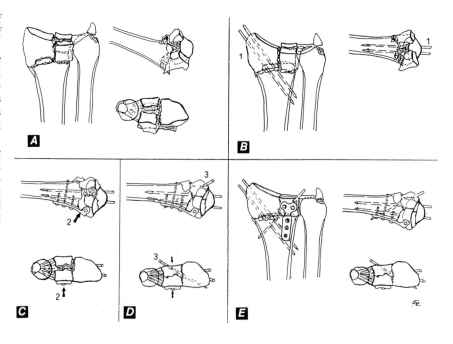

Figure 7.24. A schematic representation of the surgical tactics in the management of displaced four-part articular fractures (C3.1). A. The four-part fracture consists of the styloid fragment, split lunate facet, and radial metaphysis. B. The styloid fragment is initially reduced and secured by percutaneous smooth Kirschner wires (1). C. Attention is turned to the displaced anterior fragment which is exposed through a volar approach. With larger fragments, a small buttress plate is preferred (2). D. The dorsal lunate facet fragment (3) can be reduced by manipulation onto the buttressed anterior fragment and held with percutaneously placed Kirschner wires. E. The final completed surgical tactic.

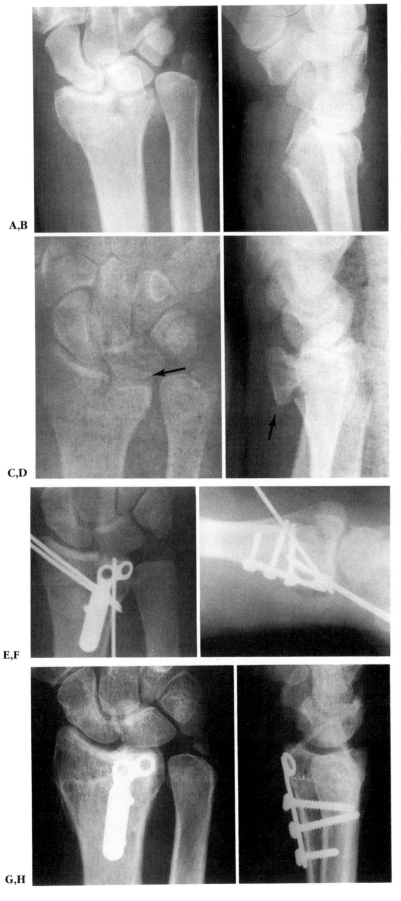

Figure 7.25. A displaced four-part articular compression fracture in a 48-year-old anesthesiologist. A,B. Anteroposterior and lateral x-rays of the initial fracture. C,D. Closed reduction and cast application was done. Note the displacement of the volar lunate facet fragment (arrow). E,F. Following reduction and percutaneous pinning of the radial styloid fragment, the volar fragment was reduced through an open technique. A small L plate was used to buttress the fragment. A provisional Kirschner wire was removed prior to wound closure. G,H. Anteroposterior and lateral x-rays at follow-up of 6 years. Slight distortion of the articular surface is evident. However, the radiocarpal articular space is well preserved. The patient is asymptomatic, although wrist motion is two-thirds of the uninjured wrist.

A,B

C,D

E,F

G,H

Figure 7.26. A multifragmented articular compression fracture with extensive soft tissue trauma associated with a high-speed motor vehicle accident in a 23-year-old. A,B. Anteroposterior and lateral x-rays of the initial fracture. Note the comminution extending into the articular surface. C,D. Following application of an external fixation device, the articular fragments were reduced through a small dorsal incision. Autogenous bone graft was placed in the metaphyseal defects. E,F. Anteroposterior and lateral x-rays at 8 weeks at the time of removal of the Kirschner wires. G,H. Anteroposterior and lateral x-rays at slightly more than 1 year follow-up. The patient had only 50 percent of wrist motion and weakened grip strength. I,J. Anteroposterior and lateral x-rays at 6 years. The patient was asymptomatic and had regained normal grip strength and 80 percent of wrist mobility.

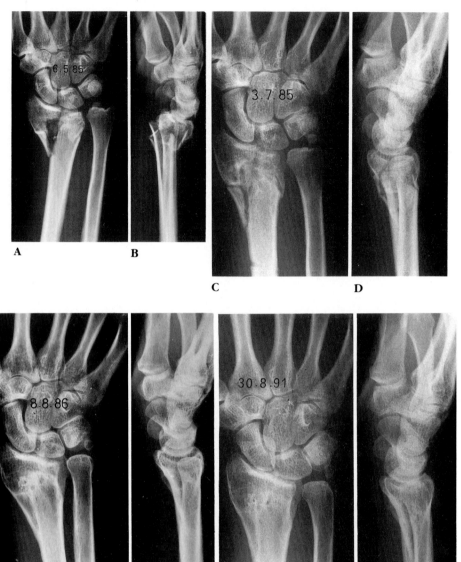

Compression Fractures: Postoperative Management

Depending upon whether or not the fracture is associated with concomitant soft tissue or ipsilateral skeletal injury, the treatment will vary from case to case. For those fractures treated by closed reduction and percutaneous pinning (group C1) without associated soft tissue swelling, a sugar tong splint is preferred for the first 2 weeks postoperatively. At that juncture, any sutures can be removed and immobilization continued with either a Muenster-type cast or a short-arm cast. If the percutaneous pins are left protruding from the skin, it is safer to create a window over the pins to avoid abrasions from the cast as well as to allow for local pin care. As with all distal radius fractures, the patients must be encouraged to mobilize their digits and attention taken to monitor any swelling that might impede digital rehabilitation. With most group C1 fractures, immobilization need only be 5 to 6 weeks. At that point, the cast can be removed but the pins left in place for an additional 2 weeks. During this time, a removable thermoplast splint is provided for support and comfort.

When an external fixator is used, digital rehabilitation must be encouraged from the onset. It is recommended to place the external fixation device to hold the wrist in a neutral position to facilitate tendon excursion. If for some reason or another the wrist was initially placed in a flexed and/or ulnar deviation position, it is advisable to change this position at 3 weeks to facilitate the digital rehabilitation. Again, with those fractures which have had percutaneous pinning or open reduction and internal fixation, it is advisable to remove the external fixation device at 5 to 6 weeks following application and apply a removable thermoplast splint for an additional 2 weeks (Fig. 7.27).

If the compression fracture is associated with a large ulnar styloid fracture with or without instability, or if a primary repair of the triangular fibrocartilage has been performed, we will choose to immobilize the forearm in approximately 45 degrees of supination for a total of 3 weeks to permit the initial healing of the soft tissue restraints about the distal radioulnar joint.

Should a repair have been undertaken of the scapholunate interosseous ligament, a more lengthy immobilization is suggested to extend a total of 8 weeks postoperatively. If, however, the associated carpal injury was a fracture that could be stably secured with internal fixation, functional wrist mobilization is begun at 5 to 6 weeks following the onset of treatment. Again, active digital mobilization should be highlighted during the postoperative period. Following fixator removal, a removable thermoplast splint would be advisable to provide additional wrist support and comfort for several weeks while the patient develops security following his or her external skeletal support.

Outcome

One of us (DLF) has compiled a clinical experience of 40 patients with articular fractures of the distal radius in which restoration of the joint surface could not be achieved solely by closed manipulative reduction or joint distraction. These patients were treated with either percutaneous pinning or open reduction. The average age in this series was 37 years and the follow-up period averaged 4 years (range, 2–8 years). Twenty-six patients were male and 14 were female. The fractures were divided into nine simple articular fractures and 31 complex articular fractures (Table 7.2). Four of the fractures were open and 36 were closed. Restoration of the articular congruity was achieved in 21 patients with percutaneous reduction. Of these, 17 were stabilized with percutaneous pinning and 4 by percutaneous pinning combined with an external fixator. The remaining 19 patients were treated with open reduction, of which 9 had internal fixation with Kirschner wires, 5 a combination of Kirschner wires and external fixation, and 5 had external fixation alone. Eleven of the 19 patients with open reduction had additional bone grafting of the metaphyseal defect. Two patients had a volar buttress plate applied to support a displaced anteromedial fragment.

Figure 7.27. A four-part articular compression fracture in a 60-year-old teacher. A,B. Initial fracture was seen on anteroposterior and lateral radiographs. C,D. Following longitudinal traction and external fixation. Note residual articular incongruity. E,F. Through a dorsal approach, the fragments were elevated and supported with smooth Kirschner wires and autogenous iliac crest bone graft. G,H. Radiographs at 5 weeks at the time of external fixation removal. (*Figure continues on facing page.*)

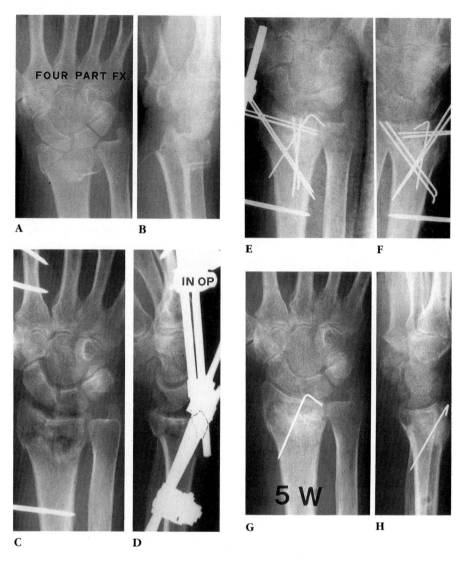

The preoperative and postoperative radiographs were assessed to include measurements of the inclination of the articular surface in both the sagittal and frontal planes, the radial shortening, and articular congruity. The radiographic follow-up showed that the fractures in 28 patients had healed with an average volar tilt of 5.6 degrees. In 4 there was no volar tilt and in 8 a residual mean dorsal tilt of 8.8 degrees. The ulnar tilt for all 40 patients averaged 18.5 degrees. Loss of correction between the postoperative and follow-up radiographs was observed in 11 patients. Importantly, these were found in cases that had metaphyseal comminution which were treated by percutaneous pinning alone with cast fixation. In contrast, the external fixator group had no loss of initial reduction observed at the time of removal of the fixator. Of the 11 patients who were noted to have loss of correction, 8 had minimal loss of the initial volar tilt, ranging from 2 to 5 degrees, while one had secondary displacement of a postoperative dorsal tilt of 2 degrees to a follow-up value of 6 degrees. Two elderly patients with a neutral postoperative tilt developed a dorsal tilt of 8 and 9 degrees. In the frontal plane, a minimal loss of correction ranging from 2 to 5 degrees was observed in 10 patients.

When the articular congruity was assessed in the follow-up radiographs, 25 patients showed no articular step-off. Fifteen others showed a joint depression

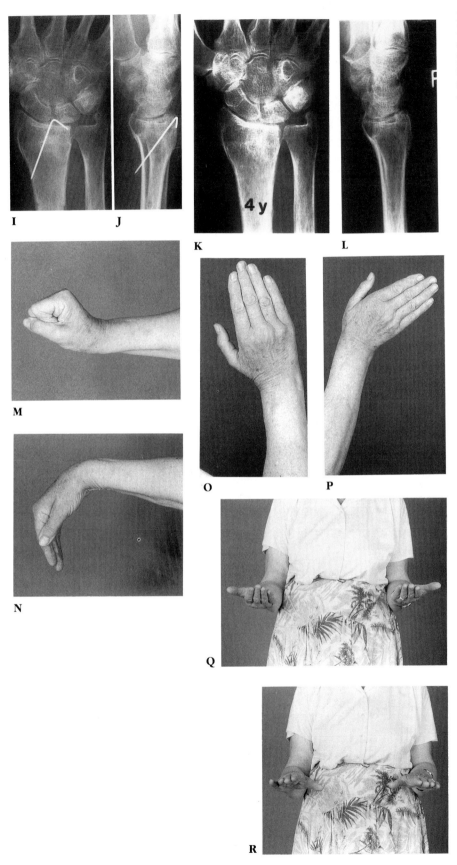

I,J Follow-up radiographs at 2 years. K,L. Follow-up radiographs at 4 years. M,N. Wrist extension and flexion at follow-up of 4 years. O,P. Wrist radial and ulnar deviation at follow-up of 4 years. Q,R. Forearm supination and pronation at follow-up of 4 years.

Table 7.2. Results of operative treatment of compression fractures.

Case	Year of treatment	Age (years)/sex	Fracture classification (Fig. 1)	Open (O)/closed (C)	Additional injuries	Type of treatment[d]	After treatment[c]	Time of immobilization	Preop Volar tilt (deg)	Preop Dorsal tilt (deg)	Preop Articular gap (mm)	Preop Articular step-off (mm)	Preop Radioulnar index (mm)	Post Volar tilt (deg)	Post Dorsal tilt (deg)	Post Ulnar tilt (deg)	Post Articular gap (mm)	Post Articular step-off (mm)	Post Radioulnar index (mm)	FU Volar tilt (deg)	FU Dorsal tilt (deg)	FU Ulnar tilt (deg)	FU Articular gap (mm)	FU Articular step-off (mm)	FU Radioulnar index (mm)	Time until union (weeks)	Extension	Flexion	Ulnar	Radial	Pronation	Supination	Power grip % loss	Key pinch % loss	Digital motion TAM (index)	Pain[b]	Working ability (%)	Complications	Occupation
1	1979	40 M	B₁₋₂	O		ORIF	STS	3		10	0	4	−1	5		15	0	0	−1	5		15	0	0	−1	6													
2	1979	20 M	B₁₋₁	C		ORIF	UPS	3	8		1	0	0	8		14	0	0	0	8		14	0	0	0	3													
3	1979	24 M	C₁₋₁	C		PRPP	VPB	4		32	0	0	6	2		22	0	0	3	3		20	0	0	3	4													
4	1979	35 F	C₁₋₂	C		PRPP	VPS	4		20	2	2	0		4	20	0	0	0		6	20	0	0	0	4													
5	1980	23 M	C₁₋₂	C		ORIF	VPS	4		7	2	2	0		2	22	0	0	0		7	11	1	0	0	5													
6	1980	28 M	C₁₋₁	C		PRPP	VPS	4		8	2	0	3	8		19	0	0	0	8		19	0	0	0	4													
7	1981	29 M	C₁₋₁	C		PRPP	VPS	4		22	2	0	2	5		25	1	0	0			23	1	0	1	4													
8	1981	24 M	C₁₋₁	C		PRPP	VPS	4		35	2	0	6	10		20	0	0	0	5		20	0	0	0	4													
9	1981	33 F	C₁₋₁	C		PRPP	VPS	4		24	2	0	2	4		16	0	0	−2	10		15	0	0	−2	4													
10	1982	20 M	B₂₋₃	O	*	ORIF	STS	4		0	0	3	0	4		24	0	0	−2	2		20	0	0	−2	4	70	60	30	13	80	85	10	5	245	None	100		Mechanic
11	1982	18 M	C₁₋₁	O		PRPP	VPS	4		14	1	0	0	5		26	0	0	0	5		22	1	0	0	4	70	55	30	12	80	85	15	5	245	None	100		Student
12	1982	38 M	C₁₋₂	C		PRPP	VPS	4		20	2	0	0	8		20	0	0	0			20	0	0	1	4	60	65	25	8	80	80	5	10	235	None	100		Mason
13	1982	28 M	C₁₋₂	C		PRPP	VPS	4		25	0	3	8	8	0	22	0	0	−1	3	0	10	0	0	+1	4	70	50	30	11	85	80	10	5	250	None	100		Painter
14	1982	22 M	C₃₋₁	C		PRPP (EF)	EF	6		14	1	0	−1	0	0	18	0	0	−2	0	0	20	0	0	−1	6	60	60	25	11	85	65	15	20	210	None	100		Police officer
15	1983	35 F	B₁₋₂	C		PRPP	VPS	4		30	0	0	0	8		26	0	0	0	8		26	0	0	0	4	65	60	25	11	85	80	10	5	245	None	100	Pintrack	Housewife
16	1983	18 M	C₁₋₁	C		PRPP	VPS	4		22	3	3	4	7		17	1	0	1	5		17	1	1	1	5	65	55	25	7	75	85	15	10	250	None	100		Farmer
17	1984	22 M	C₃₋₂	C		OREF (BG)	EF	6		14	6	5	0		7	20	2	1	0		17	20	2	1	0	6	70	50	30	11	85	80	10	5	250	Moderate	100		Truck driver
18	1984	20 M	B₂₋₂	C		ORIF (EF)	EF	6		5	0	4	2	7		20	1	0	4	7		20	1	0	4	6	60	65	25	6	65	65	10	15	265	None	100		Pianist
19	1984	19 M	B₁₋₁	C		ORIF	VPS	3	20		1	1	0	10		20	0	0	0	8		20	0	0	0	3	70	60	30	13	85	75	10	15	240	None	100		Mason
20	1984	27 M	B₂₋₂	C		ORIF	VPS	3		10	1	2	0	10	0	25	0	0	0	10	0	25	0	0	0	3	70	60	30	13	85	75	10	15	245	None	100	Pintracks (2)	Machine operator
21	1984	33 F	C₂₋₁	C		PRPP (EF)	EF	6		20	0	3	4	0	0	15	0	0	−2	0	0	15	0	0	1	6	60	55	20	6	75	75	10	5	250	None	100		Nurse
22	1984	61 F	C₁₋₁	C		PRPP	VPS	4		15	2	0	3	5		18	0	0	0	5		20	0	0	0	4	55	65	25	9	75	75	10	10	220	None	100		Housewife
23	1985	48 F	C₃₋₂	O	*	OREF (BG)	EF	7		15	5	6	0	3		18	0	0	−3	3	18	18	1	0	−3	7	60	60	25	11	75	75	20	10	240	Moderate	100		Housewife

No.	Year	Age/Sex	Class	C/O		Treatment[c,d]																											Pain[b]	Score	Complications	Occupation
24	1985	31 M	C$_{3-2}$	C		OREF (BG)	EF	7	15	4	5	5	10	18	0	0	−2	10	18	0	2	−2	8	60	55	25	7	70	70	5	15	240	Moderate	100		Carpenter
25	1985	46 M	B$_{2-2}$	C	**	ORIF BG, EF	EF	6	20	0	2	0	5	25	0	0	−2	25	0	0	2	6	65	60	30	7	80	65	15	10	260	None	100		Gym teacher
26	1985	25 M	C$_{1-1}$	C		PRPP	VPS	4	10	4	2	4	10	22	0	0	0	20	0	0	0	4	55	70	30	13	75	65	10	10	260	None	100		Mason
27	1985	32 M	C$_{1-2}$	C		PRPP (EF)	EF	6	15	0	5	4	10	12	1	0	0	10	1	0	0	6	55	65	25	10	80	70	20	10	250	Mild	100		Clerk
28	1985	70 M	C$_{1-1}$	C		PRPP	VPS	4	32	0	3	5	5	25	1	0	−1	25	1	0	−1	4	60	60	20	11	80	70	20	10	250	Mild	100		Retiree
29	1986	25 M	C$_{3-2}$	C		ORIF (BG)	VPS	4	35	1	2	−1	5	22	0	0	0	10	0	0	0	4	65	55	25	8	85	85	9	25	240	None	100 CTS		Electrician
30	1986	63 F	C$_{3-1}$	C		PRPP	VPS	4	36	2	2	9	0	16	0	0	2	9	16	0	0	2	4	60	65	25	10	80	70	15	10	235	None	100	Housewife
31	1986	56 F	C$_{3-1}$	C		PRPP	VPS	4	25	2	2	4	0	15	0	0	0	8	15	0	9	3	5	60	44	20	10	70	65	25	20	240	None	100	Housewife
32	1986	70 F	C$_{3-2}$	C		PRPP	VPS	4	30	3	2	18	10	15	2	2	4	10	15	1	1	7	1	60	55	25	12	65	70	20	10	240	None	100	Housewife
33	1986	30 M	B$_{2-2}$	C		ORIF BG, EF	EF	6	45	0	6	2	10	20	1	0	3	20	1	0	−3	6	80	75	30	15	90	90	5	10	260	None	100	Farmer
34	1986	63 F	C$_{2-3}$	C		OREF (BG)	EF	8	5	2	0	8	5	15	0	1	2	5	15	0	1	2	8	60	65	25	6	80	75	15	5	235	Mild	100 Neuroma	Housewife
35	1986	62 F	C$_{3-3}$	O	**	OREF (BG)	EF	6	15	0	3	0	0		0	0	0	0	10	0	0	0	6	60	50	25	7	70	70	25	10	255	None	100	Secretary
36	1986	73 F	C$_{3-1}$	C		ORIF BG, EF	EF	6	35	2	1	3	5	18	0	0	−1	18	0	0	0	6	55	50	15	51	55	45	35	35	190	Severe	50 OA	Housewife
37	1986	54 F	C$_{3-1}$	C		ORIF	VPS	4	32	1	1	7	5	18	1	0	0	3	18	1	0	2	4	55	55	25	9	75	65	10	10	260	None	100	Housewife
38	1986	39 M	C$_{3-2}$	C		ORIF (BG)	VPS	5	0	0	3	2	5	18	1	0	0	2	18	1	0	0	5	55	65	20	9	75	70	10	20	235	None	100	Manager
39	1986	44 M	C$_{3-1}$	C		ORIF (BG)	EF	4	0	1	2	5	5	12	0	0	0	5	12	0	0	0	4	60	60	25	8	75	75	15	5	230	None	100	Housewife
40	1986	37 M	C$_{2-1}$	C		PRPP (EF)	EF	7	5	4	7	6	6	17	3	2	2	6	17	3	2	2	7	60	50	15	9	60	40	50	30	200	Severe	50 OA, Pintracks (2)	Computer operator

* Ulnar head
** Ulnar shaft
*** Damage

OA, Osteoarthritis; CTS, carpal tunnel syndrome

a The radiographic measurements were made according to Castaing's modification of the method of Gartland and Werley. Radial deviation of the articular surface of the radius is defined as the difference between the average ulnar tilt (25°) and the radial inclination of the tilted articular surface with respect to the perpendicular to the radial shaft in the frontal plane. A negative value for ulnar tilt means that there is no ulnar inclination of the articular surface of the radius, but instead there is radial inclination so that the radial articular surface forms a negative angle with respect to the perpendicular of the radial shaft

b Pain in the wrist was graded as mild, moderate, or severe. Mild pain was present only at the extremes of the active range of motion of the wrist, and the patient was neither physically nor psychologically disturbed by the pain; moderate pain occurred during heavy manual labor and caused the patient to be disturbed physically, psychologically, or both; severe pain occurred during activities of daily living and even at rest

c STS, Sugar-tong splint; VPS, volar plaster splint; EF, external fixation

d PRPP, Percutaneous reduction, percutaneous pinning; ORIF, open reduction and internal fixation; OREF, open reduction and external fixation; (BG), bone grafting; (EF), external fixation

ranging between 1 and 3 mm. Of these 15 patients, 12 had joint depression of 1 mm, 2 had 2 mm, and one patient 3 mm. Thus 37 of the 40 patients had an articular depression of 1 mm or less at late follow-up.

At late follow-up, 12 patients exhibited radial shortening on follow-up x-rays ranging from 1 to 7 mm. In 10 of these 12 patients, the shortening did not exceed more than 3 mm.

Thirty-one of the 40 patients were evaluated for functional capacity at late follow-up. Of these, 15 had percutaneous joint reduction and 16 had an open reduction of the distal articular surface. The overall mean range of motion of the wrist for the patients reviewed was 62.5 degrees of extension (range, 55–80 degrees); 59.5 degrees of flexion (range, 50–75 degrees); 77 degrees of forearm pronation (range, 55–85 degrees); 72.5 degrees of forearm supination (range, 40–90 degrees); 25 degrees of ulnar deviation (range, 15–30 degrees); and 9.5 degrees of radial deviation (range, 5–15 degrees). The average loss of grip strength was 15 percent (range, 5–50 percent), the average loss of power pinch was 13 percent, and the average digital motion for all patients measured by the Total Active Movement Index was 240 degrees. Among these 31 patients, occasional mild pain was present in 3, moderate pain in 4, and severe pain in 2. Subjective complaints and functional results demonstrated a direct correlation with the radiographic findings. It was found that a residual dorsal tilt was responsible for loss of palmar flexion and a radial shortening of more than 4 mm associated with decreased forearm rotation. Radiocarpal pain with articular incongruity was detected in 3 of the 4 patients with residual moderate pain and in one of the 2 patients with severe pain. Of the latter 2 patients, one developed a rapid posttraumatic arthrosis with narrowing of the joint space in spite of an anatomic reduction of the articular surface. Ultimately this patient required a total wrist arthroplasty 2 years following injury. The rapid onset and progression of the arthrosis in this patient with an anatomically reduced joint space would suggest either that there was a major articular injury at the time of the trauma or that a subclinical low-grade infection occurred following the open reduction (Case 36). The other patient who developed substantial articular changes demonstrated proximal migration of the lunate as a result of settling of the dorsomedial fragment with an articular step-off of 3 mm (Case 40).

With the exception of the 2 patients with complaints of severe pain, all of the patients returned to their prior occupation without any disability noted for their work requirements. Additionally, none complained of limitation on activities of daily living.

Additional problems that should be noted included one patient who required later release of the median nerve in the carpal tunnel, 5 patients who were treated for pin tract infections which resolved with removal of the pins, and one iatrogenic lesion of a branch of the superficial radial nerve.

The conclusions when reviewing this group of patients confirm the fact that anatomic reduction of the joint surface as well as prevention of secondary

Table 7.3. Articular compression fractures.

Pitfalls	Pearls
Inadequate reduction "die-punch" fragment	Percutaneous elevation with pointed awl. Use of large pointed reduction clamp
Displaced anterior lunate facet fragments	Open reduction with volar ulnar approach, buttress plate, and bone graft
Late loss of articular reduction	Autogenous bone graft. Leave Kirschner wire for minimum of 8 weeks

intraarticular displacement not only will lead to functional outcome but also will avoid problems of posttraumatic arthrosis. In this particular group of patients, in whom anatomic reduction of the joint surface could not be obtained by closed manipulation alone, half the patients had their articular realignment achieved with percutaneous manipulation and the other half with open reduction (Table 7.3).

References

1. Axelrod TS, Mcmurtry RY: Open reduction and internal fixation of comminuted intraarticular fractures of the distal radius. *J Hand Surg* 15A: 1–10, 1990.
2. Axelrod TS, Paley D, Green J, Mcmurtry RY: Limited open reduction of the lunate facet in comminuted intraarticular fractures of the distal radius. *J Hand Surg* 13A: 372–377, 1988.
3. Bartosh RA, Saldaña MJ: Intraarticular fractures of the distal radius. A cadaveric study to determine if ligamentotaxis restores palmar tilt. *J Hand Surg* 15A: 18–21, 1990.
4. Bradway J, Amadio PC, Cooney WP III: Open reduction and internal fixation of displaced, comminuted intraarticular fractures of the distal end of the radius. *J Bone Joint Surg [Am]* 71A: 839–847, 1989.
5. Callendar GW: Fractures injuring joints. Fractures interfering with the movements at the wrist and with those of pronation and supination. Saint Banthdomewis Hospital Reports, pp. 281–298, 1865.
6. Castaing J: Les fractures récentes de l'extrémité inférieure du radius chez l'adulte. *Rev Chir Orthop* 50: 581–696, 1964.
7. Clancey CJ: Percutaneous Kirschner wire fixation of Colles' fractures: A prospective study of thirty-two cases. *J Bone Joint Surg [Am]* 66A: 1008–1014, 1984.
8. Clyburn TA: Dynamic external fixation for comminuted intraarticular fractures of the distal end of the radius. *J Bone Joint Surg [Am]* 69A: 248–254, 1987.
9. Cole JM, Obletz BE: Comminuted fractures of the distal end of the radius treated by skeletal transfixion in plaster cast: An end-result study of thirty-three cases. *J Bone Joint Surg [Am]* 48A: 931–945, 1966.
10. Colles A: On the fracture of the carpal extremity of the radius. *Edinburgh Med Surg J* 10: 181–184, 1814.
11. Cooney WP III: Distal radial fractures: External fixation. In: *Fractures of the Hand and Wrist*, edited by Barton NJ Edinburgh, London, Melbourne, New York: Churchill Livingstone, 1988, pp. 290–301.
12. Cooney WP III, Linscheid RL, Dobyns JH: External pin fixation for unstable Colles' fractures. *J Bone Joint Surg [Am]* 61A: 840–845, 1979.
13. Cotton FJ: Fractures of the lower end of the radius. *Ann Surg* 32: 194–218, 1900.
14. DePalma AF: Comminuted fractures of the distal end of the radius treated by ulnar pinning. *J Bone Joint Surg [Am]* 34A: 651–662, 1952.
15. Dowling JJ, Sawyer B Jr: Comminuted Colles' fractures. Evaluation of a method of treatment. *J Bone Joint Surg [Am]* 43A: 657–668, 1961.
16. Edwards GS: Intraarticular fractures of the distal part of the radius. Treatment with the small AO external fixator. *J Bone Joint Surg. [Am]* 73A: 1241–1250, 1991.
17. Fernandez DL: Avant-bras segment distal. In: *Classification AO des Fractures des Os Longs*, edited by Müller ME, Nazarian S, Koch P. Berlin, Heidelberg, New York: Springer-Verlag, 1987, pp. 106–115.
18. Fernandez DL: Current management of intraarticular fractures of the distal radius. In: *Wrist Disorders*, edited by Nakamura R and Linscheid R. Tokyo: Springer-Verlag, 1993.
19. Fernandez DL, Geissler WB: Treatment of displaced articular fractures of the radius. *J Hand Surg* 16A: 375–384, 1991.
20. Fernandez DL, Jakob RP, Büchler U: External fixation of the wrist. Current indications and techniques. *Ann Chir Gyn* 72: 298–302, 1983.
21. Gartland JJ, Werley CW: Evaluation of healed Colles' fractures. *J Bone Joint Surg. [Am]* 33A: 895–907, 1951.
22. Geissler WB, Fernandez DL: Percutaneous and limited open reduction of the articular surface of the distal radius. *J Orthop Trauma* 5: 255–264, 1991.
23. Hastings H II, Leibovic S: Indications and techniques of open reduction: Internal fixation of distal radius fractures. *Orthop Clin North Am* 24: 309–326, 1993.
24. Huresh Z, Volpin G, Hoener D, Stein H: The surgical treatment of severe comminuted intraarticular fractures of the distal radius. *Clin Orthop Rel Res* 263: 147–153, 1991.

25. Jakim I, Pieterse HS, Sweet MBE: External fixation for intraarticular fractures of the distal radius. *J Bone Joint Surg [Am]* 73B: 302–306, 1991.

26. Jupiter JB, Lipton H: The operative treatment of intraarticular fractures of the distal radius. *Clin Orthop Rel Res* 292: 1–14, 1993.

27. Knirk JL, Jupiter JB: Intraarticular fractures of the distal end of the radius in young adults. *J Bone Joint Surg [Am]* 68A: 647–659, 1986.

28. Kopylov P, Johnell O, Redlund-Johnell I, Bengner U: Fractures of the distal end of the radius in young adults: A 30-year follow-up. *J Hand Surg* 18B: 45–49, 1993.

29. Leung KS, Shen WY, Tsang HK, Chiu KH, Leung PC, Hung LK: An effective treatment of comminuted fracture of the distal radius. *J Hand Surg* 15A: 11–17, 1990.

30. Melone CP Jr: Open treatment for displaced articular fractures of the distal radius. *Clin Orthop Rel Res* 202: 103–111, 1986.

31. Melone CP Jr: Distal radius fractures: Patterns of articular fragmentation. *Orthop Clin North Am* 24: 239–254, 1993.

32. Missakian ML, Cooney WP III, Amadio PC, Glidewell HL: Open reduction and internal fixation for distal radius fractures. *J Hand Surg* 17A: 745–755, 1992.

33. Mortier JP, Baux S, Uhl JF, Mimoun M, Mole B: L'importance du fragment postero-interne et son brochage spécifique dans les fractures de l'extremité inférieur. *Ann Chir Main* 2: 219–229, 1983.

34. Mortier JP, Kuhlmann JN, Richet C, Baux S: Brochage horizontal cubito-radial dans les fractures de l'extremité inférieure du radius comportent un fragment postero-interne. *Rev Chir Orthop* 72: 567–571, 1986.

35. Morton R: A radiographic survey of 170 cases clinically diagnosed as "Colles' fracture." *Lancet* March: 731–732, 1907.

36. Mudgal CS, Jones WA: Scapholunate diastasis: A component of fractures of the distal radius. *J Hand Surg* 15B: 503–505, 1990.

37. Petit JL: *Complete Works of J.L. Petit.* Paris, 1844.

38. Pilcher LS: Fractures of the lower extremity or base of the radius. *Ann Surg* 65: 1–25, 1917.

39. Porter ML, Tillman RM: Pilon fractures of the wrist. *J Hand Surg* 17B: 63–68, 1992.

40. Pouteau C: *Oeuvres posthumes de M. Pouteau. Mémoire, contenant quelques réflexions sur quelques fractures de l'avant-bras sur les luxations incomplètes du poignet et sur le diastasis.* Paris: Ph-D Pierres, 1783.

41. Raskin KB, Melone CP Jr: Unstable articular fractures of the distal radius: Comparative techniques of ligamentotaxis. *Orthop Clin North Am* 24: 275–286, 1993.

42. Rogers SC: An analysis of Colles' fracture. *Br Med J* 1: 807–809, 1944.

43. Scheck M: Long-term follow-up of treatment of comminuted fractures of the distal end of the radius by transfixation with Kirschner wires and cast. *J Bone Joint Surg [Am]* 44A: 337–351, 1962.

44. Seitz WH, Froimson AI, Leb R, Shapiro JD: Augmented external fixation of unstable distal radius fracture. *J Hand Surg* 16A: 1010–1016, 1991.

45. Seitz WH, Putnam MD, Dick HM: Limited open surgical approach for external fixation of distal radius fractures. *J Hand Surg* 15A: 288–293, 1990.

46. Stevens JH: Compression fractures of the lower end of the radius. *Ann Surg* 71: 594–618, 1920.

47. Szabo RM, Weber SC: Comminuted intraarticular fractures of the distal radius. *Clin Orthop Rel Res* 230: 39–48, 1988.

48. Villar RN, March D: Three years after Colles' fracture. A prospective review. *J Bone Joint Surg [Am]* 69B: 635–638, 1987.

49. Voillemire: *Arch Gen Med* 13: 261, 1842.

50. Wagner HE, Jakob RP: Operative Behandlung der distalen Radiusfrakturen mit Fixateur externe. *Unfallchirurgie* 88: 473–480, 1985.

51. Weber SC, Szabo RM: Severely comminuted distal radius fractures as an unsolved problem: Complications associated with external fixation and pins and plaster techniques. *J Hand Surg* 11A: 157–165, 1986.

Chapter Eight

Radiocarpal Fracture-Dislocation

co-authored with Richard Ghillani, M.D.

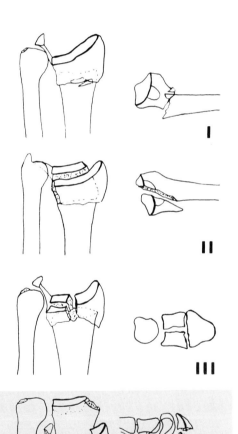

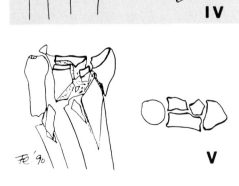

The fracture may be transverse or oblique, and at a distance of six lines, an inch, or an inch and a half from the articulating extremity of the bone: but the nearer the fracture is to the joint, the more closely does the consecutive displacement resemble an active dislocation.

B. Dupuytren, M.D. 1847

A Practical, Treatment Oriented Classification of Fractures of the Distal Radius and Associated Distal Radioulnar Joint Lesions.
Diego L. Fernandez, M.D. PD

FRACTURE TYPES (ADULTS) BASED ON THE MECHANISM OF INJURY		CHILDREN FRACTURE EQUIVALENT	STABILITY/ INSTABILITY: high risk of secondary displacement after initial adequate reduction	DISPLACEMENT PATTERN	NUMBER OF FRAGMENTS	ASSOCIATED LESIONS	RECOMMENDED TREATMENT
TYPE I BENDING FRACTURE OF THE METAPHYSIS		DISTAL FOREARM FRACTURE SALTER II	STABLE UNSTABLE	NON-DISPLACED DORSALLY (Colles-Pouteau) VOLARLY (Smith) PROXIMAL COMBINED	ALWAYS 2 MAIN FRAGMENTS + VARYING DEGREE OF METAPHYSEAL COMMINUTION (instability)	UNCOMMON carpal ligament, fractures, median, ulnar nerve, tendons, ipsilat., fx upper extremity, compartment syndrome	CONSERVATIVE (stable fxs) PERCUTANEOUS PINNING (extra- or intrafocal) EXTERNAL FIXATION (exceptionally BONE GRAFT)
TYPE II SHEARING FRACTURE OF THE JOINT SURFACE		SALTER IV	UNSTABLE	DORSAL RADIAL VOLAR PROXIMAL COMBINED	TWO-PART THREE-PART COMMINUTED	LESS UNCOMMON	OPEN REDUCTION SCREW-/PLATE FIXATION
TYPE III COMPRESSION FRACTURE OF THE JOINT SURFACE		SALTER III, IV, V	STABLE UNSTABLE	NON-DISPLACED DORSAL RADIAL VOLAR PROXIMAL COMBINED	TWO-PART THREE-PART FOUR-PART COMMINUTED	COMMON	CONSERVATIVE CLOSED, LIMITED, ARTHROSCOPIC ASSISTED, OR EXTENSILE OPEN REDUCTION PERCUTANEOUS PINS COMBINED EXTERNAL AND INTERNAL FIXATION BONE GRAFT
TYPE IV AVULSION FRACTURES, RADIO CARPAL FRACTURE DISLOCATION		VERY RARE	UNSTABLE	DORSAL RADIAL VOLAR PROXIMAL COMBINED	TWO-PART (radial styloid ulnar styloid) THREE-PART (volar, dorsal margin) COMMINUTED	FREQUENT	CLOSED OR OPEN REDUCTION PIN OR SCREW FIXATION TENSION WIRING
TYPE V COMBINED FRACTURES (I - II - III - IV) HIGH-VELOCITY INJURY		VERY RARE	UNSTABLE	DORSAL RADIAL VOLAR PROXIMAL COMBINED	COMMINUTED and/or BONE LOSS (frequently intraarticular, open, seldom extraarticular)	ALWAYS PRESENT	COMBINED METHOD

Fracture of the distal radius: associated distal radioulnar joint (DRUJ) lesions.

	Patho-anatomy of the lesion	Degree of joint surface involvement	Prognosis	Recommended treatment
Type 1 Stable (following reduction of the radius the DRUJ is congruous and stable)	 A Avulsion fracture tip ulnar styloid B Stable fracture ulnar neck	None	Good	A+B Functional aftertreatment Encourage early pronation-supination exercises Note: Extraarticular unstable fractures of the ulna at the metaphyseal level or distal shaft require stable plate fixation
Type II Unstable (subluxation or dislocation of the ulnar head present)	 A Substance tear of TFCC and/or palmar and dorsal capsular ligaments B Avulsion fracture base of the ulnar styloid	None	• Chronic instability • Painful limitation of supination if left unreduced • Possible late arthritic changes	A Closed treatment Reduce subluxation, sugar tong splint in 45° of supination four to six weeks A+B Operative treatment Repair TFCC or fix ulnar styloid with tension band wiring Immobilize wrist and elbow in supination (cast) or transfix ulna/radius with k-wire and forearm cast
Type III Potentially unstable (subluxation possible)	 A Intraarticular fracture of the sigmoid notch B Intraarticular fracture of the ulnar head	Present	• Dorsal subluxation possible together with dorsally displaced die punch or dorso-ulnar fragment • Risk of early degenerative changes and severe limitation of forearm rotation if left unreduced	A Anatomic reduction of palmar and dorsal sigmoid notch fragments. If residual subluxation tendency present immobilize as in type II injury B Functional aftertreatment to enhance remodelling of ulnar head If DRUJ remains painful: partial ulnar resection, darrach or sauvé-kapandji procedure at a later date

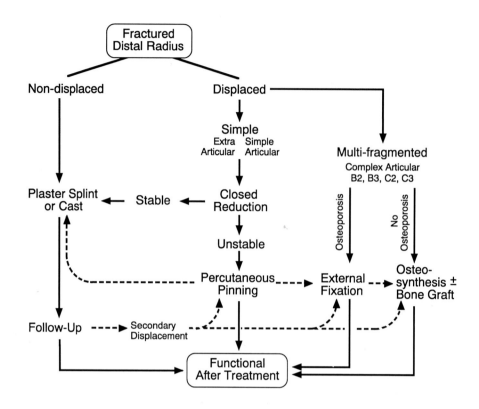

Introduction

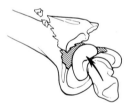

This group of uncommon but complex distal radius fractures is characterized principally by the presence of a complete dislocation of the radiocarpal joint. The dislocation may be in either a dorsal or a palmar direction, with the distal radius fracture(s) involving the marginal cortical rims, the radial styloid, or both. It is commonplace also to find a fracture of the ulnar styloid (Fig. 8.1).

Although they represent one of a host of injury patterns that have been identified involving the radiocarpal joint,[3,4,7,9,10,13,16–22,24–28,33,37,39–41,44,45] these injuries are to be differentiated from both the Type II shearing fracture of the distal radius (Chapter 6) and patterns of perilunate ligamentous injuries that have a radial styloid component.[17,22,24,25,26,28] In the Type II shearing fracture, the displaced portion of the articular surface of the distal end of the radius remains in contact with the proximal carpal row, still attached by the intact

Figure 8.1. Anteroposterior, lateral, and oblique radiographs revealing a Type IV radiocarpal fracture-dislocation. Note the characteristic findings of complete radiocarpal dislocation, marginal rim fractures, and styloid process fractures of both radius and ulna.

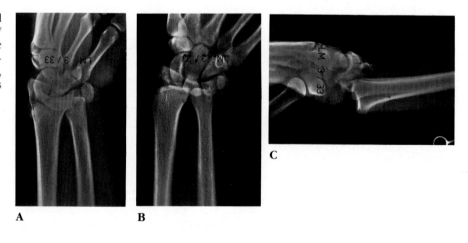

radiocarpal capsular ligaments. Furthermore, the displaced distal radial fragment represents a substantial portion of the articular surface, in contrast to the small marginal rim fractures commonly found in the Type IV fracture-dislocations Although in some instances intercarpal interosseous ligament injury in addition to extrinsic radiocarpal ligament damage will be found, the Type IV fracture-dislocations are likely the result of a somewhat different mechanism than the perilunate patterns of injury. As such, the functional outcome of the Type IV fractures without interosseous ligament injury is likely to be more favorable than that of the perilunate fracture-dislocation.

Incidence

Radiocarpal fracture-dislocations are most often the result of high-energy trauma and are uncommon. Given the fact that the experience in the literature has been generally in the form of single case reports or small series of patients,[1,3–9,12,15,21,23,27,29,31,32,34,35,37,42,46] the incidence of these as compared to other fractures of the distal radius has never been accurately determined. In a retrospective review of 112 carpal fracture-dislocations, Dunn identified six radiocarpal fracture-dislocations: three dorsal, two volar, and one in which the carpal bones were themselves fractured and dislocated in a number of directions.[9]

Despite being uncommon, the injury was recognized as early as 1838 by Malle, identifying a volar radiocarpal fracture-dislocation, and shortly thereafter by both Marjolin and Voillemier, who each identified dorsal radiocarpal fracture-dislocations (see Chapter 1). As was the standard of that era, their observations were made from examination of post-mortem specimens. The complexity of these injuries could be highlighted as well from a case described in 1926 by Destot, who identified a patient who died from overwhelming sepsis following an open radiocarpal fracture-dislocation.[7]

Mechanism of Injury

Although the cases described by nineteenth-century investigators were associated with falls from a height or vehicular trauma, the report of Böhler in 1930 may have been among the earliest to shed light on the mechanism producing these lesions.[5] In Böhler's case, an open dorsoulnar radiocarpal dislocation was produced when the individual's hyperextended wrist was struck by a car while his elbow was fixed against a wall. In this position the forearm would be assumed to be pronated. This position of injury has also been noted in a number of other reports (Fig. 8.2).[4,12,27,34,46]

Weiss et al., after observing a patient with an irreducible complex radiocarpal fracture-dislocation, attempted to reproduce the injury in a cadaver model.[46] They observed that an axial load, with the wrist hyperextended and ulnarly deviated and the elbow fixed, tended to produce a fracture of the scaphoid, with or without intercarpal ligament disruption, or isolated fractures of the distal end of the radius. It was only when they added a forced pronation of the forearm that they could duplicate a radiocarpal fracture-dislocation.

The studies of Johnson and of Mayfield et al. have further clarified the sequence of events that may occur with similar loading patterns.[20,24–26] Although these investigators labeled the rotational forces as "intercarpal supination," they similarly studied the effects of axial loading on the hyperextended and ulnarly deviated wrist with the forearm fixed in maximal

Figure 8.2. The proposed mechanism for most radiocarpal fracture-dislocations is that of an axial force directed to a hyperextended wrist with the forearm maximally pronated and the elbow fixed. Reprinted with permission from Fernandez DL, Irreducible radiocarpal fracture dislocation, *Journal of Hand Surgery*, 6: 456–461, 1981.

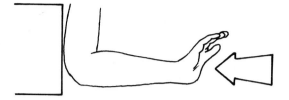

pronation. They observed two "vulnerable" zones within the carpus in which skeletal and ligamentous injury would progressively occur as the loading force was applied. What is noteworthy from their studies in attempting to understand the events that occur to produce Type IV fracture-dislocation is the observation that in forced ulnar deviations and extension, tension is produced on the radial volar ligaments, which can produce avulsion fractures of the volar lip of the radius or radial styloid (Fig. 8.3).

It is evident that these radiocarpal injuries are the product of a number of factors. These include the anatomy of the articulating units; the strength and elasticity of the ligaments; the magnitude, rate of loading, and position of the force of injury of the hand and forearm; and the underlying bony structure.[20] We have postulated the mechanism of the Type IV radiocarpal fracture-dislocations as follows: a major torsional and hyperextension force on the hyperpronated forearm with the hand and wrist in ulnar deviation results in avulsion of the strong volar radiocarpal as well as the ulnocarpal ligaments. This, in turn, allows the carpus to displace dorsally. If the radiocapitate ligament remains intact, the radial styloid will be avulsed as the impact continues. The ulnar styloid will be avulsed by the ulnar collateral ligament and volar ulnocarpal ligaments. This will then present as a radiocarpal fracture-dislocation with the carpal relationships intact. Moneim, Bolger, and Omer termed this a Type I radiocarpal fracture-dislocation.[27] The radiographic hallmark of this is the fact that the relationship of the proximal row carpal bones is undisturbed due to the presence of intact interosseous scapholunate and lunotriquetral interosseous ligaments (Fig. 8.4A and B).

In some instances, the mechanism of injury must resemble more closely that observed by Mayfield, Johnson, and Kilcoyne, in which some of the interosseous ligaments are disrupted leading to intercarpal dissociation.[26] Monheim and co-workers termed these Type II radiocarpal fracture-dislocations.[27] These injuries represent a more complex pattern and will offer a graver prognosis for full functional restoration.[4,5,22,27,31,46]

Figure 8.3. Forced ulnar deviation and extension of the wrist with the forearm maximally pronated produces tension on the volar radiocarpal ligaments and can produce avulsion fractures of the radial styloid (A) as well as the volar rim of the radius (B). (Reprinted with permission, Mayfield J, Johnson RP, Kilcoyne RK. Carpal dislocations: pathomechanics and progressive periulnar instability. *J Hand Surg* 5: 226–241, 1980.)

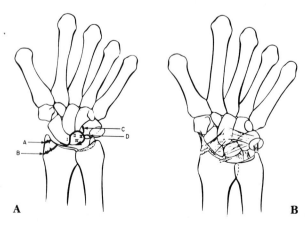

A   B

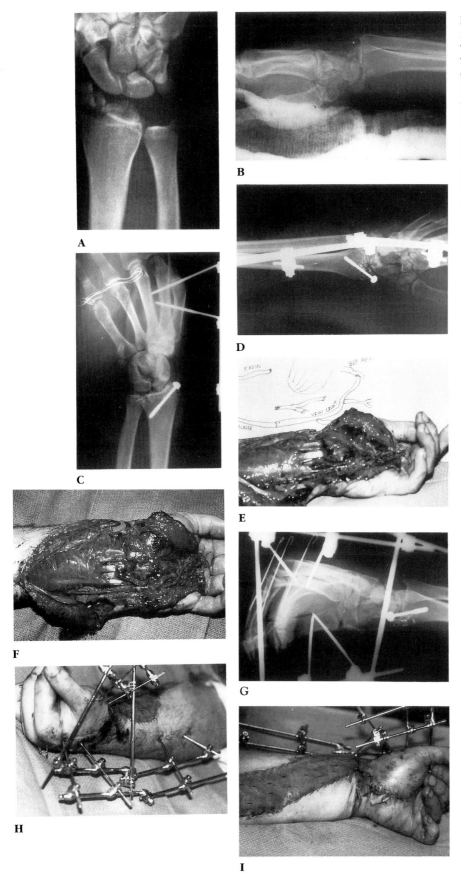

Figure 8.4. A 28-year-old man was involved in a high-speed motor vehicle accident in which the car rolled over his hand and wrist. Upon admission his hand was ischemic and insensate. (Reprinted with permission, *Journal of Hand Surgery*, CV Mosby.) A,B. Anteroposterior and lateral radiographs of the volar radiocarpal fracture-dislocation. C,D. Following longitudinal traction and application of external fixation, the anteroposterior radiograph demonstrates the avulsion fragments of the radial styloid and volar rim of the distal radius. The entire radiocarpal capsular ligaments were attached to their fragments. Note the normal relationships of the carpal bones to each other. The fragments were reapproximated with a screw through the styloid and small wire intraosseous sutures. E,F. Both the radial and ulnar arteries were found transected. The arterial inflow was reestablished using a long vein graft to reconstruct the superficial palmar arch. G,H. The external fixation was extended to include his thumb to maintain an adequate first web space as well as to provide traction on the thumb metacarpal to avoid displacement of a trapezial fracture. I. The volar forearm compartment was released and the wound covered by a split-thickness skin graft.

In both Types I and II, disruption of the volar radiocarpal capsular ligament will also result in a tendency for the carpus to translocate in an ulnar direction and may be more likely to occur if the ligaments are not repaired at the time of the initial treatment.[12,32,33]

Treatment Considerations

The Type IV radiocarpal fracture-dislocations represent graver injuries than the vast majority of distal radius fractures. The most frequent etiologies include falls from large heights, motor vehicle injuries, and industrial accidents.[1–6,8,11–13,15,17–19,21,23,27,28,30–32,34,35,37,42–44,46] It is not surprising that associated injuries either within the same limb or elsewhere are not uncommon. In one study involving 10 open radiocarpal fracture-dislocations in 9 patients, associated fractures or injuries to other organ systems were found in every patient.[31]

A careful assessment not only of the presence and extent of any associated overlying soft tissue wound but also of the integrity of the neurovascular structures is necessary upon the initial evaluation of the patient. In some instances, the extreme deformity will produce a mechanical occlusion of the arterial inflow, which can be rapidly restored by an expeditious relocation of the radiocarpal alignment by longitudinal traction.[27,37] If the circulation remains impaired, local vascular thrombosis or even a more proximal injury must be considered (Fig. 8.4A–I).

For very much the same reason, the neurologic status must be documented, as neurapraxic lesions to both median and ulnar nerves are commonplace.[12,13,27,31,37] Along these lines, the surgeon should be mindful of the possibility of elevation of the compartment pressures in the forearm, the hand, or both.

The extent of the injury patterns is often difficult to assess on the initial radiographs. An anteroposterior and lateral radiograph with the radiocarpal fracture-dislocation reduced and longitudinal traction applied is recommended (Fig. 8.5A–H).

Although several reports have suggested a role for closed reduction and cast immobilization for these fracture-dislocations,[5,9,10,15,27,29,35] it has been our preference all along to approach these complex injuries operatively (Fig. 8.6A–H). It goes without saying that the operative approach is mandatory in those cases that prove irreducible,[12,46] that are associated with open joint injury,[12,31] or that are associated with neurovascular deficits or compartment syndrome.[27,31,37]

After the patient is taken to the operating room following induction of anesthesia, the radiocarpal dislocation is generally readily reduced by longitudinal traction accompanied at times by rotation of the hand and wrist. We prefer to apply an external fixation frame holding the radiocarpal joint distracted to facilitate the operative reposition of the capsular ligaments and avulsion fractures.[14]

Through an extensile volar incision, the median and ulnar nerves are both inspected and the canal of Guyon and carpal tunnel opened. In the presence of an open wound, the original wound is extended proximally and distally in an extensile manner (Fig. 8.6A–N). Through the large rent in the palmar capsule, the radiocarpal joint is inspected and irrigated to remove any cartilaginous or bony debris. The scapholunate and lunotriquetral interosseous ligaments are inspected and repaired with interosseous suture if they are found to be disrupted. Stay sutures are placed into the volar capsule, but at this point they

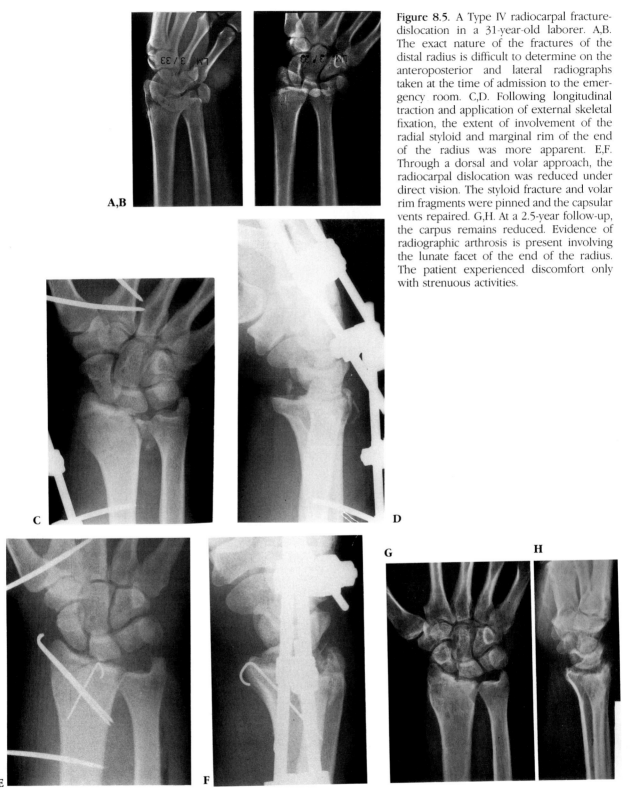

Figure 8.5. A Type IV radiocarpal fracture-dislocation in a 31-year-old laborer. A,B. The exact nature of the fractures of the distal radius is difficult to determine on the anteroposterior and lateral radiographs taken at the time of admission to the emergency room. C,D. Following longitudinal traction and application of external skeletal fixation, the extent of involvement of the radial styloid and marginal rim of the end of the radius was more apparent. E,F. Through a dorsal and volar approach, the radiocarpal dislocation was reduced under direct vision. The styloid fracture and volar rim fragments were pinned and the capsular vents repaired. G,H. At a 2.5-year follow-up, the carpus remains reduced. Evidence of radiographic arthrosis is present involving the lunate facet of the end of the radius. The patient experienced discomfort only with strenuous activities.

are not tied back to the radius. It is critical to try to leave any bony fragments attached to the capsule, as these will facilitate reposition and hasten healing of the capsular defect.

The radial styloid fragment, if present, can now be reduced under direct vision. Fixation is ordinarily satisfactory with one or two smooth Kirschner

Figure 8.6. A 20-year-old man was admitted with an open irreducible radiocarpal fracture-dislocation. A,B. Anteroposterior and lateral roentgenographs of the injury reveal widespread disruption of the radiocarpal joint. Note that the carpal bones appear to have maintained their alignment. The radial and ulnar styloid processes are displaced. C,D. Postoperative anteroposterior and lateral radiographs show the anatomic reduction of the radiocarpal joint and Kirschner wire fixation of the radial styloid and volar ulnar lip of the radius. Tension band fixation was also applied to the displaced ulnar styloid process. E,F. The radiographic appearance 1 year postinjury. Note the normal carpal alignment with some flattening of the radial articular surface of the lunate due to subchondral impaction at the time of the injury. G,H. Function at 2 years: full digital motion and normal sensibility. I,J. Excellent radial and ulnar deviation. K,L. Excellent wrist extension, some reduction in wrist flexion. M,N. Slight limitation of forearm supination, full forearm pronation. Reprinted with permission from Fernandez DL, Irreducible radiocarpal fracture dislocation, *Journal of Hand Surgery*, 6: 456–461, 1981.

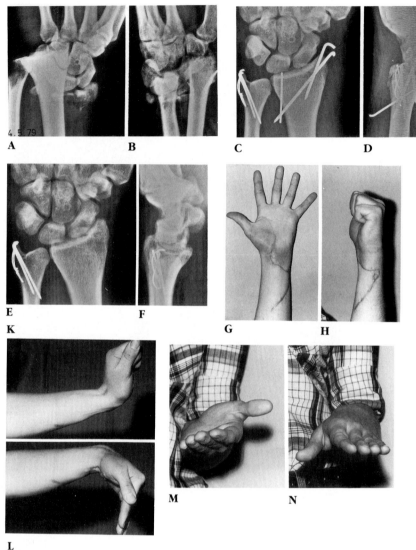

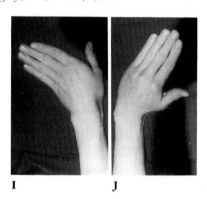

wires placed percutaneously through the tip of the styloid. At this juncture, the volar capsule is reapproximated either through intraosseous suture or by reapproximating the small attached volar marginal rim fractures of the radius.

Should this injury include displacement of the dorsal of the radius, the bony fragments rim can be reapproximated through a dorsal extensile approach. The internal fixation of the marginal fracture fragments is dependent on the fragment size. Ordinarily, smooth Kirschner wires, wire loop sutures, or small screws prove adequate. In some instances in which the metaphysis of the radius has been impacted, the defects are filled with cancellous bone graft and supported with a buttress plate (Fig. 8.7A–E).

In most instances, we have elected operatively to reduce and internally to stabilize associated displaced ulnar styloid fractures in order both to improve the stability of the radiocarpal joint and to offset the possibility of late radioulnar joint instability.[38]

At the conclusion of the surgery, attention must be taken to assess the forearm and hand soft tissue compartments. If the distal radioulnar joint is stable and an external fixateur is in place, no further immobilization will be necessary. If, however, concern exists regarding the soft tissues of the distal

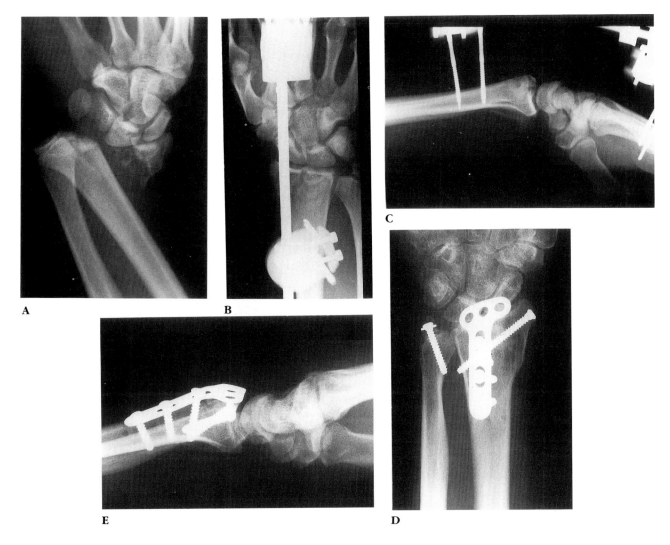

C

E   **D**

radioulnar joint, we prefer to immobilize the forearm in midsupination with an above-elbow sugar tong splint for 3 weeks.

As a general rule, the external fixation frames are left in place for 6 to 8 weeks, depending on the extent of initial injury, the stability of the reduction, and the presence of intracarpal ligament injury. In the face of the latter, 8 weeks of external fixation is preferred.

Outcome

Despite the fact that Type IV radiocarpal fracture-dislocations are more complex injuries, favorable results can be obtained in many instances with early operative intervention, with the goal of restoring both the skeletal and the soft tissue anatomy.

Although it is difficult to glean much in the way of outcome from the literature, given the various methods of treatment, several predictive features can be recognized. When the radiocarpal fracture-dislocation also involves intercarpal dissociation (Moneim et al., Type II), residual alteration in the carpal kinematics can result in residual loss of wrist mobility and strength.[4,27,31,37] Every effort should be taken to anatomically reduce the radial styloid as well as to repair scapholunate or lunatotriquetral ligament tears.

Figure 8.7. A 26-year-old house painter fell two stories, sustaining a complex open radiocarpal fracture-dislocation. A. The initial anteroposterior radiograph reveals the extensive radiocarpal dislocation. B,C. His initial treatment at a local hospital involved irrigation and debridement of the open joint, reduction of the dislocation, and the application of an external fixation device. Reduction could only be held with the wrist palmar flexed. Severe pain developed. D,E. He was brought to surgery where the median and ulnar nerves were decompressed and the volar capsular defect repaired. Through a dorsal approach, the dorsal rim fragments were repositioned and supported with both cancellous graft and a dorsal plate. The ulnar styloid was also secured with a cannulated screw. At 1 year he has excellent function.

Figure 8.8. A dorsal radiocarpal fracture-dislocation in a young laborer. A,B. The radiocarpal fracture-dislocation is well seen in the initial anteroposterior and lateral radiographs. C,D. The patient was treated with open reduction and internal fixation of the radial and dorsal marginal fragments along with a volar capsular repair. E,F. At 2 years the patient is functioning reasonably well. Note the ulnar translocation of the carpus on the end of the radius with only half the lunate articulating with the lunate fossa.

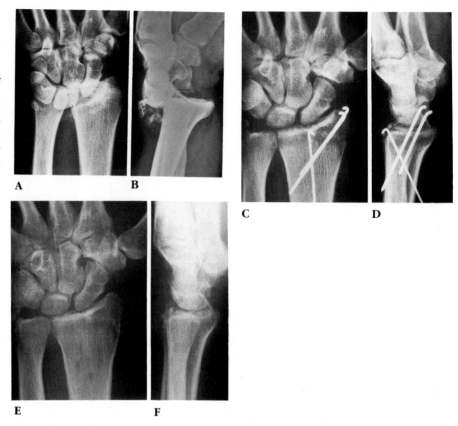

A second factor that can lead to residual impairment is residual neurologic dysfunction.[31] A careful preoperative neurologic assessment and operative decompression of both the median and the ulnar nerves is recommended, particularly given the higher energy of injury.

Complications

Along with the problems noted above, one particular problem that can occur involves residual ulnar translocation of the carpus on the end of the radius. There is, by definition, an increased space between the radial styloid and scaphoid with displacement of the lunate over the distal ulnar.[3,32,33,41] Often less than one-half of the lunate's articular surface remains in the lunate fossa of the distal radius (Fig. 8.8A–F). Taleisnik defined Type I ulnar translocations, which are completely isolated ulnar carpal translocations, as compared to Type II ulnar translocations, which are associated with a scapholunate dissociation.[40] Unfortunately, early enthusiasm with ligamentous reconstruction has not proven justified by experience, and symptomatic ulnar translocation may require radiolunate arthrodesis.

References

1. Baker DM: Modern day chauffeur's fracture. A fracture-dislocation of the radiocarpal joint. *Orthop Rev* 5: 47–51, 1976.
2. Bell MJ: Perilunar dislocation of the carpus and an associated Colles' fracture. *Hand* 15: 262–266, 1983.
3. Bellinghousen HW, Gilula LA, Leroy VY, Weeks PM: Post-traumatic palmar carpal subluxation. A report of two cases. *J Bone Joint Surg [Am]* 65A: 998–1006, 1983.

4. Bilos ZJ, Pankovich AM, Yelda S: Fracture-dislocation of the radiocarpal joint. *J Bone Joint Surg [Am]* 59A: 198–203, 1977.
5. Böhler L: Verrenungen der Handgelenke. *Acta Chir Scand* 67: 154–177, 1930.
6. Bounds TB: Bilateral radiocarpal dislocation. A case report. *Orthopaedics* 5: 42–45, 1982.
7. Destot E: *Injuries of the Wrist. A Radiological Study.* New York: PB Hoeber, 1926.
8. Dodd CAF: Triple dislocation in the upper limb. *J Trauma* 27: 1307, 1987.
9. Dunn AW: Fractures and dislocations of the carpus. *Surg Clin North Am* 52: 1513–1518, 1972.
10. Fahey JH: Fractures and dislocations about the wrist. *Surg Clin North Am* 37: 19–40, 1957.
11. Fehring TK, Milek MA: Isolated volar dislocation of the radiocarpal joint. A case report. *J Bone Joint Surg [Am]* 66A: 464–466, 1984.
12. Fernandez DL: Irreducible radiocarpal fracture-dislocation and radioulnar dissociation with entrapment of the ulnar nerve, artery, and flexor profundus II-V. *J Hand Surg* 6: 456–461, 1981.
13. Fernandez DL, Ghillani R: External fixation of complex carpal dislocations. A preliminary report. *J Hand Surg* 12A: 335–347, 1987.
14. Fernandez DL, Jakob RP, Büchler U: External fixation of the wrist. Current indications and techniques. *Ann Chir Gyn* 72: 298–302, 1983.
15. Freund LG, Ovesen J: Isolated dorsal dislocation of the radiocarpal joint. *J Bone Joint Surg [Am]* 59A: 277, 1977.
16. Gilula LA: Carpal injuries: Analytic approach and case exercises. *Am J Roentgenol* 133: 503–517, 1979.
16A. Gilula LA, Weeks PM: Post-traumatic ligamentous instabilities of the wrist. *Radiology* 129: 641–651, 1978.
17. Green DP, O'Brien, ET: Classification and management of carpal dislocations. *Clin Orthop Rel Res* 149: 55–72, 1980.
18. Green DP, O'Brien ET: Open reduction of carpal dislocation. Indications and operative techniques. *J Hand Surg* 3: 250–265, 1978.
19. Herzberg C, Comtet JJ, Linscheid RL: Perilunate dislocations and fracture-dislocations: A multi-center study. *J Hand Surg* 18A: 768–779, 1993.
20. Johnson RP: The acutely injured wrist and its residuals. *Clin Orthop Rel Res* 149: 33–44, 1980.
21. Lenen D, Riot O, Caro P, Lefèvre D, Courtois B: Luxation-fractures de la radio-carpienne: Etude clinique de six cas et revue générale. *Ann Chir Main* 10: 5–12, 1991.
22. Linscheid RL, Dobyns JH, Beabout JW, Bryan RS: Traumatic instability of the wrist. Diagnosis, classification, and pathomechanics. *J Bone Joint Surg [Am]* 54A: 1612–1632, 1972.
23. Matthews MG: Radiocarpal dislocation with associated avulsion of the radial styloid and fracture of the shaft of the ulnar. *Injury* 18: 70–71, 1987.
24. Mayfield JK: Mechanism of carpal injuries. *Clin Orthop Rel Res* 149: 45–54, 1980.
25. Mayfield JK, Johnson RP, Kilcoyne RF: Carpal dislocations: Pathomechanics and progressive perilunar instability. *J Hand Surg* 5: 226–241, 1980.
26. Mayfield JK, Johnson RP, Kilcoyne RF: The ligaments of the human wrist and their functional significance. *Anat Rec* 186: 417–428, 1976.
27. Monheim MS, Bolger JT, Omer GE: Radiocarpal dislocation—classification and rationale for management. *Clin Orthop Rel Res* 192: 199–209, 1985.
28. Monheim MS, Hofammann KE, Omer GE: Transscaphoid perilunate fracture-dislocation. Results of open reduction and pin fixation. *Clin Orthop Rel Res* 190: 227–235, 1984.
29. Moore DP, McMahon BA: Anterior radiocarpal dislocation: An isolated injury. *J Hand Surg* 13B: 215–217, 1988.
30. Mullan GB, Lloyd GJ: Complete carpal disruption of the hand. *Hand* 12: 39–43, 1980.
31. Nyquist SR, Stern PJ: Open radiocarpal fracture-dislocations. *J Hand Surg* 9A: 707–710, 1984.
32. Penny WH, Greene TG: Volar radiocarpal dislocation with ulnar translocation. *J Orthop Trauma* 2: 322–326, 1988.
33. Rayhack J, Linscheid RL, Dobyns JH, Smith JH: Post-traumatic ulnar translation of the carpus. *J Hand Surg* 12A: 180–189, 1987.
34. Reynolds ISR: Dorsal carpal dislocation. *Injury* 12: 48–49, 1980.
35. Rosado AP: A possible relationship of radiocarpal dislocation and dislocation of the lunate bone. *J Bone Joint Surg [Br]* 48B: 504–506, 1966.

36. Rosenthal DI, Schwartz M, Phillips WC, Jupiter JB: Fracture of the radius with instability of the wrist. *Am J Roentgenol* 141: 113–116, 1983.
37. Schoenecker P, Gilula LA, Shively RA: Radiocarpal fracture-dislocation. *Clin Orthop Rel Res* 197: 237–244, 1985.
38. Shaw JA, Bruno A, Paul EM: Ulnar styloid fixation in the treatment of post-traumatic instability of the radioulnar joint. A biomechanical study with clinical correlation. *J Hand Surg* 15A: 712–720, 1990.
39. Taleisnik J: The ligaments of the wrist. *J Hand Surg* 1: 110–118, 1976.
40. Taleisnik J: *The Wrist*. Philadelphia: Churchill Livingstone, 1985.
41. Taleisnik J: Post-traumatic carpal instability. *Clin Orthop Rel Res* 149: 73–82, 1980.
42. Thomsen ST, Søren FJ: Palmar dislocation of the radiocarpal joint. *J Hand Surg* 14A: 627–630, 1989.
43. Varodompin N, Pichit L, Pirapong P: Isolated dorsal radiocarpal dislocation: Case report and literature review. *J Hand Surg* 10A: 708–710, 1985.
44. Wagner CJ: Fracture-dislocations of the wrist. *Clin Orthop Rel Res* 15: 181–196, 1959.
45. Wagner CJ: Perilunar dislocations. *J Bone Joint Surg [Am]* 38A: 1198–1207, 1956.
46. Weiss C, Laskin RS, Spinner M: Irreducible radiocarpal dislocation. A case report. *J Bone Joint Surg [Am]* 52A: 562–564, 1970.

Chapter Nine

Combined Fractures of the Distal Radius—Type V

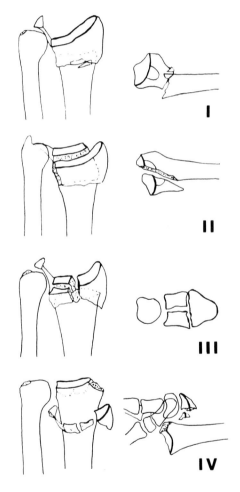

On May 6, 1855, Catherine A, age 56, ran out of a public-house, where she had been drinking, and threw herself beneath the wheels of a passing cab. Her left wrist was crushed. Mr. Stanley amputated by double flaps, just below the elbow. On examining the forearm the muscles about the wrist were found to be greatly lacerted. Of the arteries, the ulna was torn across one inch above the pisiform bone. The nerves were uninjured. Both bones were extensively comminuted just above their carpal ends, and the fracture of the radius extended into the wrist joint. On the eleventh day she died from tetanus.

G.W. Callender 1865

A Practical, Treatment Oriented Classification of Fractures of the Distal Radius and Associated Distal Radioulnar Joint Lesions.
Diego L. Fernandez, M.D. PD

FRACTURE TYPES (ADULTS) BASED ON THE MECHANISM OF INJURY	CHILDREN FRACTURE EQUIVALENT	STABILITY/ INSTABILITY: high risk of secondary displacement after initial adequate reduction	DISPLACEMENT PATTERN	NUMBER OF FRAGMENTS	ASSOCIATED LESIONS carpal ligament, fractures, median, ulnar nerve, tendons, ipsilat., fx upper extremity, compartment syndrome	RECOMMENDED TREATMENT
TYPE I — BENDING FRACTURE OF THE METAPHYSIS	DISTAL FOREARM FRACTURE — SALTER II	STABLE — UNSTABLE	NON-DISPLACED DORSALLY (Colles-Pouteau) VOLARLY (Smith) PROXIMAL COMBINED	ALWAYS 2 MAIN FRAGMENTS + VARYING DEGREE OF METAPHYSEAL COMMINUTION (instability)	UNCOMMON	CONSERVATIVE (stable fxs) PERCUTANEOUS PINNING (extra- or intrafocal) EXTERNAL FIXATION (exceptionally BONE GRAFT)
TYPE II — SHEARING FRACTURE OF THE JOINT SURFACE	SALTER IV	UNSTABLE	DORSAL RADIAL VOLAR PROXIMAL COMBINED	TWO-PART THREE-PART COMMINUTED	LESS UNCOMMON	OPEN REDUCTION SCREW-/PLATE FIXATION
TYPE III — COMPRESSION FRACTURE OF THE JOINT SURFACE	SALTER III, IV, V	STABLE — UNSTABLE	NON-DISPLACED DORSAL RADIAL VOLAR PROXIMAL COMBINED	TWO-PART THREE-PART FOUR-PART COMMINUTED	COMMON	CONSERVATIVE CLOSED, LIMITED, ARTHROSCOPIC ASSISTED, OR EXTENSILE OPEN REDUCTION PERCUTANEOUS PINS COMBINED EXTERNAL AND INTERNAL FIXATION BONE GRAFT
TYPE IV — AVULSION FRACTURES, RADIO CARPAL FRACTURE DISLOCATION	VERY RARE	UNSTABLE	DORSAL RADIAL VOLAR PROXIMAL COMBINED	TWO-PART (radial styloid ulnar styloid) THREE-PART (volar, dorsal margin) COMMINUTED	FREQUENT	CLOSED OR OPEN REDUCTION PIN OR SCREW FIXATION TENSION WIRING
TYPE V — COMBINED FRACTURES (I · II · III · IV) HIGH-VELOCITY INJURY	VERY RARE	UNSTABLE	DORSAL RADIAL VOLAR PROXIMAL COMBINED	COMMINUTED and/or BONE LOSS (frequently intraarticular, open, seldom extraarticular)	ALWAYS PRESENT	COMBINED METHOD

Fracture of the distal radius: associated distal radioulnar joint (DRUJ) lesions.

Patho-anatomy of the lesion	Degree of joint surface involvement	Prognosis	Recommended treatment
Type I **Stable** (following reduction of the radius the DRUJ is congruous and stable) A Avulsion fracture tip ulnar styloid B Stable fracture ulnar neck	None	Good	A+B Functional aftertreatment Encourage early pronation-supination exercises Note: Extraarticular unstable fractures of the ulna at the metaphyseal level or distal shaft require stable plate fixation
Type II **Unstable** (subluxation or dislocation of the ulnar head present) A Substance tear of TFCC and/or palmar and dorsal capsular ligaments B Avulsion fracture base of the ulnar styloid	None	• Chronic instability • Painful limitation of supination if left unreduced • Possible late arthritic changes	A Closed treatment Reduce subluxation, sugar tong splint in 45° of supination four to six weeks A+B Operative treatment Repair TFCC or fix ulnar styloid with tension band wiring Immobilize wrist and elbow in supination (cast) or transfix ulna/radius with k-wire and forearm cast
Type III **Potentially unstable** (subluxation possible) A Intraarticular fracture of the sigmoid notch B Intraarticular fracture of the ulnar head	Present	• Dorsal subluxation possible together with dorsally displaced die punch or dorso-ulnar fragment • Risk of early degenerative changes and severe limitation of forearm rotation if left unreduced	A Anatomic reduction of palmar and dorsal sigmoid notch fragments. If residual subluxation tendency present immobilize as in type II injury B Functional aftertreatment to enhance remodelling of ulnar head If DRUJ remains painful: partial ulnar resection, darrach or sauvé-kapandji procedure at a later date

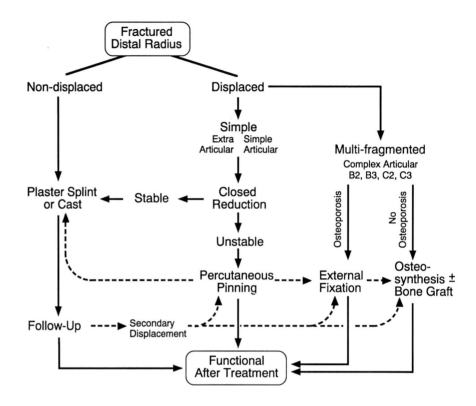

Type V—Combined Fractures of the Distal Radius

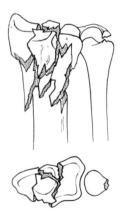

This group of fractures of the distal end of the radius includes those injuries made more complex by either the fracture pattern itself or by associated ipsilateral skeletal or soft tissue trauma, or those resulting from high-energy impact such as a fall from a height, automobile accident, crush trauma, or gunshot wound.[2,7–9,17–19,21,32–34,37,41] Most often the fracture pattern is that of a complex intra- and extraarticular injury with comminution extending into the radial shaft. In some instances, however, the articular surface may be intact although the metaphysis has experienced massive comminution or bone loss, such as that which might occur from a gunshot wound. These fractures have a high incidence of associated soft tissue injuries, compartment syndrome, and ipsilateral fractures or dislocations of the upper limb (Fig. 9.1A–H).

Complex Fracture Patterns

The Type V injury cannot be easily fit into standard fracture classifications. The subgroup C3.3 identifies the complex articular and metaphyseal injury that can be found in some of the Type V injuries (Fig. 9.2). Yet, this injury type may include fractures with primarily longitudinal fracture lines, those associated with bone loss, or complex fractures of the distal ulna (Fig. 9.3A–E). In reality, the distinguishing features of this type of fracture may relate more to associated skeletal or soft tissue injuries than to the actual distal radius fracture pattern.

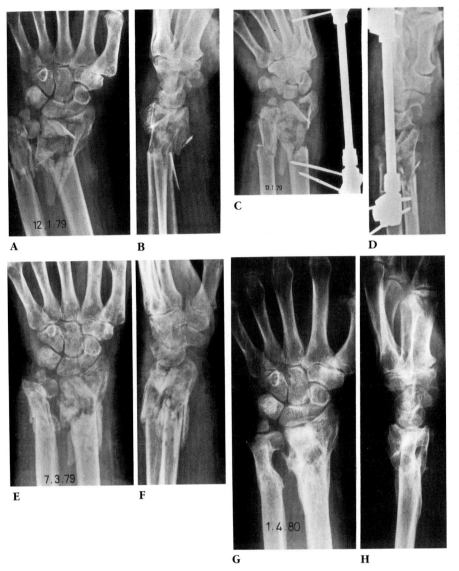

A   B   C   D

E   F

G   H

Figure 9.1. A complex fracture Type V pattern without extensive intraarticular, metaphyseal, and diaphyseal comminution in an active 80-year-old patient. A,B. The anteroposterior and lateral radiographs of the injury reveal extensive articular and more proximal disruption. This would be classified as an subgroup C3.3. Note the extensive distal ulna fracture. C,D. With longitudinal traction the fragments were manipulated to attempt to gain acceptable length and alignment. One of the earliest AO/ASIF prototype fixatures was used. E,F. At 8 weeks the external fixateur was removed. The alignment remained surprisingly acceptable. G,H. At 16 months the patient has regained full function including that of the distal radioulnar joint without pain.

Ipsilateral Skeletal and Ligament Injury

It should not be surprising that complex distal radius fractures resulting from high-energy impact may be only one part of a constellation of injuries to the ipsilateral limb. Although the goals of treatment of the Type V radius fracture parallel those of the other radius fractures, the ultimate outcome may reflect the sequelae of the associated injuries.

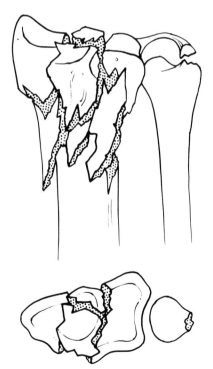

Figure 9.2. The subgroup C3.3 is representative of the high-energy Type V fractures.

Figure 9.3. A complex metaphyseal-diaphyseal fracture in a laborer which occurred following a fall from a height. A volar forearm compartment syndrome was evident upon presentation. A,B. Anteroposterior and lateral radiographs of the complex metaphyseal-diaphyseal fracture. This would be considered subgroup A3.3. C. The fracture was reduced and held with external skeletal fixation. Note that one pin was placed across the metaphysis to stabilize the distal longitudinal extension of the fracture. An anterior forearm compartment fasciotomy was done. D,E. At 1 year an anatomic result is noted. Full function was restored.

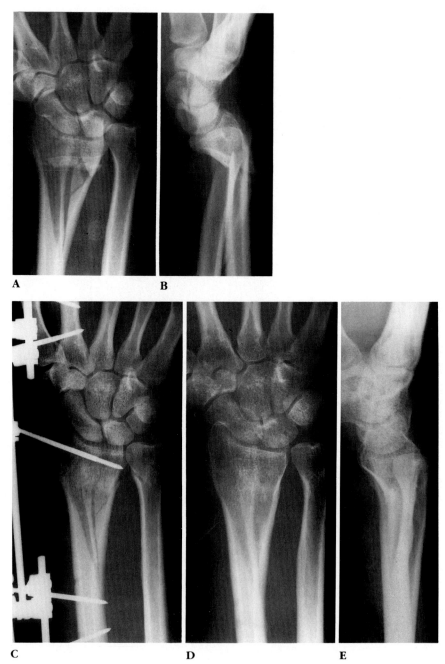

Fractures Associated with Complex Carpal Trauma

Whereas the vast majority of isolated distal radius fractures occur from low-impact falls in the older age population, the combination of distal radius fracture with a carpal injury is likely to be found in a younger individual from a high-energy impact.[1,10,15,17,20,35,36,38,43,45,46,48]

The mechanism of each injury pattern has been investigated by a number of workers.[10,11,21,24] Most would agree that both fracture of the distal radius and carpal fracture or ligament injury are most often the result of a fall or impact on the outstretched hand with the wrist in extension. The specific features of what type and direction of forces leads to a combined injury pattern has yet to be clearly defined. If one accepts the bending theory of Lewis as the most common injury pattern for fractures of the distal radius[21] (see Chapter 2), it is reasonable to postulate that as the energy of injury continues, the radius fracture is impacted, leading to increased tension on the volar radiocarpal ligaments. As the only motion is now in the radiocarpal and midcarpal joints, disruption of the volar ligaments allows for the scaphoid to impact on the dorsal lip of the radius or to separate from the lunate, leading to supination between the carpal bones. This, in turn, may result in the capitate moving out from the lunate, and even in ulna-sided intercarpal ligament disruption.[1]

In some instances, a distal radius fracture may be seen in association with a nondisplaced scaphoid fracture that can be treated by external plaster support.[26,43] This approach is best reserved for the elderly patient or those refusing surgical intervention, as the duration of immobilization may be considerable.

In most situations of combined complex carpal injuries and distal radius fractures, it is the authors' preference to treat the distal radius fracture operatively; in most instances, the treatment includes an external fixator to help reduce the axial load of the capitate onto the injured proximal carpal row. This, in turn, helps to maintain normal carpal alignment during the initial stages of ligament healing. As the majority of associated carpal fractures involve the scaphoid, we also tend to treat these with internal fixation, especially if the fracture is displaced.

For those intraarticular fractures of the distal radius which cannot be anatomically reduced by longitudinal traction with or without percutaneous manipulation of the articular fragments (see Chapter 7), the fracture fragments are approached through a dorsal or palmar incision, depending on the direction of the displacement of the fracture fragment (Fig. 9.4A–J). In the presence of metaphyseal comminution or defects, cancellous bone grafts are of extreme importance to accelerate union and provide a mechanical buttress of the articular fragments.

Once the articular surface has been accurately reduced and stabilized, internal fixation of the carpal fractures or ligament reconstruction is completed. The scaphoid fracture may be stabilized by Herbert screws placed through the dorsal capsulotomy from a proximal to a distal direction or a cannulated screw or Herbert screw placed through a volar approach (Fig. 9.5A–J).

Associated scapholunate ligament tears without carpal fracture may not be readily recognized on the initial radiographs.[29,30] A characteristic sign called the axial scaphoid shift sign (see Chapter 5) is likely to become apparent following reduction of the radius fracture and application of the longitudinal traction using the external fixation frame (Fig. 9.6A–G). We prefer to repair the scapholunate ligament with nonabsorbable intraosseous sutures (Fig. 9.7A–D). If the scaphoid has a tendency to rotate palmarward, a smooth Kirschner wire should be passed into the scaphoid and lunate and perhaps the scaphocapitate joint and kept in place for upwards of 8 weeks.

It is important to release the distraction through the external fixation across the wrist at the completion of the distal radius surgery. If this is not done, it may be more difficult to anatomically fix the fractured scaphoid or reduce this scapholunate diastasis.

Figure 9.4. A 35-year-old man fell off a staging sustaining a complex intercarpal injury along with a distal radius fracture. A,B. Initial anteroposterior and lateral radiographs reveal a complex carpal injury along with a four-part intraarticular fracture of the distal radius. C,D. Initial reduction and pinning of the radius fracture. A "naviculocapitate" injury can be identified. Note persistence of a displaced volar articular fragment of the distal radius. E,F. Anteroposterior and lateral radiographs after open reduction and internal fixation of the radius, fixation of the scaphoid with a Herbert screw directed from proximal to distal, fixation of the capitate fracture with a Herbert screw and one Kirschner wire, and application of an external fixator. G,H. Anteroposterior and lateral radiographs at 2-year follow-up. The scaphoid has united in a malposition and mild arthrosis is noted in the radiocarpal and radioulnar joint. (Reprinted with permission. Fernandez DL: Technique and results of external fixation of complex carpal injuries. *Hand Clinics* 9: 631–632, 1993. Philadelphia: WB Saunders.) (*Figure continues on facing page.*)

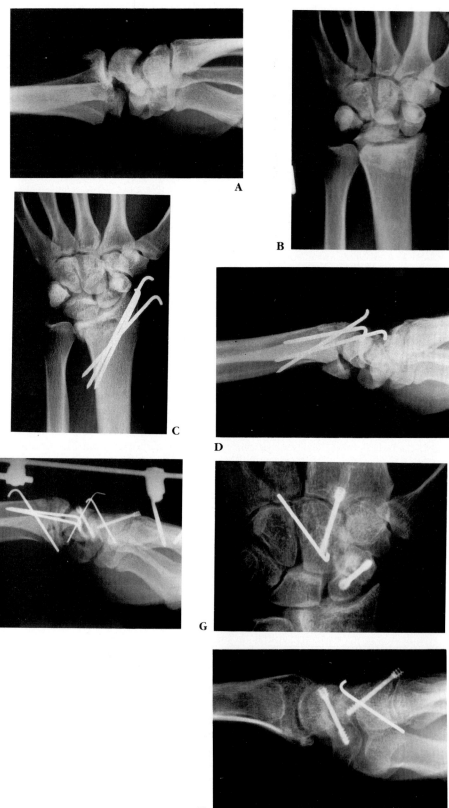

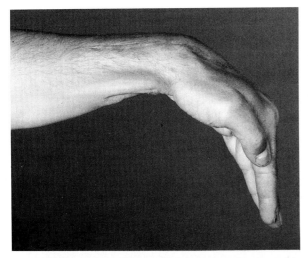

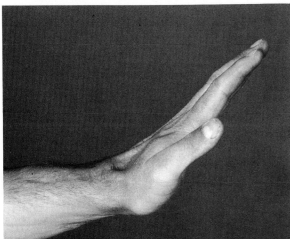

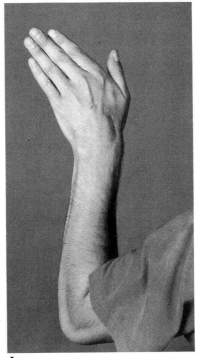

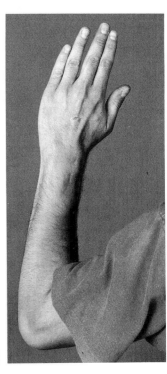

J

I,J. Some limitation is seen in functional wrist motion. However, the patient is pain-free and fully functional.

I

Proximal Skeletal and Articular Injury

Fractures of the distal end of the radius associated with a more proximal skeletal or articular injury or both may well have communicating features leading to extensive injury patterns. Odena in 1952 coined the term "bipolar fracture-dislocation" of the forearm.[32] This produced injuries which at times could resemble a combined Galeazzi and Monteggia lesion, disrupting both the proximal and distal radioulnar articulations.[12,27] The disruption of the associated soft tissue structures rather than the fractures of the distal radius and more proximal structures will prove to be the ultimate source of disability for many of these injuries.[4–6,47]

One of the authors (JBJ) reported on 10 cases of complex forearm injuries of which 8 had fractures of the distal radius (Table 9.1).[19] In conjunction with these, there was disruption of the distal radioulnar joint in 9, proximal radioulnar joint in 8, elbow dislocation in 3, radial head fracture in 7, and fracture of either the radius or ulnar diaphysis in 7. Associated ipsilateral skeletal injuries included a humeral shaft, trochlea, scaphoid, and proximal

Figure 9.5. An 18-year-old college student fell two stories out of her dormitory window. An intraarticular distal radius fracture was associated with a displaced scaphoid fracture. A,B. Anteroposterior and lateral radiographs of the intraarticular distal radius fracture and displaced scaphoid fracture. C,D. Anteroposterior and lateral radiographs of the initial treatment consisting of Herbert screw fixation of the scaphoid, percutaneous pinning of the distal radius, and external fixation spanning the wrist. E–H. Four months postinjury, excellent function returned. I,J. Follow-up radiographs reveal the scaphoid and distal radius to be healed in excellent alignment.

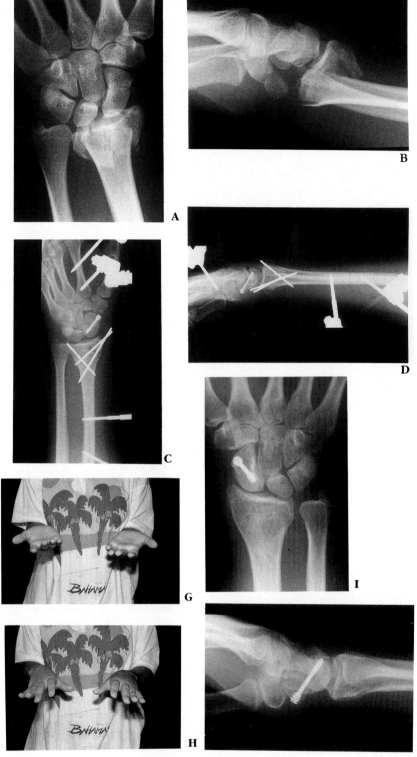

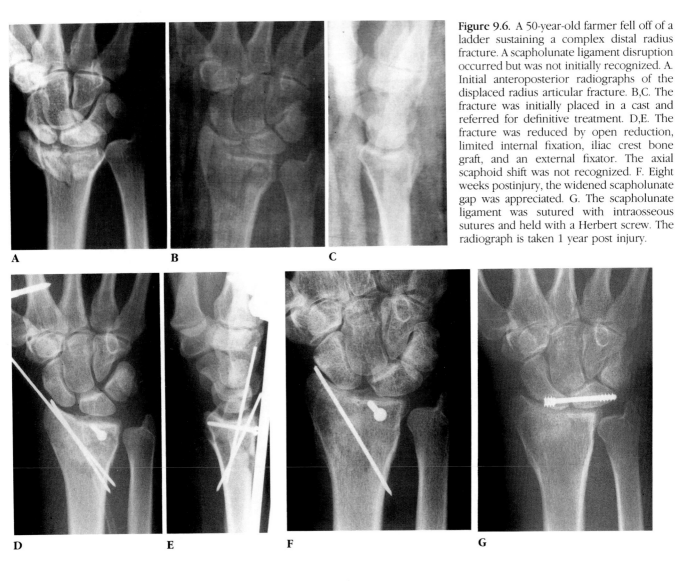

Figure 9.6. A 50-year-old farmer fell off of a ladder sustaining a complex distal radius fracture. A scapholunate ligament disruption occurred but was not initially recognized. A. Initial anteroposterior radiographs of the displaced radius articular fracture. B,C. The fracture was initially placed in a cast and referred for definitive treatment. D,E. The fracture was reduced by open reduction, limited internal fixation, iliac crest bone graft, and an external fixator. The axial scaphoid shift was not recognized. F. Eight weeks postinjury, the widened scapholunate gap was appreciated. G. The scapholunate ligament was sutured with intraosseous sutures and held with a Herbert screw. The radiograph is taken 1 year post injury.

Figure 9.7. A combined intraarticular distal radius fracture with associated injury to the scapholunate interosseous ligament. A. Following application of the external fixator, a dorsal incision is made. B. The displaced articular fragments are elevated under direct vision. Note that the scapholunate interval appears disrupted. C. Intraosseous nonabsorbable suture is placed between the scaphoid and lunate. D. Following tying of the intraosseous suture, cancellous iliac crest graft is packed into the metaphyseal defect of the radius.

Table 9.1. Complex forearm and radius injury.

Case no.	Age (yrs)	Sex	Limb (dominant)	Mechanism of injury	Injury components	Initial treatment	Secondary treatment
1	24	F	Left	Motorcycle	Midshaft ulna fx Fracture-dislocation: radial head Fracture of radial neck Fracture distal radius Fracture of scaphoid Fracture capitate Fracture pisiform Fracture ulnar styloid DRUJ disruption	ORIF ulna ORIF radial head and neck ORIF distal radius External fixation ORIF scaphoid	Screw fixation, ulnar styloid
2	28	M	Left	Industrial accident	Fracture proximal ulna Fracture-dislocation radial head Proximal RU joint injury Distal radius fracture Disruption of DRUJ Fracture ulnar styloid	ORIF ulna Silicone radial head replacement K wire distal ulna to radius	
3	63	F	Left	Fall	Fracture proximal ulna Fracture-dislocation radial head Disruption of proximal rad oulnar joint Distal radius fracture Disruption of DRUJ Opposite limb distal radius fracture	ORIF ulna ORIF radial head External fixation distal radius External fixation	
4	45	M	(Right)	Fall	Fracture proximal ulna Fracture-dislocation radial head Disruption proximal RU joint Disruption of DRUJ	ORIF ulna Open reduction radial head External fixation Distal radius	
5	22	M	(Right)	Industrial	Trochlea fracture Elbow dislocation Fracture ulna middle Radial head dislocation Fracture midradius Disruption DRUJ	Reduction of elbow ORIF trochlea ORIF ulna ORIF radius Reduction of radial head	

	Age	Sex	Side	Mechanism	Injuries	Treatment
6	40	M	(Right)	Airplane crash	*Right* Segmental fracture radius Open fracture of ulna Radial head fracture-dislocation Disruption DRUJ Compartment syndrome	ORIF radius ORIF ulna Excision radial head fragment Fasciotomy Skin graft
					Left Comminuted radius Fracture Open fracture distal ulna	ORIF radius K wire ulna
7	40	M	Left	Fall	Elbow dislocation Radial head fracture Disruption of proximal RU joint Open distal radius fracture Disruption DRUJ	Reduction elbow dislocation Debridement of radius External fixation
8	25	M	Left	Fall	Disruption proximal RU joint Diaphyseal ulna fracture Comminuted distal radius fracture Disruption DRUJ Compartment syndrome	ORIF ulna Reduction proximal RU joint ORIF distal radius Compartment release Skin graft
9	35	M	(Right)	Fall	Fracture-dislocation of elbow Disruption proximal RU joint Disruption of DRUJ Fracture-dislocation PIP joint	Silicone radial head Repair medial collateral ligament of elbow Ulnar nerve transposition Percutaneous pin distal radius Reduction of PIP joint and splint
10	28	M	(Right)	Industrial accident	Open humerus fracture Open segmental ulna fracture Comminuted proximal radius fracture Disruption proximal RU joint Disruption DRUJ	ORIF humerus: plate ORIF ulna ORIF radius Reduction of RU joints Skin graft

ORIF, Open reduction internal fixation; DRUJ, distal radioulnar joint; PIP, proximal interphalangeal joint; RU, radioulnar.

Figure 9.8. A 24-year-old woman with a complex ipsilateral upper limb injury from a motorcycle accident. (Reprinted with permission. Jupiter J: Multiple fractures in a single extremity, *Journal of Hand Surgery,* CV Mosby Co.) A,B. The presenting radiographs reveal a complex fracture-dislocation at the elbow with a radial head and neck fracture, proximal ulnar diaphysis fracture, intraarticular distal radius fracture, and a fracture of the scaphoid, capitate, and triquetrum. C. The radial head and neck were treated with stable internal fixation. D. The distal radius was approached through a dorsal incision and the die-punch fragment elevated and pinned. E. The scaphoid fracture was fixed with two Kirschner wires and local bone graft. F. An external fixator was used to support the complex wrist and distal radius fracture. G,H. Full elbow flexion and extension were achieved. I,J. Nearly full wrist extension and flexion were present. K,L. The fracture healed with good restoration of the articular surfaces.

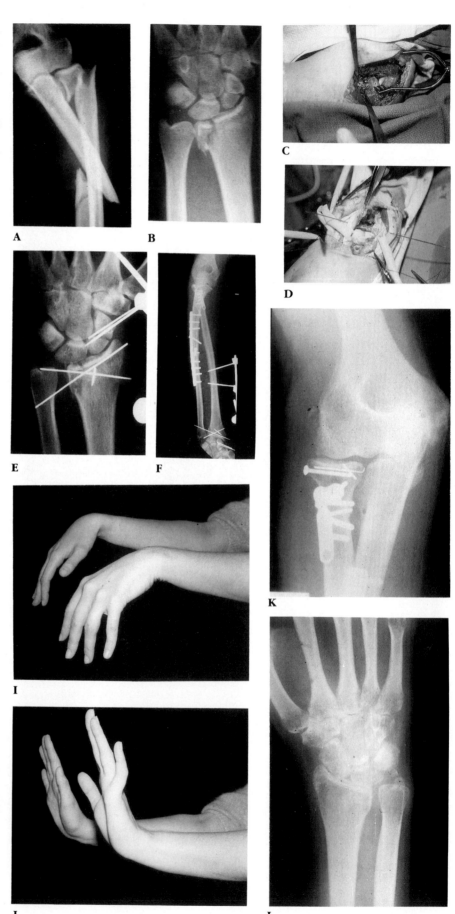

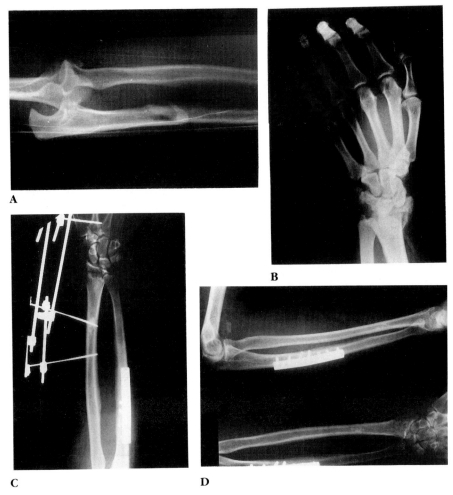

A

B

C   D

Figure 9.9. A 45-year-old construction worker fell on his outstretched right arm. A,B. A closed fracture of the proximal ulnar was associated with a complex fracture-dislocation of the elbow, disruption of both proximal and distal radioulna joints, and a complex fracture of the distal radius. C. The distal radius was reduced by longitudinal traction and placed in external skeletal fixation. The ulna was treated with a plate and screws and the disrupted proximal radioulna joint was reduced under direct vision. D. The radiographs at 6 months show anatomic restoration of the distal radius and reduction of the distal and proximal radioulnar joints.

interphalangeal joint fracture-dislocation in one case each. Three forearm fractures were open, and elevated forearm compartment pressure was found in two other cases (Fig. 9.8A–I).

The distal radius fractures were treated by open reduction and internal fixation in 4 cases, external skeletal fixation in 5, percutaneous Kirschner wire fixation in 2, and a plaster splint in one (Fig. 9.9A–D).

In follow-up, the average elbow flexion was 135 degrees and the average extension was 11 degrees. The average forearm pronation was 57 degrees and the average supination was 55 degrees. In 6 patients the distal radioulnar joint was unstable at follow-up, averaging 18 months. The average wrist extension was 64 degrees and the average flexion was 58 degrees (Table 9.2).

Fractures with Bone Loss

In certain instances, a combined Type V fracture will feature metaphyseal bone loss with the distal articular surface either intact or capable of being restored sufficiently to avoid an arthrodesis. This is sometimes the case with a gunshot injury or that due to machinery. As most of these will require initial open wound care, external fixation proves the method of choice for the primary skeletal stabilization.[36] Once wound control has been accomplished and the soft tissue coverage secured, restoration of the defect with autogenous iliac crest graft can be accomplished. Care should always be directed at trying to maintain the integrity of the distal radioulnar joint (Fig. 9.10A–F).

Table 9.2. Complex forearm and radius injury.

Case no.	Outcome			Radiograph	Functional rating
	Elbow flexion/ extension	Forearm pronation/ supination	Wrist extension/ flexion		
1	135/0°	80/40°	65/60°	Fractures healed; widened DRUJ	Excellent
2	140/0°	60/80°	60/60°	Healed fractures; nonunion ulnar styloid	Excellent
				Marginal compression of silicone implant	
3	130/5°	50/30°	70/60°	Fractures healed; malunion proximal ulna	Satisfactory
4	125/20°	20/30°	40/40°	Fractures healed; heterotopic bone at elbow	Unsatisfactory
5	130/10°	80/80°	60/60°	Fractures healed	Excellent
6	130/30°	45/80°	60/50°	Fractures healed	Satisfactory
7	150/20°	75/75°	70/70°	Fractures healed; grade I posttraumatic arthritis of radiocarpal joint	Satisfactory
8	150/5°	80/80°	75/50°	Fractures healed; Grade I arthritis radiocarpal joint	Excellent
9	130/20°	80/70°	60/50°	Fractures healed	Satisfactory
10	135/5°	5/15°	80/80°	Fractures healed; synostosis proximal forearm, disrupted DRUJ	Unsatisfactory

DRUJ, distal radioulnar joint.

Figure 9.10. A complex open distal radius fracture in a 46-year-old male injured by a press. A,B. The initial radiograph reveals extensive metaphyseal bone loss. Surprisingly, his neurovascular status remained intact and the radiocarpal articular surface was spared. C. External fixation was applied which maintained the length of both the radiocarpal orientation and the soft tissue alignment. D,E. At 6 weeks post injury, an intercalary iliac crest graft was placed.

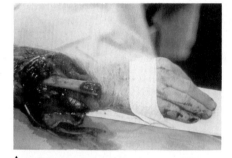

A

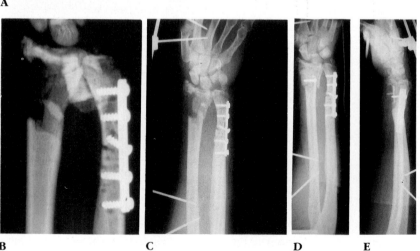

B   C   D   E

Fracture with Neurovascular Injury

These Type V fractures are characterized by their association with nerve or vascular disruption. As one might expect, they are likely to be the result of high-energy injury, and more often than not, they are associated with soft tissue injury, bone loss, and even forearm compartment syndrome (Fig. 9.11A–H).

When ischemia of the hand is present, definitive fixation of the distal radius fracture should be considered prior to revascularization (Fig. 9.12A–C). Given that the fractures are often comminuted, associated with bone loss and soft tissue loss, and require careful postoperative monitoring, external fixation is commonly added (Fig. 9.13A–G). When crushing injury involves the hand,

Figure 9.11. A high-energy combined Type V fracture from a motorcycle accident. A Gustillo Grade II soft tissue injury was present on the dorsal surface. The brachial artery was disrupted at the elbow. A,B. Anteroposterior and lateral radiographs show the extensive injury pattern with the marked destruction of the articular surface. Note that the fracture extends proximally into the diaphysis of the radius. C,D. The ipsilateral limb was injured as well with a severely displaced open olecranon fracture and brachial artery disruption. The elbow was unstable. Following debridement, fasciotomy, and artery repair, the olecranon was secured with a tension band. An external fixator was required to span the unstable elbow. E,F. Following debridement of the open distal radius, the ulnar was stabilized with a four-hole 3.5-mm dynamic compression plate. The radius was brought out to length and also stabilized with an external fixator. Anteroposterior and lateral postoperative x-ray at 5 weeks. G,H. The wrist was salvaged with a radioscapholunate fusion using bicortical iliac crest bone graft. A distal ulna resection was also done at the time. The patient returned to work requiring full bimanual function.

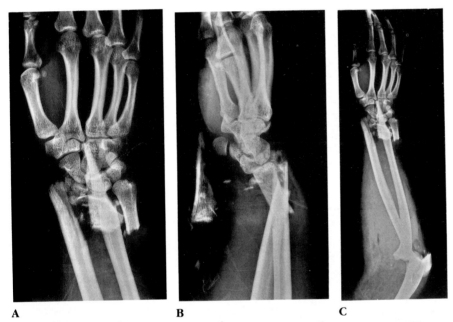

A   B   C

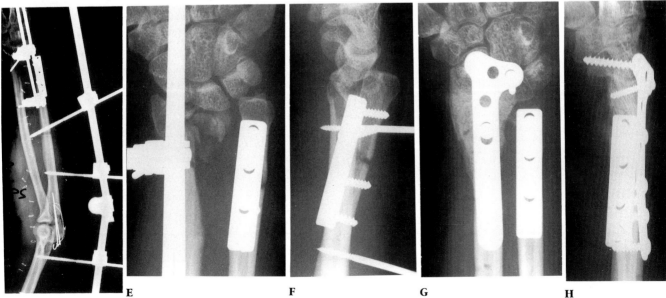

E   F   G   H

D

Figure 9.12. A 40-year-old male had his dominant hand and arm caught in a machine, resulting in an incomplete amputation of his hand. A. The hand was incompletely severed through the mid-palm. B. The radiograph reveals proximal fractures of both the distal radius and the ulnar. C. Both fractures were stabilized with plates and screws prior to revascularization of the hand.

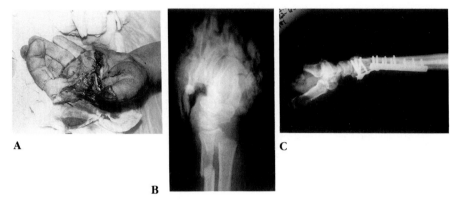

Figure 9.13. A 43-year-old woman sustained a mutilating injury to her left hand and wrist from the propeller of a motor boat. A. The initial radiographs reflect the extreme amount of skeletal disruption. B. Extensive soft tissue injury was present, including both neurovascular bundles and all of the flexor tendons. C. Following debridement the hand was realigned and revascularized. D. Extensive internal and external fixation was used. E. A free serratus flap was placed to cover the extensive soft tissue defect. F,G. At 4 months postinjury a wrist arthrodesis was performed using a long plate and autogenous iliac crest bone graft.

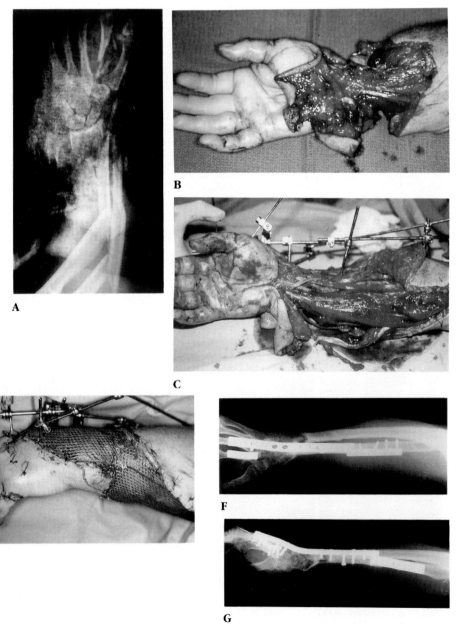

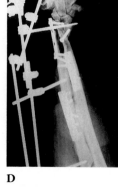

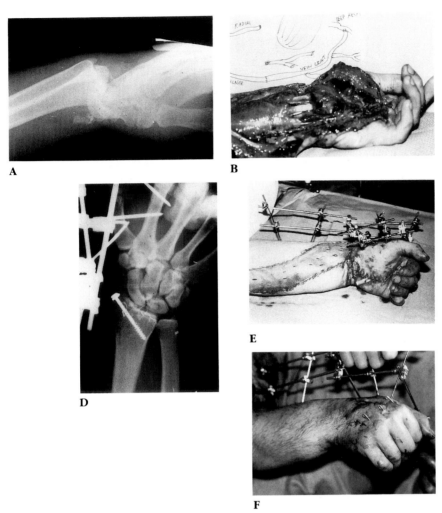

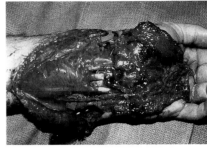

Figure 9.14. A high-energy injury resulting in a complex Type IV fracture-dislocation but also complete occlusion of both the radial and ulnar arteries. The hand was ischemic. A. The lateral radiograph reveals the complex skeletal injury. B. Upon exploration of the soft tissue injury it was apparent that the entire arterial supply of the hand had been disrupted. C. Using a vein graft the arterial supply was restored. Prior to this the fracture-dislocation had been stabilized and an external fixator applied. D. The radiograph of the external fixator in place. Note the pins in the second and first metacarpal to help maintain the width of the first web space. E. A split-thickness skin graft was applied to cover the forearm which had its volar compartments released. F. An additional view of the external fixation construction. The metacarpophalangeal joints were temporarily pinned in flexion to maintain the resting length of the collateral ligaments.

addition of pins into the first metacarpal will help maintain the first web space (Fig. 9.14A–F).

In the setting of isolated median or ulnar nerve dysfunction, judgment should be made according to the nature of the injury, extent of sensory or motor loss, and associated soft tissue loss (Fig. 9.15A–O). It has been the authors' preference to explore and decompress the median and ulnar nerves at the level of the distal forearm and wrist when nerve dysfunction is associated with these high-energy Type V injuries (Fig. 9.16A–J).

Compartment Syndrome

A number of conditions are associated with elevated pressure within the soft tissue compartments of the forearm. These include, among others, forearm fractures,[14] constricting dressings or casts,[13] burns,[40] vascular injuries,[28] and any condition that can lead to a reduced volume or increased pressure within the forearm compartment.[22,39] Although distal radius fractures are common, including those due to high-velocity injury, it is of interest that relatively few cases of associated forearm compartment syndromes have been reported.[3,23,25,31,41,49]

Although some reports have implicated constricting casts,[3] hematoma block,[49] or Bier's block,[16] the more commonly described condition is the

Figure 9.15. A 24-year-old house painter fell off a scaffolding onto his outstretched left hand. On presentation, dense sensory loss was noted in the distribution of both median and ulnar nerves. His distal forearm was tense and the volar compartment pressure measurement was 70 mm Hg. A,B. Initial anteroposterior and lateral radiographs reveal a complex intraarticular fracture with both dorsal and palmar displacement. C. The lesion was initially approached volarly. The forearm compartments as well as the median and ulnar nerves were decompressed. A large fragment from the anterior lunate facet was found displaced, rotated, and compressing both the ulnar nerve and the artery (arrow). D. Following provisional stabilization of the anterior fragment, a dorsal incision was made to facilitate reconstruction of the lunate facet. The dorsal fragment was still found to be attached to the dorsal radioulnar ligament. E. The fragments were held with multiple Kirschner wires and a loop wire was passed through a drill hole in the volar radius and through the volar capsule to hold the lunate facet fragment. F,G. External fixation permitted early functional aftercare beginning on the initial postoperative day. (*Figure continues on facing page.*)

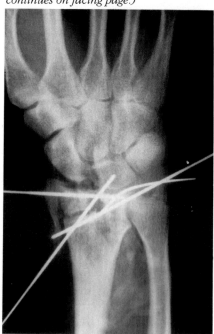

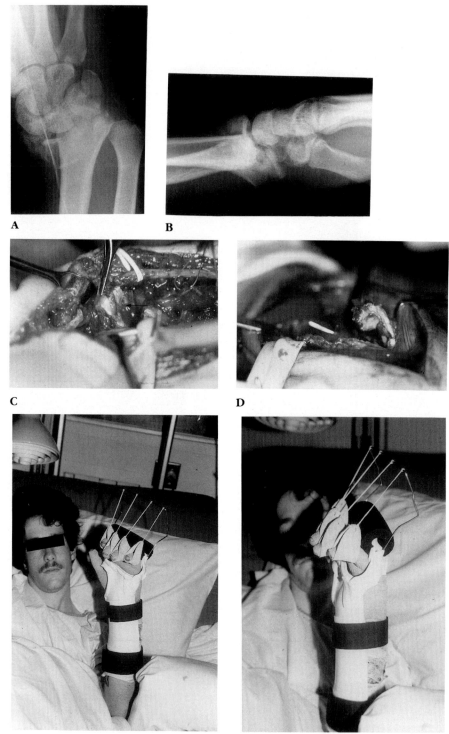

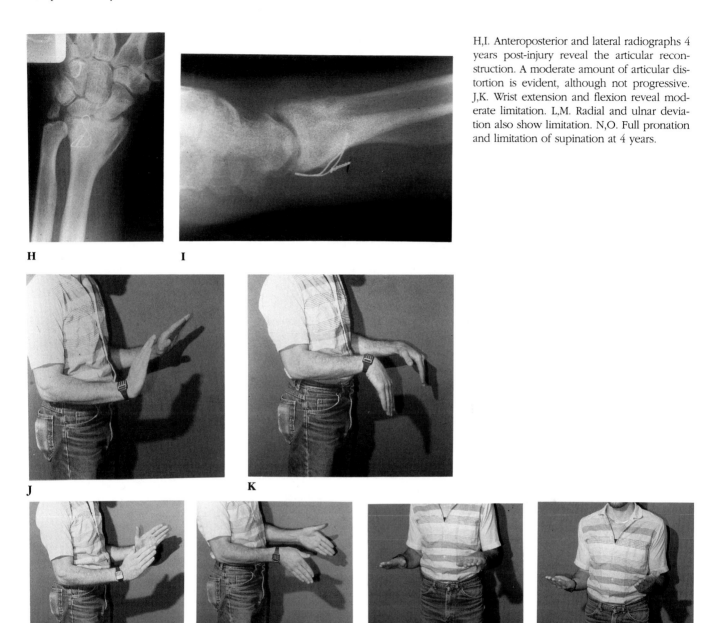

H,I. Anteroposterior and lateral radiographs 4 years post-injury reveal the articular reconstruction. A moderate amount of articular distortion is evident, although not progressive. J,K. Wrist extension and flexion reveal moderate limitation. L,M. Radial and ulnar deviation also show limitation. N,O. Full pronation and limitation of supination at 4 years.

delayed onset of signs and symptoms of elevated compartment pressure after initial treatment of the fracture. Furthermore, a fracture in a younger individual from a high-velocity impact is more likely to develop the compartment-related problem.[42,44] Stockley, Harvey, and Getty reported on a series of five cases of compartment syndromes with distal radius fractures.[44] All were due to high-energy trauma in a younger group of patients—all male. What was also noteworthy is the fact that none of their patients had any signs or symptoms upon presentation. Rather, the diagnosis of elevated forearm compartment pressure was not made in some cases until upwards of 48 hours following the initial treatment.

Simpson and Jupiter have reviewed a similar experience of eight fractures in five patients which also featured a delayed onset of signs and symptoms of a forearm compartment syndrome (Fig. 9.17A–R).[42] Four patients were male and one female, with an average age of 32 years. All fractures were associated with a higher-energy injury (Table 9.3). The fractures were initially reduced using a

Figure 9.16. A combined Type V injury associated with extensive soft tissue trauma in a 36-year-old man injured on a motorcycle. A,B. The initial anteroposterior and lateral radiographs demonstrate the extensive displacement at the fracture. C,D. Following decompression of the median nerve, the fracture was reduced using both longitudinal traction and direct manipulation of the fragments. E,F. A second debridement was performed, at which time the defect in the radius was filled with autogenous iliac crest bone graft. Note as well the stabilization of the ulna with a contoured third tubular plate. G,H. Anteroposterior and lateral radio graphs 6 weeks postinjury at the time of removal of the external skeletal fixation.

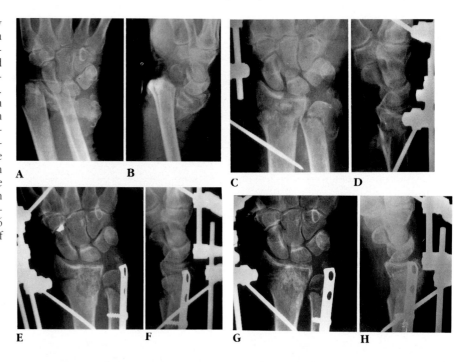

Figure 9.17. A 24-year-old male fell from a roof sustaining bilateral complex distal radius fractures and a left zygoma fracture. His initial treatment was a closed reduction and sugar tong splint application. Signs and symptoms of a forearm compartment syndrome developed approximately 30 hours postinjury. A–D. Anteroposterior and lateral radiographs of the initial fractures. E. The left forearm compartment was released through a volar approach with release of the canal of Guyon and carpal tunnel. F,G. The left complex intraarticular fracture was fixed with a volar buttress plate, tension wire, oblique Kirschner wire across the radial styloid, and cannulated screw to hold the lunate facet. External fixation was also used. H,I. The right extraarticular fracture was fixed with a percutaneous Kirschner wire and external fixation. Both volar wounds were covered with split-thickness skin grafts. J,K. Anteroposterior and lateral radiographs of the healed fracture at 12 weeks postinjury. N–Q. Full functional recovery was noted at a very early stage. These pictures were at 12 weeks postinjury.

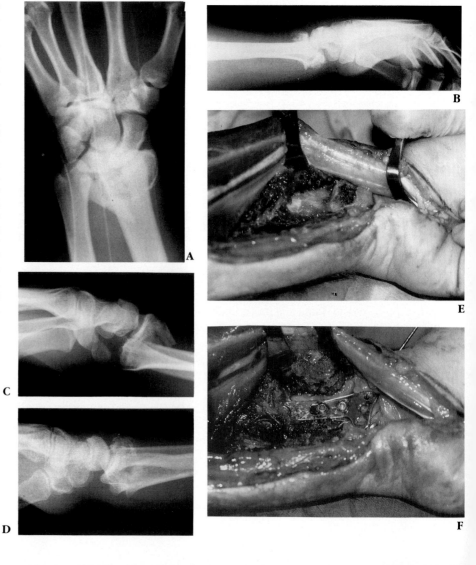

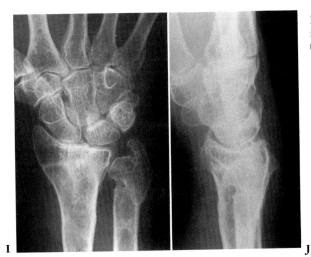

I,J. At 3 year follow-up, excellent anatomy is maintained. The patient noted few functional difficulties.

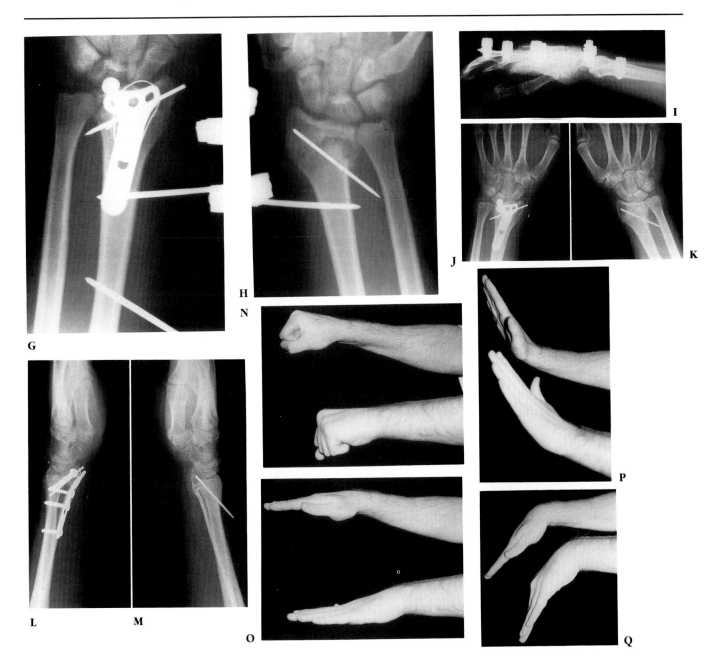

Table 9.3. Radius fracture and compartment syndrome.

Case no.	Patient	Age (yrs)	Gender	Limb (*Dominant)	Mechanism	Associated injuries	Delayed onset	Compartment Pressure (mm Hg)	Fracture classification AO/ASIF	Fracture classification Fernandez	Treatment
1	1	45	M	L	Fall from 20 feet	None	20 h	90	C1.2	Combined compression/shearing	External fixation Volar T plate Percutaneous pins
2	1	45	M	R*	Fall from 20 feet	None	20 h	85	C3.1	Combined compression/shearing	External fixation Volar T plate Percutaneous pins
3	2	31	M	L	Fall from 30 feet	L subtrochanteric femur fracture	18 h	65	C3.2	Combined compression/shearing	External fixation
4	3	26	M	L	Fall from 20 feet	Closed head injury; L zygoma fracture	30 h	—	C3.2	Combined compression/shearing	External fixation Volar T plate Percutaneous pins Tension band wire
5	3	26	M	R(*)	Fall from 20 feet	Closed head injury; L zygoma fracture	30 h	—	C1.2	Shearing	External fixation Percutaneous pins
6	4	34	M	R(*)	Motorcycle accident	Ipsilateral scapholunate diastasis	24 h	70	C3.1	Combined compression/shearing	External fixation Volar T plate Percutaneous pins Scapholunate pins
7	5	23	F	L	Fall from 8 feet	None	48 h	70	C3.3	Combined compression/shearing	External fixation Percutaneous pins
8	5	23	F	R(*)	Fall from 8 feet	None	48 h	90	C3.1	Combined compression/shearing	External fixation Percutaneous pins

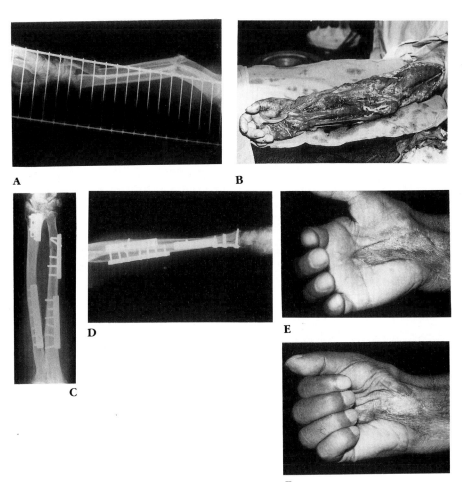

Figure 9.18. A 60-year-old man had his right dominant hand caught in machinery that rolled hot plastic sheets. He presented with a swollen arm with compromised arterial inflow to his hand. A. The lateral radiographs with his arm supported on a metal splint. The fractures included transverse fractures of the proximal radius and ulna, an oblique fracture of the distal third of the ulna, and a comminuted fracture of the distal radius extending into the radio-carpal joint. B. Through an extensile anterior exposure, fasciotomies of the superficial and deep flexor compartments were done. The fractures were stabilized through this anterior approach. C,D. Anteroposterior and lateral radiographs 16 weeks post-operatively showing the anatomic reduction and stable internal fixation. Two small plates, including a 3.5-mm plate and third tubular plate, supported the reduction of the distal radius. E,F. Good flexion resulted with a residual flexion contracture due to ischemia of the extrinsic forearm flexion muscles. Note the split-thickness graft required to cover the extensive forearm wound.

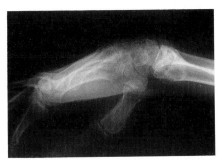

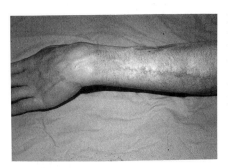

Figure 9.19. A 28-year-old male with a complex distal radius fracture and delayed onset of compartment syndrome. A. At 6 months postinjury, the lateral radiograph reveals a flexed wrist with articular disruption. B. The clinical appearance at 6 months postinjury. C,D. The definitive treatment required to restore a functional position and digital mobility was a wrist arthrodesis.

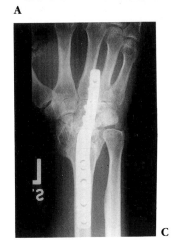

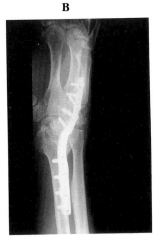

hematoma block in five and a Bier's block in three. Each fracture was initially immobilized in sugar tong above-elbow splints.

The signs and symptoms consistent with elevated pressure in the forearm compartment were not appreciated for at least 18 hours, and in one case 52 hours, following initial treatment. Forearm compartment pressure measured in six of eight fractures with pressures in the volar flexor compartment ranged from 65 to 90 mm Hg.

In each case, the forearms were decompressed using a Henry approach to the volar forearm. Fracture fixation was accomplished using a volar buttress plate in four cases and external skeletal fixation in all eight. Adjuvant percutaneous Kirschner wires were also used in seven of eight cases. It was possible to secondarily close the volar wounds in six and to cover them with a split thickness skin graft in two fractures (Fig. 9.18A–F).

At a minimum follow-up of 12 months, most patients had recovered good to excellent function. One patient, however, did not, and was left with contracted flexor tendons and a stiff and painful wrist. He ultimately elected to have a wrist arthrodesis (Fig. 9.19A–D).

References

1. Bell MJ: Perilunar dislocation of the carpus and an associated Colles' fracture. *Hand* 15: 262–266, 1983.
2. Bickerstoff DR, Bell MJ: Carpal malalignment in Colles' fractures. *J Hand Surg* 143: 155–160, 1989.
3. Cooney W, Dobyns JH, Linscheid RL: Complications of Colles' fractures. *J Bone Joint Surg* 62A: 613–619, 1980.
4. Curr JF, Coe WA: Dislocation of the inferior radioulna joint. *Br J Surg* 34: 74–77, 1946.
5. Edwards GS, Jupiter JB: Fractures with acute distal radioulna joint dislocation. The Essex-Lopresti lesion revisited. *Clin Orthop* 234: 61–69, 1988.
6. Essex-Lopresti P: Fracture of the radial head with distal radioulna joint dislocation. *J Bone Joint Surg* 33B: 244–47, 1951.
7. Fernandez DL: Techniques and results of external fixation of complex carpal injuries. *Hand Clin* 9: 625–637, 1993.
8. Fernandez DL, Ghillani R: External fixation of complex carpal dislocations: A preliminary report. *J Hand Surg* 12A: 335–347, 1987.
9. Fernandez DL, Jakob RP, Büchler U: External fixation of the wrist. Current indications and technique. *Ann Chir Gyn* 72: 298–302, 1983.
10. Fisk GR: The wrist: Review article. *J Bone Joint Surg* 66B: 396–407, 1984.
11. Frykman GK: Fracture of the distal radius including sequelae—shoulder hand finger syndrome. Disturbance in the distal radioulna joint and impairment of nerve function. A clinical and experimental study. *Acta Orthop Scand Suppl* 108: 1–155, 1967.
12. Galeazzi R: Ueber ein besonderes Syndrom bei Verletzungen im Bereich der Unterarmknocken. *Arch Orthop Unfallchir* 35: 557–562, 1934.
13. Garfin SR, Mubarak SJ, Evans KL, et al: Qualification of intracompartmental pressure and volume under plaster casts. *J Bone Joint Surg* 63A: 449–453, 1981.
14. Gelberman RH, Garfin SR, Hergenroeder P, et al: Compartment syndromes of the forearm: Diagnosis and treatment. *Clin Orthop* 161: 252–262, 1981.
15. Green WB, Anderson WJ: Simultaneous fracture of the scaphoid and radius in a child. Case report. *J Pediat Orthop* 2: 191–194, 1982.
16. Hastings H, Misamore G: Compartment syndrome resulting from intravenous regional anesthesia. *J Hand Surg* 12: 559–562, 1987.
17. Jenkins R, Jones R: Simultaneous Colles' and scaphoid fractures. *Am J Emerg Med* 4: 229–235, 1986.
18. Jupiter JB: The management of fractures in one upper extremity. *J Hand Surg* 11A: 279–282, 1986.
19. Jupiter JB, Kour AK, Richards RR, Nathan J, Meinhard B: The floating radius in bipolar fracture-dislocation of the forearm. *J Orthop Trauma* 8: 99–106, 1994.
20. Kristiansen B: Simultaneous Colles' fracture and fracture of the carpal scaphoid. *Ugeskrift Læger* 144: 799, 1982.
21. Lewis RM: Colles' fracture—causative mechanism. *Surgery* 27: 427–436, 1950.

22. Matsen FA: Compartmental syndrome: A united concept. *Clin Orthop* 113: 8–14, 1975.
23. Matthews LS: Acute volar compartment syndrome secondary to distal radius fracture in an athlete. *Am J Sports Med* 11: 6–7, 1983.
24. Mayfield JK, Johnson RP, Kilcoyne, RF: Carpal dislocations: Pathomechanics and progressive perilunar instability. *J Hand Surg* 5: 226–241, 1980.
25. McQuillan WM, Nolan B: Ischaemia complicating injury. *J Bone Joint Surg* 50B: 482–488, 1968.
26. Moeller BN: Simultaneous fracture of the carpal scaphoid and adjacent bones. *Hand* 15: 258–261, 1983.
27. Monteggia GB: *Instituzione Chirurgiche*, 2nd ed. G Maspero: 1813.
28. Mubarek SJ, Hargens AR: Acute compartment syndromes. *Surg Clin North Am* 63: 539–565, 1983.
29. Mudgal CS, Hastings H: Scapholunate diastasis in fractures of the distal radius. *J Hand Surg* 18B: 725–729, 1993.
30. Mudgal CS, Jones WA: Scapholunate diastasis: A component of fractures of the distal radius. *J Hand Surg* 15B: 503–505, 1990.
31. Naito M, Ogata K: Acute volar compartment syndrome during skeletal traction in distal radius fracture. *Clin Orthop* 24: 234–237, 1989.
32. Odena IC: Bipolar fracture-dislocation of the forearm. *J Bone Joint Surg* 34A: 968–976, 1952.
33. Porter ML, Tillman RM: Pilon fractures of the wrist. *J Hand Surg* 17B: 63–68, 1992.
34. Putnam M, Walsh T: External fixation of open fractures of the upper extremity. *Hand Clin* 9: 613–623, 1993.
35. Richards RR, Ghose T, McBroom RJ: Ipsilateral fractures of the distal radius and scaphoid treated by Herbert screw and external skeletal fixation. A report of two cases. *Clin Orthop* 282: 219–221, 1992.
36. Riggs SA, Cooney W: External fixation of complex hand and wrist fractures. *J Trauma* 23: 332–341, 1983.
37. Rosenthal DI, Schwartz M, Phillips WC, Jupiter JB: Fractures of the radius with instability of the wrist. *Am J Roentgenol* 141: 113–116, 1983.
38. Ruster D, Nepieralsk, K: Zur pathogenese von Navikularefrakturen unter Berücksichtung der Kombination mit Brüchen am distalen Unterarmende. *Beiträge Orthop Traumatol* 19: 155–160, 1972.
39. Rydholm U, Werner CO, Ohlin P: Intracompartment forearm presssure during rest and exercise. *Clin Orthop* 175: 213–215, 1983.
40. Saffle JR, Zeluff GR, Warden GD: Intramuscular pressure in the burned arm: Measurement and response to escharotomy. *Am J Surg* 140: 825–831, 1980.
41. Shall J, Cohn BT, Froimson AI: Acute compartment syndrome of the forearm in association with fracture of the distal end of the radius. *J Bone Joint Surg* 68A: 1451–1454, 1986.
42. Simpson NS, Jupiter J: Delayed presentation of compartment syndrome following distal radius fracture. Unpublished.
43. Smith JT, Keeve JP, Bertin KC, Mann RJ: Simultaneous fracture of the distal radius and scaphoid. *J Trauma* 28: 676–679, 1988.
44. Stockley I, Harvey IA, Getty CJM: Acute volar compartment syndrome of the forearm secondary to fractures of the distal radius. *Injury* 19: 101–104, 1986.
45. Stother IG: A report of 3 cases of simultaneous Colles' and scaphoid fractures. *Injury* 7: 185–188, 1976.
46. Tountas AA, Waddell JP: Simultaneous fractures of the distal radius and scaphoid. *J Orthop Trauma* 1: 312–316, 1988.
47. Trousdale RT, Amadio PC, Cooney WP, Morrey BF: Radioulna dissociation. *J Bone Joint Surg* 74: 1486–1497, 1992.
48. Trumble TE, Benirschke S, Vedder NB: Ipsilateral fractures of the scaphoid and radius. *J Hand Surg* 18A: 8–14, 1993.
49. Younge D: Haematoma block for fractures of the wrist: A cause of compartment syndrome. *J Hand Surg* 14B: 194–195, 1989.

Chapter Ten

Malunion of the Distal End of the Radius

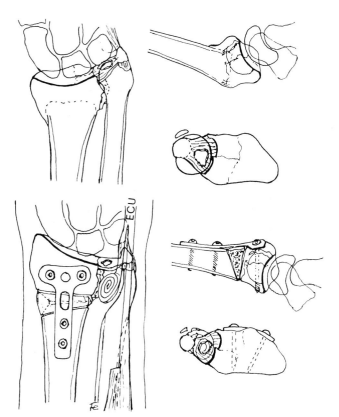

Fractures of the radius within two inches of the wrist, where treated by the most eminent surgeons, are of very difficult management so as to avoid all deformity; indeed, more or less deformity may occur under the treatment of the most eminent surgeons, and more or less imperfection in the motion of the wrist or radius is very apt to follow for a longer or shorter time. Even when the fracture is well cured, an anterior prominence at the wrist, or near it, will sometimes result from the swelling of the soft parts.

As the above opinion of Professor Mott coincides with my own observations, both in Europe and in this city, as well as with many of our most distinguished surgical authorities, I venture to hope that it may assist in removing some of the groundless and ill-merited aspersions which are occasionally thrown on the members of our profession by the ignorant or designing.

Boston Med. Surg. J. XXV, p. 289

Figure 10.1. The "natural history" of an unstable extraarticular dorsal bending fracture. A,B. The initial anteroposterior and lateral radiographs demonstrate wide displacement of the distal fragment. The radiographs fail to accurately depict the comminution of the dorsal metaphyseal cortical and cancellous bone. C,D. Initial anteroposterior and lateral radiographs following fracture reduction and plaster immobilization. E,F. As early as 1 week postreduction, the radiographs demonstrate loss of reduction, with the distal fragment beginning to displace in a dorsal and radial direction. G,H. At 6 weeks following fracture, the fracture has nearly returned to its original position. I,J. At 8 weeks postinjury, extreme displacement has occurred with deformity involving both the radiocarpal and radioulnar articulations.

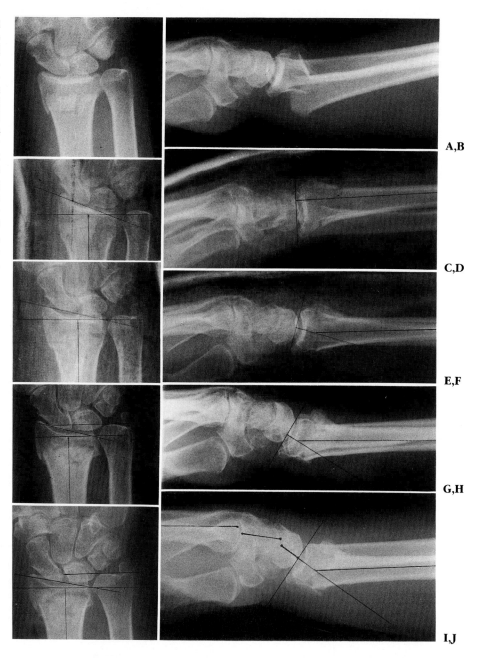

A,B

C,D

E,F

G,H

I,J

Union with deformity continues to be the most common complication following fracture of the distal end of the radius.[7,31,32] Malunion may be extraarticular, characterized by metaphyseal angulation and loss of radial length; intraarticular, involving distortion of the either the radiocarpal or the radioulnar joints or both; or a combination of the two.

The most commonly observed cause of an extraarticular malunion is secondary displacement of the initial fracture reduction due to deficient cancellous bone in the metaphysis (Fig. 10.1A–J). In contrast, failure to restore articular congruity within 1 to 2mm of anatomic restoration can result in arthritic changes and subsequent disability.[26]

The need for operative correction of a symptomatic, malunited fracture of the distal radius has been long recognized. Distal ulnar resection attributed to Darrach following his description of the procedure in 1913[8] had in fact been noted by Desault in 1791[9] and by Moore in 1880.[36]

Surgical correction through the radial deformity was described early by Ghormley and Mroz in 1932.[20] In describing four corrective osteotomies, they observed that this procedure, with or without a bone graft, could help improve the external appearance of the deformity. In 1935 Durman also reported on satisfactory results following radial osteotomy, also in four patients.[10,11] Durman obtained bone graft from the distal end of the proximal radial fragment which was then fit transversely into the osteotomy. By making one end of the graft wider, he was able to correct the radial deformity. In 1937 Campbell published an important paper on the subject of radial osteotomy.[5] In his approach, the radius was osteotomized transversely approximately 1 inch above the radiocarpal joint through a surgical approach between the brachioradialis and extensor pollicis brevis tendons. He employed bone graft harvested from the medial border of the distal ulnar proximal to the distal radioulnar joint. This graft was inserted into the dorsoradial defect of the opening osteotomy. Campbell observed that this approach offered an enhanced appearance and function compared to osteotomy without bone graft interposition. Hobart and Kraft in 1941[21] published results of osteotomy of the distal radius with graft obtained from the resected distal ulnar or from the proximal radius as described by Dorman. In the same year, Milch described his technique of "cuff resection of the ulnar," which involved a shortening osteotomy of the distal ulnar for a malunited distal radius fracture characterized by severe shortening.[35] In 1945 Speed and Knight[46] analyzed the results of their experience with osteotomy of malunited Colles' fractures in 60 patients. They recommended the use of intramedullary bone pegs or dual onlay grafts to avoid loss of the operative correction, especially in the setting of extreme deformity or underlying osteoporosis. They also suggested that corrective osteotomy be avoided in the presence of wrist or digital stiffness.

Merle d'Aubigné and Joussement, also in 1945,[33] described a multiple-facet curved osteotomy in the sagittal plane designed to restore radial length without the need for an interpositional bone graft. The results of the procedure were later analyzed by Merle d'Aubigné and Tubiana, noting a satisfactory outcome in 27 patients.[34] The distal ulnar was resected in 17 of the 27 wrists. Although the authors concluded that their curved-facet osteotomy along with resection of the distal ulnar offered better cosmetic and functional results than the Darrach resection alone, the disadvantage of their procedure proved to be the prolonged period of postoperative immobilization in plaster. They also observed that the cosmetic correction was not as evident when substantial dorsal angulation was present. A similar osteotomy curved in the sagittal plane, known as the Rixford operation, was mentioned by Bunnell in 1948, although not described in detail.[4]

A posttraumatic deformity following fracture of the distal radius is not always symptomatic (Fig. 10.2). Impairment of function rather than radiologic deformity forms the basis of decision making when one approaches the patient with such a condition. This chapter will focus on the pathomechanics associated with deformity of the distal radius, indications for and surgical tactics of osteotomy, evaluation of outcome following deformity correction, and associated complications.

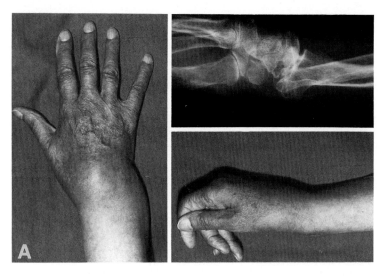

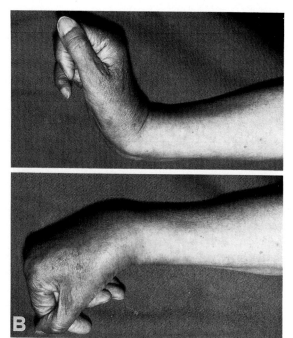

Figure 10.2. Asymptomatic malunion in a 70-year-old woman seen 30 years postfracture. A. The visible deformity correlates well to the skeletal deformity. B. A functional arc of wrist extension and flexion was retained. There was little residual discomfort.

The Anatomic Correlation of a Malunited Fracture of the Distal Radius

A malunited extraarticular fracture of the distal end of the radius is more often than not a complex deformity. The most common deformity following a dorsal bending fracture includes loss of the volar tilt of the articular surface in the sagittal plane, loss of the ulnar inclination in the frontal plane, loss of length, and a supination deformity of the distal fragment with respect to the proximal diaphysis (Fig. 10.3A–C).[13] In addition, the distal fragment may be displaced in radial or ulnar translation as well as by a dorsopalmar shift in the sagittal plane.

It has been observed in clinical studies that there is a certain relationship between the quality of the anatomic result and the overall wrist function.[18–21,23,31,50] It should not therefore be difficult to appreciate the fact that a multidirectional deformity will affect the function not only of the radiocarpal but also of the radioulnar and midcarpal articulations.

At the radiocarpal articulation, deformity will have a negative influence on the arc of flexion and extension. With a dorsal deformity, patients will experience loss of palmar flexion and at times exaggerated wrist extension with respect to the contralateral uninjured wrist (Fig. 10.3B). The load transmission from the carpus to the radius is displaced, reducing the overall articular contact surface. This, in turn, will represent a potential for the development of symptomatic, posttraumatic arthrosis (Fig. 10.3B).[30,40,50] A third problem is to be found with dorsal displacement of the carpus with intact intercarpal ligamentous support. This in effect represents a radiocarpal instability with dorsal translation of the entire carpus. It is more likely to be present when the dorsal angulation of the distal end of the radius is greater than 35 degrees. The wrist will prove stable only when the hand is extended, causing the carpus to return to a reduced position. Active wrist flexion will increase the dorsal subluxation of the carpus, with pain developing at the radiocarpal articulation (Fig. 10.4).

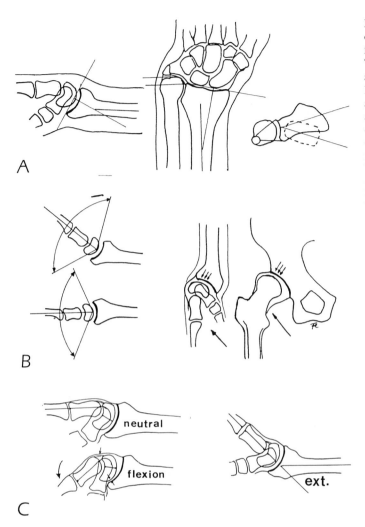

Figure 10.3. Diagrammatic representation of problems associated with a malunited fracture of the distal end of the radius. A. The deformity most commonly involves the sagittal, frontal, and coronal planes. B. Dorsal displacement of the flexion–extension arc of motion as well as dorsal carpal subluxation is compared to a prearthritic deformity with a subluxated dysplastic hip. C. Adaptive carpal instability nondissociative malalignment with a malunited dorsal bending (Colles') fracture. (Reprinted with permission. Fernandez DL: Reconstructive procedures for malunion and post-traumatic arthritis. *Orthop Clin N America* 24: 343, 1993. WB Saunders: Philadelphia.)

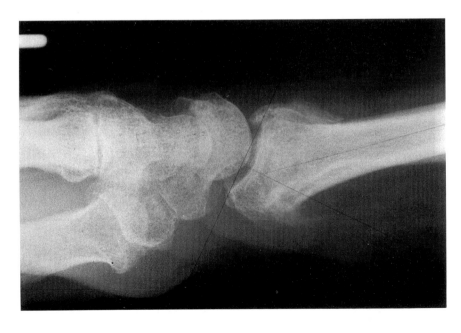

Figure 10.4. Lateral radiograph demonstrating a malunited dorsally displaced bending (Colles') fracture with dorsal carpal subluxation with a normal carpal alignment. (From Fernandez DL: Malunion of the distal radius. *AAOS Instructional Course Lectures* vol. 42, p. 100, 1993 by permission of the American Academy of Orthopaedic Surgeons.)

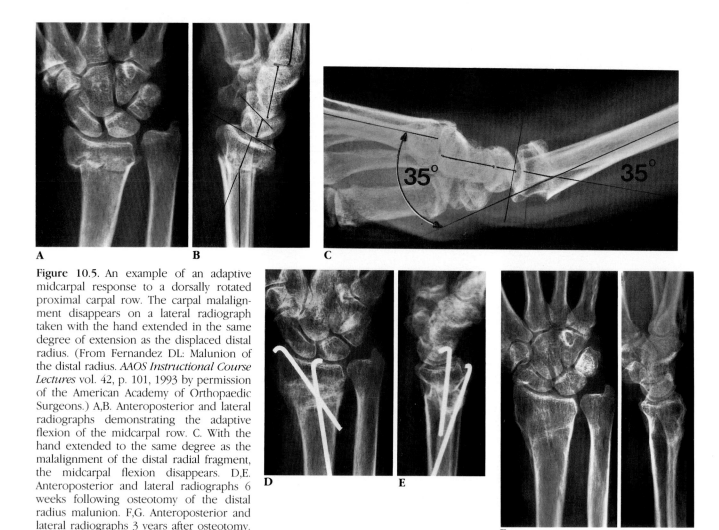

Figure 10.5. An example of an adaptive midcarpal response to a dorsally rotated proximal carpal row. The carpal malalignment disappears on a lateral radiograph taken with the hand extended in the same degree of extension as the displaced distal radius. (From Fernandez DL: Malunion of the distal radius. *AAOS Instructional Course Lectures* vol. 42, p. 101, 1993 by permission of the American Academy of Orthopaedic Surgeons.) A,B. Anteroposterior and lateral radiographs demonstrating the adaptive flexion of the midcarpal row. C. With the hand extended to the same degree as the malalignment of the distal radial fragment, the midcarpal flexion disappears. D,E. Anteroposterior and lateral radiographs 6 weeks following osteotomy of the distal radius malunion. F,G. Anteroposterior and lateral radiographs 3 years after osteotomy. Note a slight volar flexion to the lunate.

At the midcarpal articulation, the dorsal tilt of the end of the radius can result in a compensatory flexion deformity in the midcarpal joint (Fig. 10.3C). This represents an adaptive response to a dorsally rotated proximal carpal row.[28,43] The dorsal capsule of the wrist is stretched during forceful flexion, leading to pain at the midcarpal level. What is unique is that this adaptive malalignment of the carpus to the dorsal deformity of the end of the radius will not be seen in a lateral radiograph taken with the hand in the same degree of extension as the malunited distal radial fragment (Fig. 10.5A–C).

The dorsal malalignment of the distal radius can also result in an extrinsic midcarpal dynamic instability.[27,48] In this condition, a painful and audible subluxation of the midcarpus will be noted during active ulnar deviation of the wrist with the forearm in a pronated position. The dorsally rotated lunate is blocked from displacing palmarward during ulnar deviation by the dorsally tilted volar lip of the end of the radius. In those patients with associated ligamentous laxity, continued stress on the midcarpal joint will result in ligament attenuation and progressive dynamic midcarpal instability. This condition will need to be differentiated from the intrinsic palmar midcarpal instability between the triquetrum and hamate which results from laxity of the ulnar fibers of the palmar arcuate ligament and presents with an ulnar sag of the carpus.[27]

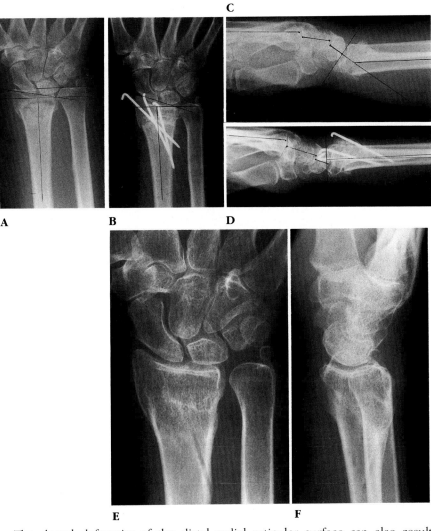

Figure 10.6. Fixed DISI instability in a 30-year-old secretary. A,B. Anteroposterior views before and after osteotomy. C,D. Lateral radiographs before and after osteotomy reveal that the carpus remains malrotated despite correction of the radial malunion. E,F. The healed osteotomy with continued DISI instability pattern.

The dorsal deformity of the distal radial articular surface can also result in a fixed carpal malalignment in dorsiflexion—a dorsal intercalary segment instability (DISI). For practical purposes, the DISIs associated with malunited dorsally angulated distal radial fractures may be divided into two types:

Type I A lax, reducible dorsal carpal malalignment that can be improved or totally corrected by radial osteotomy. This is more likely to be seen in younger patients with ligamentous laxity and good preoperative carpal motion (Fig. 10.5).

Type II A DISI deformity in which there is a fixed non-reducible dorsal carpal malalignment that cannot be improved by radial osteotomy (Fig. 10.6).

The third articulation that is affected by a malunited fracture is the distal radioulnar joint. The function of this joint can be impaired as a sequela of the distal radial fragment healing in either dorsal or volar angulation or shortening in reference to the distal ulnar, producing an incongruity of the joint surfaces in the sagittal, frontal, and horizontal planes (Fig. 10.7A). Several studies have identified the association of radial shortening with impaired function.[6,19,30,50]

Radial shortening results in mechanical impingement of the triangular fibrocartilage. During normal rotation of the forearm, the triangular fibrocartilage will "sweep" uniformly over the articular head of the distal ulnar. With shortening of the distal radius in relation to the distal ulnar, the triangular fibrocartilage is tightened and relatively blocked in both an anterior and

Figure 10.7. Schematic representation of the anatomic problems which will affect the distal radioulnar joint with a malunited distal end of the radius. A. The radioulnar incongruity is depicted in the sagittal, frontal, and horizontal planes. B. There may be mechanical impingement of the triangular fibrocartilage complex in an ulnar plus variance. C. Three common problems identified at the distal radioulnar joint include ulnocarpal abutment, instability, and a "fibrous" union of the ulnar styloid fracture without instability.

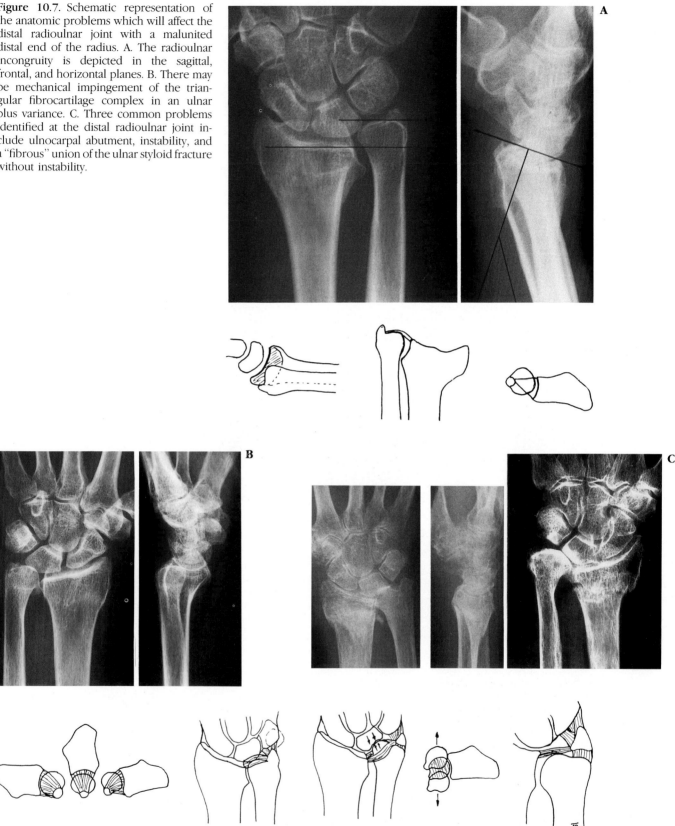

posterior position with respect to the head of the ulnar (Fig. 10.7B). This will result in impedance of the arc of forearm rotation. Longstanding radial shortening has also been shown to lead to ulnocarpal impingement with attrition wear in the center of the triangular fibrocartilage and ulnar head impaction onto the lunate (Fig. 10.7C). The correlation of a relative change in the normal relationships between the distal ulnar and radius has been shown to have a demonstrable effect on the transmission of force from the carpus to the end of the radius.[24,38] Dorsal tilt of the articular surface not only shifts the load distribution in the radiocarpal joint dorsally but also increases the load on the distal ulnar.[45]

Anteroposterior instability of the ulnar head may coexist with distal radius malunions due to loss of articular congruity between the ulnar and the distal radius and rupture or secondary elongation of the triangular ligament. Castaing[6] evaluated 440 distal radius fractures, noting a nonunion of the ulnar styloid in 77.5 percent of cases. By the same token, however, the presence of an ulnar styloid nonunion did not affect overall results. This was attributed to the feeling that the ulnar styloid had in fact healed, with a fibrous union between the ulnar head and triangular fibrocartilage complex (Fig. 10.7C). Although distal radioulnar joint instability does not appear to correlate directly with a nonunion of the ulnar styloid, some have suggested that ulnar styloid fractures should be treated with internal fixation when found to be associated with radioulnar joint instability.[44]

Fractures extending into the sigmoid notch can lead to posttraumatic arthrosis if incongruity remains after union. This may manifest itself with painful forearm rotation (Fig. 10.8A and B).

In addition to the above-described articular problems, malunion of the distal radius, particularly with the loss of ulnar inclination in the frontal plane, may direct the carpal tunnel into a radial direction, angulating the flexor tendons and thereby decreasing their mechanical advantage. This will result in a decrease in grip strength. Radial deviation will also result in limitation of ulnar

Figure 10.8. Schematic of other identified problems with the distal radioulnar joint. A. Incongruity following a displaced fracture involving the sigmoid notch. B. Incongruity following a displaced ulnar head fracture. C,D. Malunited Smith's fracture demonstrates increased palmar tilt and pronation deformity of the end of the radius with dorsal subluxation of the distal ulnar head.

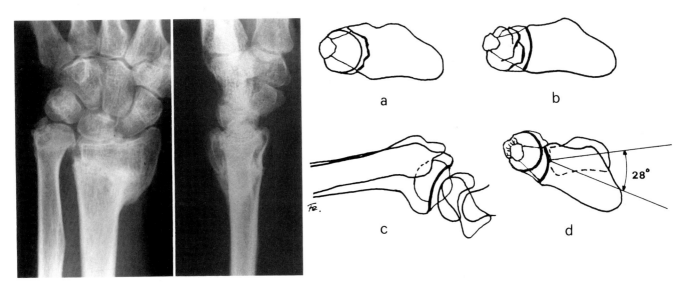

deviation of the wrist. Dorsal tilt of the distal fragment will favor a compensatory, spontaneous flexion deformity of the wrist with extensor tendon tightness, resulting in a slight degree of hyperextension of the proximal interphalangeal joints.[4] The extension posture of the distal radius can also cause entrapment neuropathy of the median nerve.[41] Lastly, bony irregularities and step-offs in the floors of the dorsal extensor compartments may lead to attrition tendinitis and rupture, in particular of the extensor pollicis longus.

The malunited palmar bending fracture (Smith's fracture) will present with an increased palmar tilt and a pronation deformity of the distal fragment that favors dorsal subluxation of the ulnar head (Fig. 10.8C,D).[12] This will lead to limitation of active wrist extension and limitation of forearm supination. In contrast to malunion with dorsal angulation, midcarpal instability or carpal malalignment following Smith's fractures has not been reported to date (Fig. 10.9).

Intraarticular malunion with residual incongruity of the articular surface greater than 2 mm has been shown to be associated with a significant incidence of secondary osteoarthritis at both the radiocarpal and the radioulnar levels.[26] Several patterns of articular involvement have been noted. Posttraumatic collapse of the lunate facet (die-punch fracture) is usually associated with a palmar rotation of the lunate, often resulting in a volar intercalary segment carpal instability (VISI) (Fig. 10.10). Malunited shearing (Barton's) fractures will lead to chronic volar or dorsal carpal subluxation. Lastly, some intraarticular fractures with unrecognized associated scapholunate tears heal with joint incongruence and a perilunate instability pattern. Because of primary articular involvement, pain as well as functional limitation is usually found to be more severe in the malunited articular fracture than in the extraarticular malunion (Fig. 10.11).

Preoperative Evaluation

A number of factors enter into the decision making for the surgical treatment of a distal radius malunion. These include the extent of functional wrist impairment, severity of pain, radiographic findings, and clinical appearance. The examination should attempt to determine if associated pain is located at the radiocarpal, midcarpal, or distal radioulnar joints. The presence or absence of distal radioulnar joint instability must be determined. The grip strength when compared to the uninjured side will often reflect the degree of deformity and associated functional impairment.

Standardized biplanar radiographs of both wrists are ordinarily adequate to identify the degree of deformity and preoperatively plan an osteotomy.[13,14,16] Carpal malalignment, ulnar variance, and the inclination of the articular surface will necessitate comparison with the opposite wrist to quantitate accurately.[38] Computerized tomography (CT) may be of use in evaluating the presence of posttraumatic subluxation or incongruence of the distal radioulnar joint or rotational malalignment of the distal radius.[25,37] The latter can be accurately measured by superimposing tracings of symmetrical CT cut of both forearms in neutral rotation. The proximal cuts should include the bicipital tuberosity and the distal cut should include Lister's tubercle as bony reference points. The difference of rotation between the uninjured and the injured side represents the true bony rotational malalignment.

The computerized tomograms can be especially useful in cases in which both intraarticular and extraarticular corrections are planned. Three-dimensional reformatting of CT images may enhance the understanding of

Figure 10.9. Typical deformity following malunion of a palmar bending fracture (Smith's fracture). Anteroposterior and lateral radiographs demonstrating radial shortening, palmar tilt, and pronation deformity of the distal radial fragment and an apparent dorsal subluxation of the distal radioulnar joint.

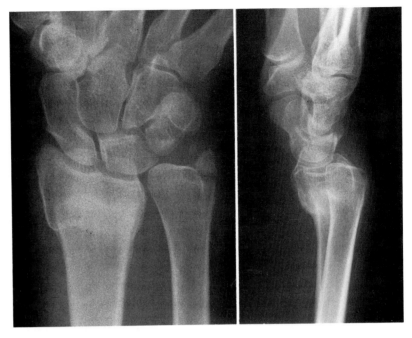

Figure 10.10. Malunited die-punch injury in a 30-year-old pharmacist. Note the VISI intercarpal deformity.

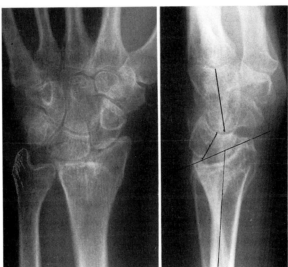

Figure 10.11. A severe intraarticular malunion resulted in persistent pain and nearly complete loss of radiocarpal motion.

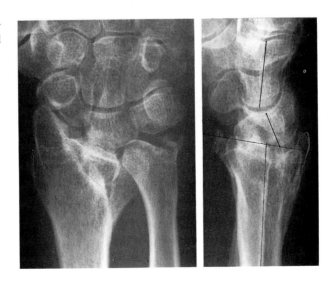

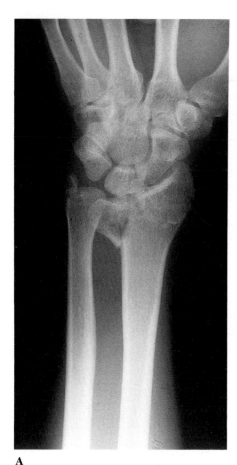

A

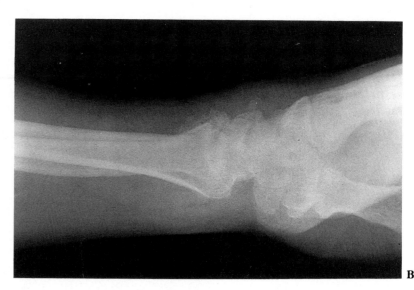

B

Figure 10.12. The use of computer-generated bone models is illustrated in this complex intra- and extraarticular deformity in a 65-year-old general surgeon seen 3 months following a complex distal radius fracture. (Illustration reprinted courtesy of CV Mosby Co., St. Louis. *J Hand Surg* 17: 406–415, 1992.) A,B. Anteroposterior and lateral radiographs of the initial fracture. (*Figure continues on facing page.*)

some complex deformities,[29,49,52] although the spatial reconstruction required during a corrective osteotomy may not be readily predicted from these reformatted images. The advent of computer-assisted design (CAD) and computer-assisted manufacturing (CAM) technology has resulted in the capability to produce three-dimensional solid models of distal radius malunions to facilitate a preoperative understanding of the true deformity.

One of us (JBJ) reported in 1992 on the use of computer-generated bone models in the planning of osteotomy of complex deformities associated with malunited fractures of the distal radius.[22] In each case, deformity was present in the frontal, sagittal, and horizontal planes. In addition, two patients had intraarticular radiocarpal deformities (Fig. 10.12A–I). The surgical procedure could be readily performed on the solid models, with the dimensions of the required bone graft as well as the size, slope, and placement of the internal fixation accurately planned in advance.

Unfortunately, there are no fixed parameters to determine the surgical indications for corrective osteotomy. It is quite evident that alteration of the flexion-extension arc of motion is seen with a sagittal tilt of more than 25 degrees. By the same token, in those patients with underlying "ligamentous laxity," a dorsal tilt of 10 to 15 degrees can result in a symptomatic midcarpal instability. Fourrier and co-workers, in an analysis of 64 malunions of the distal radius, correlated the functional impairment with the residual deformity of the distal radius. They concluded the lower limits of deformity at which symptoms are likely to be present would be a radial deviation between 20 and 30 degrees, a sagittal tilt between 10 and 20 degrees, and radial shortening between 0 and 2 mm. In addition, experimental evidence would suggest that a sagittal tilt between 20 and 30 degrees should be viewed as a prearthrotic condition.[30,40,45]

The distal radioulnar joint will also require careful radiologic evaluation.[39] Abnormalities will influence decision making as to the need for a simultaneous procedure at the distal radioulnar joint at the time of the radial osteotomy. Wrist arthroscopy or magnetic resonance imaging may provide further information as to the status of the triangular fibrocartilage. The presence of

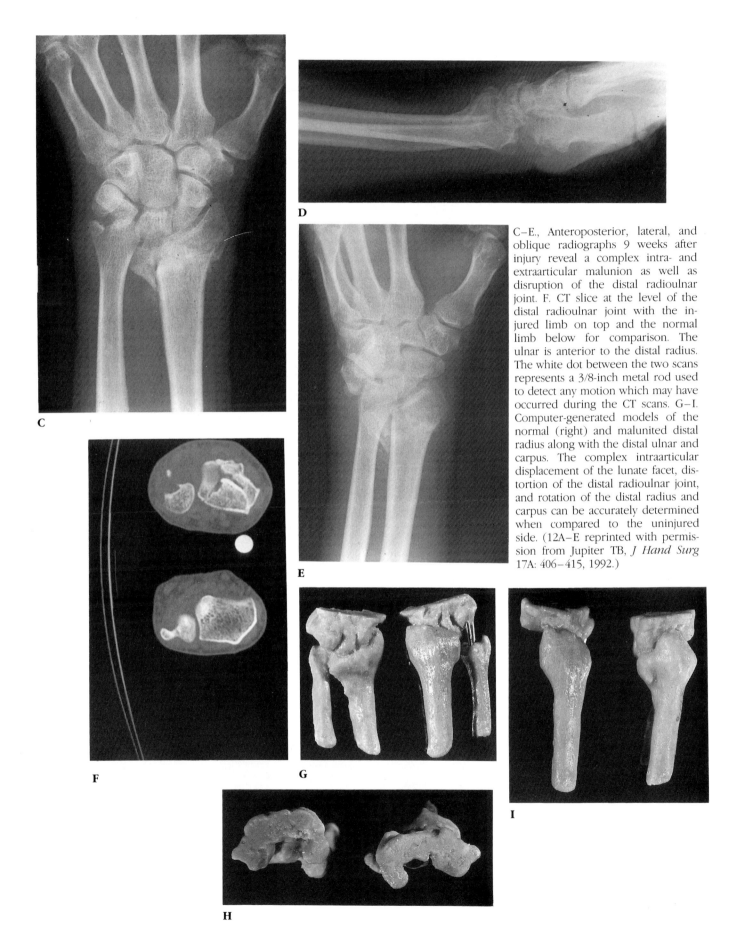

C–E., Anteroposterior, lateral, and oblique radiographs 9 weeks after injury reveal a complex intra- and extraarticular malunion as well as disruption of the distal radioulnar joint. F. CT slice at the level of the distal radioulnar joint with the injured limb on top and the normal limb below for comparison. The ulnar is anterior to the distal radius. The white dot between the two scans represents a 3/8-inch metal rod used to detect any motion which may have occurred during the CT scans. G–I. Computer-generated models of the normal (right) and malunited distal radius along with the distal ulnar and carpus. The complex intraarticular displacement of the lunate facet, distortion of the distal radioulnar joint, and rotation of the distal radius and carpus can be accurately determined when compared to the uninjured side. (12A–E reprinted with permission from Jupiter TB, *J Hand Surg* 17A: 406–415, 1992.)

Table 10.1. Distal radius osteotomy: *relative indications.*

Limitation of function
Pain
Midcarpal instability
Distal radioulnar joint disruption
Prearthrotic articular incongruity

degenerative changes at the distal radioulnar joint, especially with restriction of forearm rotation, will usually require an additional procedure on the ulnar side of the wrist in order to guarantee a good functional result.[2,3,12,17]

Based upon our experience of over 120 osteotomies of malunited fractures of the distal end of the radius, the authors' indications for radial osteotomy are

Figure 10.13. A 30-year-old male fell from a roof sustaining a compex intraarticular fracture of his dominant distal radius. The fracture was complicated by a compartment syndrome. Ultimately, painful arthrosis was felt a contraindication to osteotomy and a realignment and wrist arthrodesis performed. A,B. Anteroposterior and lateral radiographs of the healed malunited fracture demonstrating distortion of the radiocarpal joint with carpal malalignment and a fixed flexion deformity. C,D. The clinical presentation revealed a dysfunctional hand and wrist due to the soft tissue contracture. E,F. A wrist arthrodesis was performed resulting in considerable functional improvement.

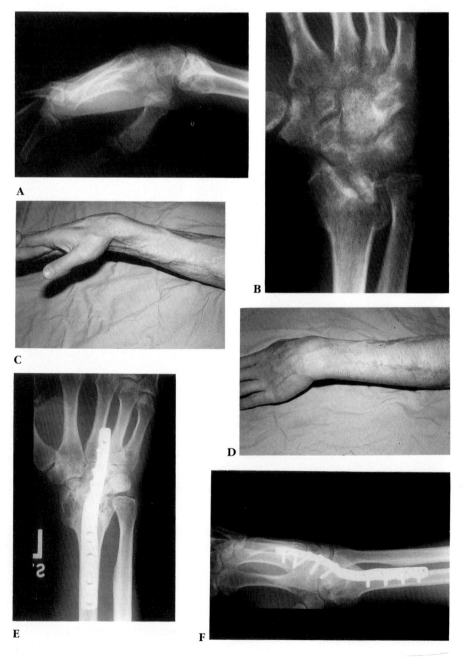

Table 10.2. Distal radius osteotomy: *contraindications.*

Advanced degenerative articular changes
Fixed carpal malalignment
Limited functional capabilities
Extensive osteoporosis

based upon the presence of limitation of function, severity of pain, midcarpal instability, associated distal radioulnar problems, and a substantial deformity with radiographic findings such as prearthrotic deformity, mechanical imbalance of the carpus, and incongruence of the distal radioulnar joint, which represent a menace for the future of wrist function (Table 10.1).

The contraindications for corrective osteotomy of the distal radius include advanced degenerative changes in the radiocarpal and intercarpal joints, fixed carpal malalignment, limited functional capabilities of the hand due to underlying neurologic dysfunction, and extensive osteoporosis (Fig. 10.13A–F).[46] In reality, age is not nearly as much a contraindication as it was thought to be in the past, provided the quality of bone is adequate and the patient is physiologically active (Table 10.2).

Timing

Optimally, an osteotomy should be considered as soon as the soft tissues demonstrate an absence of trophic changes, the radiographs reveal limited or no osteopenia, and wrist mobility is adequate. With those features in mind, the authors have developed an interest in intervening operatively in malpositioned fractures of the distal radius at an early stage. The theoretical advantages of this include decreased likelihood of deformity; correction through an immaturely healed fracture site, thus limiting the problems of soft tissue contracture and radioulnar joint dysfunction; and limitation of the economic and physiologic impact on the individual.

One of us (JBJ) followed two groups of patients who had had osteotomies of malunions following fracture of the distal radius. One group of 10 had osteotomy an average of 8.2 weeks following fracture ("nascent" malunion), while a comparable group of ten had osteotomy an average of 39.9 weeks postfracture ("mature" malunion). While the overall outcome was following osteotomy in each group was relatively the same, it was quite evident that performing the osteotomy at an earlier stage facilitated both radial realignment and realignment of the distal radioulnar joint. Perhaps most importantly, the total duration of disability was considerably decreased: the time back to work postfracture averaged 21 weeks in the nascent group compared to 70 weeks in the mature group. (Table 10.3 and Fig. 10.14A–F).

Technique: "Nascent" Malunion

The surgical approach is by necessity on based on the direction of displacement of the distal fragment. Careful preoperative planning as well as the use of intraoperative Kirschner wires to mark the angle of deformity is essential to guarantee an accurate angular correction and simplify the procedure.

Table 10.3A. "Nascent" malunion: preosteotomy data.

Case #	Sex	Age	Limb (dominant)	Occupation	Mechanism of injury	Date of injury	Primary treatment	Fracture type	Wrist motion Extension/normal	Flexion/normal	Ulnar deviation/normal	Radial deviation/normal	Forearm motion Pronation/normal	Supination/normal	Grip (kg) normal
1	M	41	Left	Photographer	Fall from a standing height	07-20-91	Closed reduction, cast	Four-part bending Colles'	40/60	40/60	15/30	5/15	60/80	80/80	20/55
2	M	65	Left	Surgeon	Fall from a standing height	07-14-89	Closed reduction, cast	Complex intra- and extraarticular bending Colles'	30/70	30/60	10/30	15/15	40/80	80/80	10/35
3	F	20	Left (bilateral fractures)	Student	Motor vehicle accident	04-13-91	Closed reduction, cast	Die-punch bending Colles'				Still in cast			
4	M	27	Left (bilateral fractures)	Contractor	Motor vehicle accident	04-24-91	Closed reduction, cast	Die-punch bending Colles'				Still in cast			
5	M	41	(Right)	Executive	Sport	01-26-87	Open reduction internal fixation	Shear volar impacted lunate facet	5/60	10/65	0/30	5/20	40/80	45/80	20/45
6	M	54	Left (bilateral fractures)	Executive	Fall from a height	08-02-92	Closed reduction, cast	Bending Colles'				In cast			
7	M	34	Left	Firefighter	Fall from a height	03-14-83	Closed reduction, cast	Bending Colles'				In cast			
8	M	39	(Right) (bilateral fractures)	Contractor	Fall from a height	03-26-84	Closed reduction, external fixation	Complex intraarticular bending Colles'				In external fixation			
9	M	47	(Right)	Bus driver	Fall from a height	05-01-84	Closed reduction, cast	Bending Colles', intraarticular				In cast			15/50
10	M	48	(Right)	Military	Fall from a height	03-16-93	Closed reduction, cast	Bending Colles'	60/60	50/60	15/30	10/15	70/80	35/80	20/65

Case No.	Appearance	Level pain Radiocarpal	Radioulnar	Radiograph Dorsal tilt	Volar tilt	Shortening (mm)	Ulnar inclination	Intraarticular	Time injury to osteotomy (wks)
1	+++	+	+	10°	—	5	12°	—	13
2	+++	++	+++	45°		11	11°	Lunate facet	14
3	+++	In cast	In cast	20°		4	12°		7
4	++	In cast	In cast	13°		8	10°	Die-punch	6
5	+	++	+	—		2	11°	Displaced lunate facet	8
6	+	In cast	In cast	20°		4	5°		6
7	++	In cast	In cast	30°		9	8°		6
8	++	++	+	20°		5	10°	Displaced lunate facet	6
9	+++	++	—	20°		8	10°	Displaced lunate facet	6
10	++	++	+++	30°		6	20°		10

+ = mild
++ = moderate
+++ = severe

Table 10.3B. "Mature" nonunion: preoperative data.

Case No.	Sex	Age	Limb (dominant)	Occupation	Mechanism of injury	Date of injury	Primary treatment	Fracture type	Wrist motion				Forearm motion		Grip (kg) normal
									Extension/ normal	Flexion/ normal	Ulnar deviation/ normal	Radial deviation/ normal	Pronation/ normal	Supination/ normal	
11	F	26	(Right)	Insurance agent	Fall from a height	12-29-91	Closed reduction and external fixation	Open complex	-25/65	30/60	-10/30	25/15	70/80	0/80	2/25
12	F	60	Left	Bookkeeper	Fall from a standing height	09-10-89	Closed reduction and cast	Bending Colles'	0/50	50/50	0/30	25/10	30/80	30/80	0/20
13	M	29	(Right)	Carpenter	Fall from a height	06-04-88	Closed reduction and cast	Complex intra- and extraarticular bending Colles'	40/60	40/60	-5/25	35/15	80/80	20/80	15/45
14	M	34	Left	Laborer	Fall from a height	11-05-89	Closed reduction and cast	Bending Colles'	40/65	25/50	0/25	30/10	60/80	70/80	25/65
15	F	27	(Right)	Housewife	Moton vehicle accident	09-09-89	Closed reduction and cast	Bending Colles'	20/70	20/65	15/30	10/20	60/80	20/80	10/25
16	M	29	Left	Carpenter	Fall from a height	07-01-84	Closed reduction, pins, and plaster	Bending Colles'	30/45	30/45	5/30	45/20	45/80	50/80	18/38
17	F	20	(Right)	Laborer	Fall from a height	01-21-83	Closed reduction and cast	Bending Colles'	70/70	40/75	25/35	15/10	65/80	40/80	12/40
18	F	50	Right	Homemaker	Fall from a standing height	02-06-90	Closed reduction and cast	Bending Colles'	70/60	30/70	10/30	30/15	80/80	80/80	10/30
19	M	43	Left	Computer programmer	Moton vehicle accident	12-31-90	Closed reduction and cast	Volar shear, intraarticular impaction	50/60	40/70	15/30	10/20	95/80	20/80	25/40
20	F	58	Left	Writer	Fall from a standing height	01-29-91	Closed reduction and cast	Bending Colles'	30/80	30/70	10/30	20/10	30/80	40/80	18/35

Case No.	Appearance	Level of pain		Radiograph					Time injury to osteotomy (wks)
		Radiocarpal	Radioulnar	Dorsal tilt	Volar tilt	Shortening (mm)	Ulnar inclination	Intraarticular	
11	+++	++	++	5°		15	0°	—	36
12	++	++	—		30°	10	10°	—	35
13	+++	++	++	30°		18	-5°	Lunate facet	38
14	+	++	+	0°		16	0°	—	48
15	++	—	+++	10°		7	5°	—	48
16	+++	++	++	30°		7	-10°	—	46
17	+++	+	+	35°		8	4°	—	30
18	++	+	+	15°		17	4°	—	40
19	+++	+	—	—		6	20°	Lunate facet	42
20	++	—	+	30°		7	20°	—	36

Table 10.3C. "Nascent" malunion: postoperative data.

Case No.	Surgical exposure	Intraoperative distraction	Osteotomy site	Graft	Fixation	Immobilization Type	Duration	Time to heal (wks)	Follow-up (months)	Extension/ normal	Flexion/ normal	Wrist Motion Ulnar deviation/ normal	Radial deviation/ normal	Pronation/ normal	Supination/ normal
1	Dorsal	None	Fracture metaphysis	Cancellous	T plate	Splint	4	5	20	50/60	40/65	25/30	20/20	80/80	80/80
2	Dorsal	None	Intra- and extraarticular	Cancellous	T plate, cannulated screw	Cast	6	8	24	55/70	60/60	30/30	10/15	80/80	70/80
3	Dorsal	Yes	Fracture metaphysis	Cancellous	T plate, K wire	Splint	4	5	24	60/65	50/65	20/30	10/15	80/80	80/80
4	Dorsal	Yes	Fracture metaphysis	Cancellous	T plate	Splint	6	6	20	35/45	30/40	10/15	10/10	70/70	70/75
5	Ulnar	None	Intra- and extraarticular	Cancellous	1/4 tubular mini plate	Cast	4	5	72	55/70	40/60	20/35	6/10	80/80	80/80
6	Dorsal	Yes	Fracture metaphysis	Cancellous	T plate	Splint	4	5	12	60/60	50/60	30/30	15/15	80/80	80/80
7	Dorsal	None	Fracture metaphysis	Cancellous	T plate	Splint	4	5	120	60/60	60/60	30/30	10/15	80/80	80/80
8	Dorsal	None	Intra- and extraarticular	Cancellous	T plate	Splint	4	5	108	40/30	30/45	10/25	15/10	80/80	80/80
9	Dorsal	None	Fracture metaphysis	Cancellous	T plate	Cast	6	6	30	45/55	30/55	30/30	10/15	80/80	80/80
10	Dorsal	Yes	Fracture metaphysis	Cancellous	T plate	Cast	4	4	8	60/60	60/60	30/30	10/15	80/80	70/80

Case No.	Grip (kg)/ normal	Pain Radiocarpal	Radioulnar	Complications Deformity	Other	Implant removal	Radiograph Dorsal tilt	Volar tilt	Shortening (mm)	Ulnar inclination	Return to work Injury → work (wks)	Overall assessment
1	60/55	0	0	0		No	0		0	15	Same, 19	Excellent
2	30/35	0	0	0	EPL rupture	Yes	0		0	30	Same, 36	Good
3	18/22	0	0	0		No	0		2	20	Student	Excellent
4	30/40	+	0	0		No	5		0	18	Same, 54	Good
5	40/45	0	0	0					0	20	Same, 3	Good
6	40/40	0	0	0		No	0		0	16	Same, 10	Excellent
7	45/40	0	0	0		Yes	−5		0	22	Same, 10	Excellent
8	40/50	0	0	0		No	0		0	20	Same, 18	Excellent
9	60/50	0	0	0		Yes	0		0	22	Same, 24	Excellent
10	55/60	0	0	0		No	−5		0	20	Same, 8	Excellent

Table 10.3D. "Mature" nonunion: postoperative data.

Case No.	Grip (kg)/normal	Pain Radiocarpal	Pain Radioulnar	Complications Deformity	Complications Other	Implant removal	Radiograph Dorsal tilt	Radiograph Volar tilt	Radiograph Shortening (mm)	Radiograph Ulnar inclination	Return to work Injury → work (wks)	Overall assessment
11	15/25	–	+	+	–	–	0	–	–	10°	Same job, 30	Excellent
12	10/20	–	–	–	–	–	10°	–	–	17°	Not working	Good
13	25/40	–	–	–	–	–	0	–	–	22°	Same job, 58	Good
14	40/60	–	–	–	Delay union—2nd graft	–	0	–	–	13°	Same job, 96	Excellent
15	18/25	–	–	–	Pain—iliac donor site	–	5°	–	–	20°	Same job, 76	Excellent
16	30/40	–	–	–	–	–	0	–	–	8°	Same job, 74	Excellent
17	35/40	–	–	–	–	Yes	0	–	–	24°	Same job, 50	Excellent
18	20/30	+	–	–	–	–	4°	–	2	12°	Not working	Good
19	35/40	–	–	–	–	Yes	0	–	–	26°	Same job, 4	Good
20	24/30	–	+	–	–	–	5°	–	–	25°	Same job, 50	Good

Surgical exposure	Intraoperative distraction	Osteotomy site	Graft	Fixation	Immobilization Type	Immobilization Duration (wks)	Time to heal (wks)	Follow-up (months)	Wrist motion Extension/NL	Flexion/normal	Ulnar deviation/normal	Radial deviation/normal	Pronation/normal	Supination/normal
Dorsal	Yes	Metaphysis	Corticocancellous	T plate	Cast	6	8	12	35/6	30/60	5/30	20/30	80/80	50/80
Volar	Yes	Metaphysis	Corticocancellous	T plate	Splint	6	7	24	30/50	40/50	25/30	10/10	80/80	80/80
Dorsal	No	Metaphysis	Corticocancellous	T plate	Splint	6	10	20	45/70	50/60	30/30	10/15	80/80	70/80
Dorsal	No	Metaphysis	Corticocancellous	T plate	Cast	6	28	30	40/60	40/50	20/25	10/10	70/80	70/80
Dorsal	No	Metaphysis	Corticocancellous	T plate	Splint	4	7	30	40/70	30/65	15/30	10/20	70/80	60/80
Dorsal	No	Metaphysis	Corticocancellous	T plate	Cast	4	7	36	30/45	40/45	25/30	20/20	80/80	80/80
Dorsal	No	Metaphysis	Corticocancellous	T plate	Splint	6	6	24	70/70	60/75	25/35	10/10	80/80	80/80
Dorsal	Yes	Metaphysis	Corticocancellous	T plate	Cast	4	6	12	70/60	50/70	20/30	15/15	80/80	80/80
Volar	Yes	Intraarticular plus metaphysis	Corticocancellous	T plate	Cast	6	10	12	50/65	50/70	30/30	15/5	80/80	70/80
Dorsal	Yes	Metaphysis	Corticocancellous	T plate	Splint	6	6	20	40/80	30/70	20/30	10/10	70/80	40/80

Figure 10.14. A malunion of 9 weeks' duration in a 21-year-old woman was treated by early osteotomy. The callus was opened and the defect filled with autogenous iliac crest cancellous graft along with a plate. Excellent radiocarpal and radioulnar joint function was achieved. A. Lateral radiograph of the "nascent malunion" seen 9 weeks postfracture. B,C. The osteotomy was performed through still maturing callus and secured with a T plate and cancellous iliac crest graft. D,E. Excellent healing and function resulted.

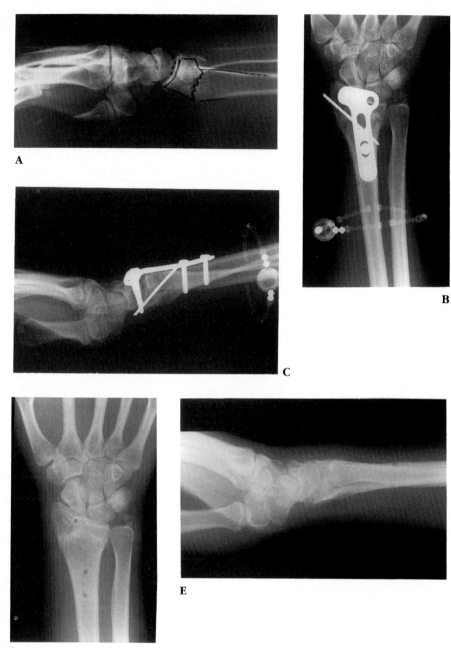

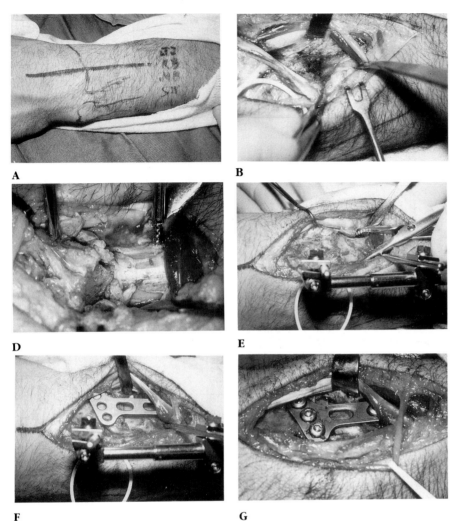

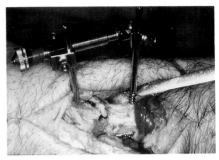

Figure 10.15. Malunited distal radius fracture seen 8 weeks postinjury in a 23-year-old man. A. The malunion is approached through a dorsal incision. Care is taken to preserve large dorsal veins. B. The extensor retinaculum is opened between the second and third extensor retinacular compartments. C. A mini distractor is placed with one Schanz pin in the distal fragment and one in the radius proximal to the malunion. D. The callus is elevated, exposing the original fracture site. E. The malunion is realigned and the defect packed with autogenous iliac crest graft to which the original fracture callus is added. F,G. The realigned distal fragment is supported with a dorsal T plate.

Since the intention is to "take down" the maturing callus, the "osteotomy" is performed at the site of the original fracture (Fig. 10.15A–G). A mini distractor is extremely useful to control lengthening and to minimize the need for more extensive elevation of the soft tissue envelope surrounding the distal radius. The callus should be saved for later combination with autogenous iliac crest cancellous graft, which will be placed in the defect that results from the realignment of the distal fragment.

In most instances, stabilization of the realignment is achieved with a T plate, although on occasion an oblique Kirschner wire and external fixation frame will be preferable.

Technique: "Mature" Extraarticular Malunion

The goals of distal radial osteotomy are to restore overall function as well as enhancing the appearance of the hand and wrist. The osteotomy should reorient the distal radial articular surface to improve normal load distribution, reestablish the kinematics of the midcarpal joint, and restore the anatomic relationships of the distal radioulnar joint. Since radial shortening is a constant

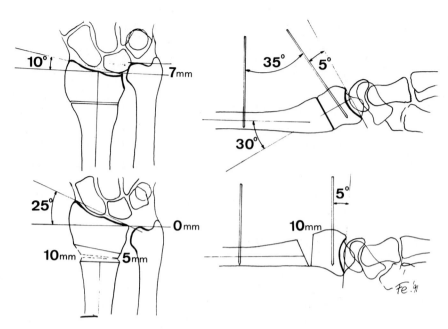

Figure 10.16. Preoperative planning of the osteotomy for a "mature" malunion. A. For correction in the frontal plane, the amount of shortening (7 mm in this example) is measured between the ulnar and ulnar corner of the radius on the anteroposterior radiograph. The lines for the measurement are perpendicular to the long axis of the radius. The ulnar tilt is reduced to 10 degrees in this example. B. In order to restore the ulnar tilt to normal (average 25 degrees), the osteotomy is opened more on the dorsoradial than on the dorsoulnar side. C. For correction in the sagittal plane, the dorsal tilt (30 degrees in this example) is measured between the perpendicular to the joint surface and the long axis of the radius on the lateral radiographs. The Kirschner wires are introduced so that they subtend the angle that corresponds to the dorsal tilt plus 5 degrees of volar tilt (30 plus 5 degrees with 35 degrees in this example). D. After the osteotomy is opened by the correct amount, the Kirschner wires lie parallel to each other. (From Fernandez DL: Malunion of the distal radius. *AAOS Instructional Course Lectures*, Vol. 42, p. 105, 1993, by permission of the American Academy of Orthopaedic Surgeons.)

component of the deformity in both malunited dorsal and palmar bending fractures, an opening wedge osteotomy which is transverse in the frontal plane and oblique (i.e., parallel to the joint surface) in the sagittal plane is recommended. Such an osteotomy will permit lengthening of the radius by as much as 10 to 12 mm as well as restoring the normal tilt in the sagittal plane, the ulnar tilt in the frontal plane, and the rotational deformity in the horizontal plane. The bony defect created by such a realignment is replaced by a corticocancellous bone graft obtained from the iliac crest.[42]

Careful preoperative planning, along with the intraoperative Kirschner wires to mark the angle of the deformity, enhances the accuracy of such a realignment (Fig. 10.16A–D). Radiographs of the opposite wrist are useful to help determine the physiologic ulnar variance for each particular patient and should be used to calculate the anticipated restoration of the radial length (Fig. 10.17A–D).

A 7-cm incision beginning 2 cm distal to Lister's tubercle and extending proximally in the forearm serves to provide more than adequate exposure. The extensor retinaculum is opened between the second and third extensor compartments with the fourth extensor compartment elevated subperiosteally off the radius (Fig. 10.18A). Approximately 2 to 2.5 cm proximal to the wrist joint, the osteotomy site is marked with an osteotome.

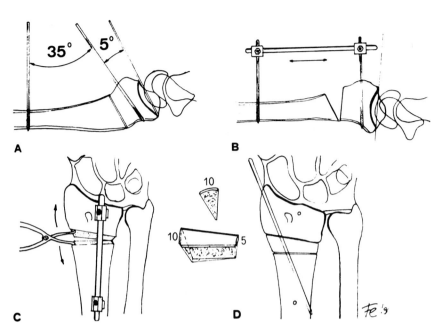

Figure 10.17. Schematic representation of the technique of osteotomy for a malunited dorsal bending fracture (Colles' fracture). A. Threaded wires subtend the angle of correction. The osteotomy is made parallel to the distal articular surface in the sagittal plane. Note the fine Kirschner wire introduced into the radiocarpal joint. B,C. The osteotomy is opened dorsally and radially with a small spreader clamp. A fixator bar helps to maintain the correction. D. An iliac graft shaped to conform to the defect is inserted, and one oblique Kirschner wire is driven through the radial styloid and grafted into the radial metaphysis. The fixator can then be removed. (From Fernandez, DL: Malunion of the distal radius. *AAOS Instructional Course Lectures*, Vol. 42, p. 105, 1993, by permission of the American Academy of Orthopaedic Surgeons.)

To assure that the osteotomy is created in the sagittal plane parallel to the joint surface, a fine Kirschner wire is introduced through the dorsal part of the capsule into the radiocarpal joint and along the articular surface of the radius. In following the preoperative plan, two 2.5-mm Kirschner wires with a threaded tip are inserted, subtending the angle of correction in the sagittal plane on both sides of the intended osteotomy (Fig. 10.18B). These wires serve not only to control intraoperative angular correction but also to help manipulate and maintain the distal fragment in the corrected position with a small external fixator bar until the graft is inserted. With careful protection of the volar soft tissues, the osteotomy is performed with the oscillating saw, taking care to avoid a complete osteotomy of the volar cortex (Fig. 10.8C). The osteotomy is then opened dorsally and radially by manipulating the wrist into flexion, as well as applying spreader clamps into the osteotomy site until the wires are parallel in the sagittal plane (Fig. 10.18D and E). At this point, a 4.0-mm external fixator bar with two clamps is placed between the two Kirschner wires to maintain the reduction of the distal fragment. Additional opening of the osteotomy along the radial side is gained by a small spreader clamp. Complete tenotomy or Z-lengthening of the brachioradialis tendon is recommended to facilitate lengthening in those malunions with severe radial deviation and shortening. In such cases, two additional Kirschner wires with threaded tips to which a distraction device can be applied can be placed in a more horizontal direction.

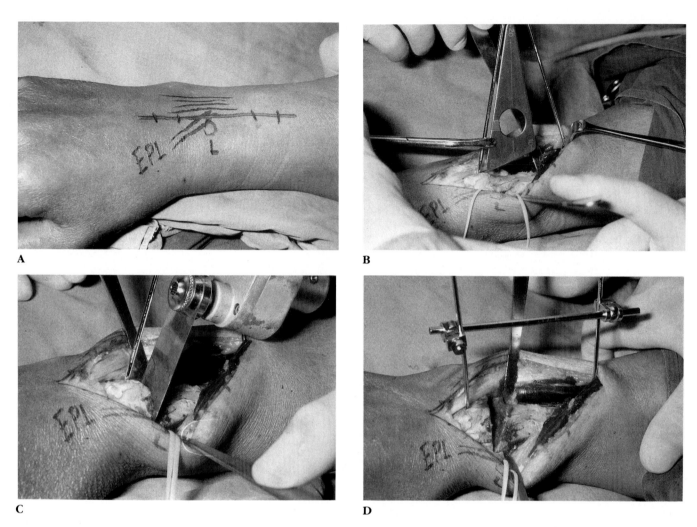

Figure 10.18. Operative technique for a malunited dorsal bending fracture. A. The skin incision is over the third extensor retinacular compartment. B. Threaded wires are placed using fixed angle guides to subtend the angle of correction in the sagittal plane. C. The osteotomy is performed with an oscillating saw parallel to the distal Kirschner wire. D. The osteotomy is opened dorsally and maintained by applying a small fixator bar between the threaded wires. (*Figure continues on facing page.*)

The iliac crest graft is shaped to conform to the dorsoradial bone defect and inserted, making certain that there is a snug fit (Fig. 10.18F). At this juncture, a 1.6- or 2.0-mm Kirschner wire is driven obliquely from the radial styloid across the graft into the proximal radius. The threaded wires and external fixator bar may now be removed. With the elbow in 90 degrees of flexion, intraoperative forearm rotation and wrist motion are controlled. Radiographic control should also be performed.

A variety of methods of stable fixation are available, including a second Kirschner wire introduced across Lister's tubercle in an oblique dorsopalmar

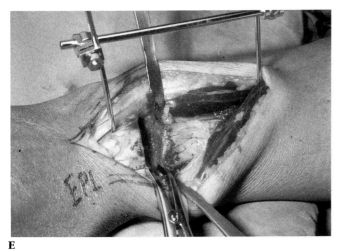

E

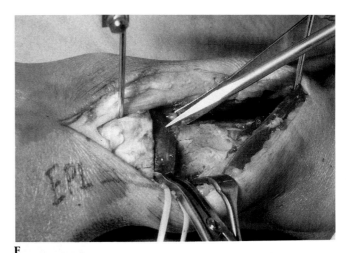

F

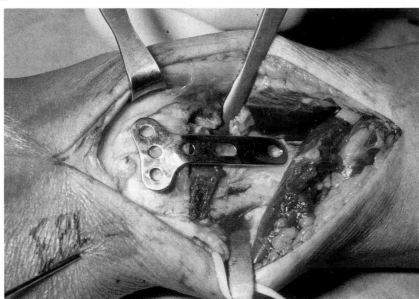

G

E. The osteotomy line is opened radially with a small spreader clamp. F. The iliac crest graft is inserted into the dorsoradial defect. G. The osteotomy is secured with a T plate with removal of the external fixator. (Reprinted with permission, Fernandez DF: Reconstructive procedures for malunion and traumatic arthritis. In: Melone C, ed. Distal radius fractures. *Orthop Clin North Am* 24: 341–336, 1993.)

direction[42] (Fig. 10.19A–E), a T plate (Figs. 10.18G and 10.21A–H), or a titanium 2.7-mm plate (Figs. 10.21A–I). The more stable support provided by plate fixation will offer the potential of early unrestricted active motion of the wrist (Fig. 10.21A–H).

During wound closure, the extensor pollicis longus tendon can be relocated back into its original location provided Lister's tubercle has been preserved. As the latter will need to be removed if a T plate is applied, in those cases the retinaculum is closed with the extensor pollicis longus tendon left above the retinaculum.

Figure 10.19. Malunited dorsal bending (Colles') fracture associated with an unstable radioulnar joint. A,B. Anteroposterior and lateral radiograph of the malunion. C. Intraoperative view showing the distal radial graft held in place with two smooth Kirschner wires. D,E. Anteroposterior and lateral radiographs showing the healed osteotomy secured with two Kirschner wires. A stabilization of the distal radioulnar joint was achieved by tightening of the triangular fibrocartilage complex by a proximal displacement osteotomy of the ulnar styloid fixed with a tension band technique.

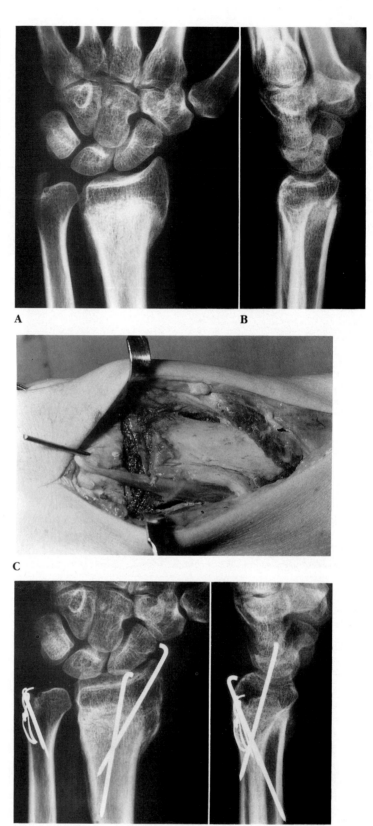

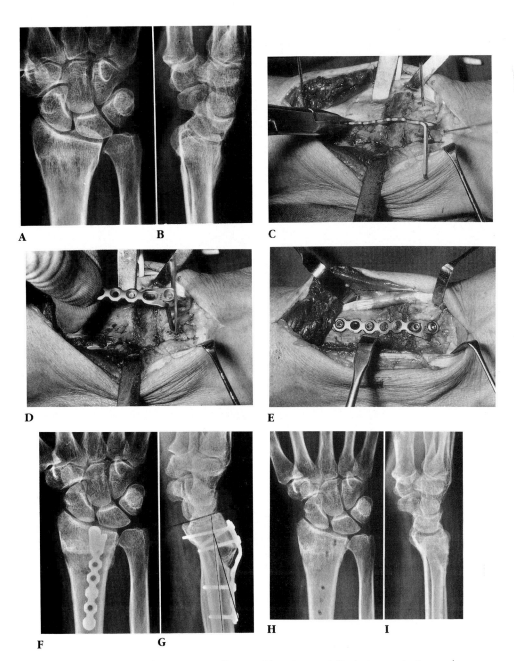

Figure 10.20. Severe malunion in a 40-year-old waitress. A,B. Anteroposterior and lateral radiographs of the dorsal malunion. C,D. Intraoperative photographs showing the interposed graft and the pre-bent titanium 2.7-mm condylar plate at its point of application. E. The plate is placed away from Lister's tubercle to prevent contact tendinitis of the extensor pollicis longus tendon. F,G. Postoperative radiographs show the graft and plate in place with correction of the preoperative deformity. H,I. Radiographs after plate removal. The carpal alignment is restored and the patient is free of pain with full forearm rotation. (Reprinted with permission, Fernandez DF: Reconstructive procedures for malunion and traumatic arthritis. In: Melone C, ed. Distal radius fractures. *Orthop Clin North Am* 24: 341–336, 1993.)

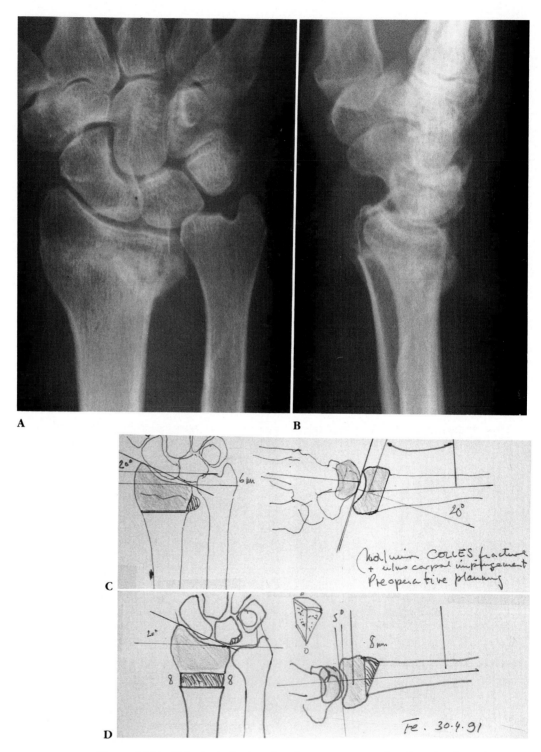

Figure 10.21. Malunited distal radius fracture associated with radioulnar disruption and ulnar abutment. A,B. Preoperative anteroposterior and lateral radiographs of the malunion. Note the abutment. C,D. Preoperative plan. (*Figure continues on facing page.*)

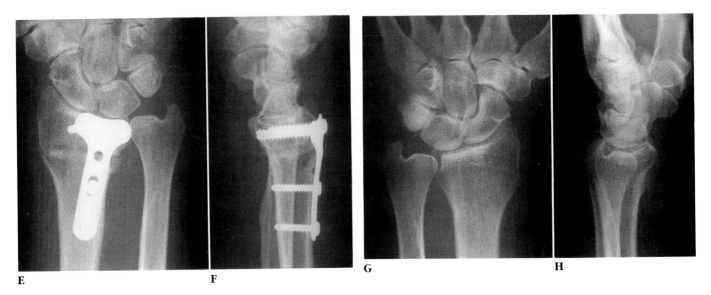

E,F. The anteroposterior and lateral radiographs following osteotomy. A T plate provided stable fixation of the interposed bone graft. G,H. Opposite wrist for comparison.

Extraarticular Palmar Malunion (Smith's Fracture)

The surgical approach to the malunited palmarly displaced bending fracture is that of the distal part of the classic Henry approach (see Chapter 4). The malunion is approached subperiosteally by reflecting the pronator quadratus muscle to the ulnar side, with the soft tissues protected with Hohmann retractors. The opening wedge osteotomy, interposed iliac crest cancellous graft, and plate application are carried out as described above for the dorsally directed malunion (Fig. 10.22A–I).

When manipulating the distal fragment into dorsiflexion, care must be taken not to overcorrect the physiologic tilt of 10 degrees. The use of a T buttress plate is important, as it will automatically derotate the pronated distal fragment by virtue of the flat surface of the plates. It is this pronation deformity that produces the apparent dorsal subluxation of the distal ulnar which is so charac teristic of malunited Smith's fractures. Dorsiflexing, derotating, and lengthening the distal fragment will help to reorient the sigmoid notch of the radius with respect to the head of the ulnar, which will restore the articular congruity of the radioulnar joint (Fig. 10.23A–H).

At times the distal fragment is not only palmarly flexed but also shortened in a radial direction. In these cases, tenotomy or Z-lengthening of the brachioradialis tendon may also be required (Fig. 10.24A–J).

One of us (DLF) reported in 1982 a series of 20 radial osteotomies for malunion following distal radius fracture, with an average follow-up of 3.5 years.[40] Using a strict scale for evaluation of outcome (Table 10.4), the results were graded as excellent in 5 patients, good in 10, fair in 4, and poor in one

Figure 10.22. Malunited volar bending (Smith's) fracture in a 45-year-old cook. Forearm rotation was substantially limited. A,B. Preoperative radiographs reveal an increased ulnar inclination, volar tilt, ulno-carpal translation, and dorsal distal radio-ulnar joint apparent subluxation. C,D. Anteroposterior and lateral radiographs of the opposite (normal) wrist for comparison. E. Preoperative plan. F,G. Postoperative anteroposterior and lateral radiographs reveal restoration of the radiocarpal and radioulnar anatomy. H,I. Two years post-operative radiographs. The patient is asymptomatic with normal forearm rotation.

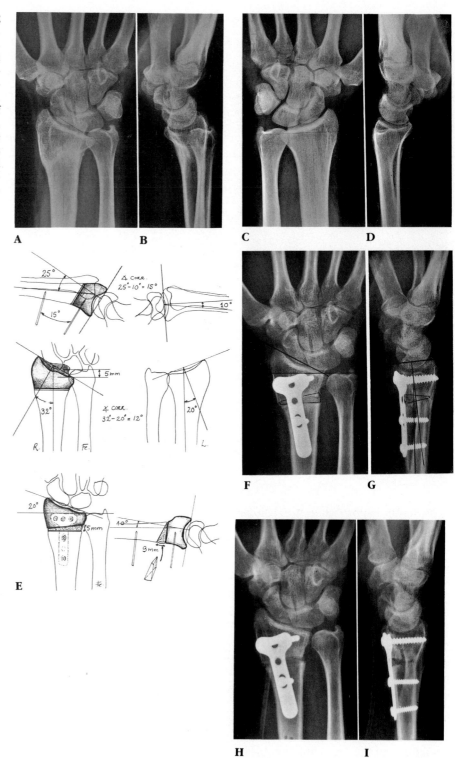

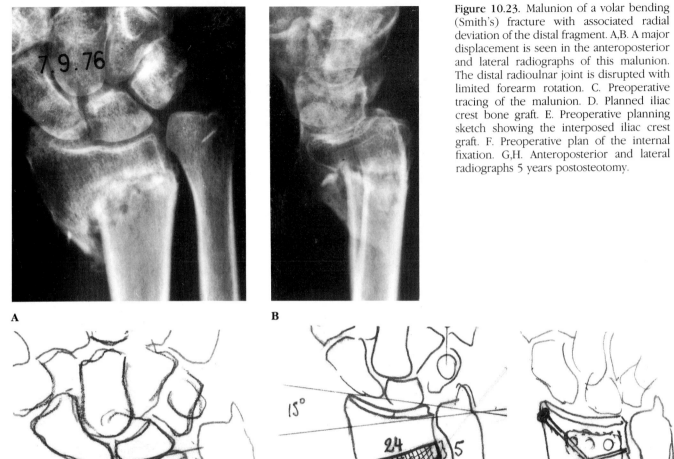

Figure 10.23. Malunion of a volar bending (Smith's) fracture with associated radial deviation of the distal fragment. A,B. A major displacement is seen in the anteroposterior and lateral radiographs of this malunion. The distal radioulnar joint is disrupted with limited forearm rotation. C. Preoperative tracing of the malunion. D. Planned iliac crest bone graft. E. Preoperative planning sketch showing the interposed iliac crest graft. F. Preoperative plan of the internal fixation. G,H. Anteroposterior and lateral radiographs 5 years postosteotomy.

Figure 10.24. Severely shortened malunion with a volar and radial deformity of the distal radial fragment. Severe limitation was noted in forearm rotation. A,B. Anteroposterior and lateral radiographs of the malunion. Note the severe disruption of the distal radioulnar joint congruity. C. Through an anterior approach the brachioradialis tendon is tenotomized. D. The osteotomy is made in line with the radial articular surface. E. The osteotomy is opened with a spreader clamp and the bone graft is held in the forceps. F. Intraoperative distraction is facilitated with a distraction device. G,H. Anteroposterior and lateral radiographs 2 weeks postoperatively. I,J. One year postoperatively the plate has been removed. Note the anatomic restoration of the sigmoid notch to the head of the distal ulnar. (Reprinted with permission, Fernandez DF: Reconstructive procedures for malunion and traumatic arthritis. In: Melone C, ed. Distal radius fractures. *Orthop Clin North Am* 24: 341–336, 1993.)

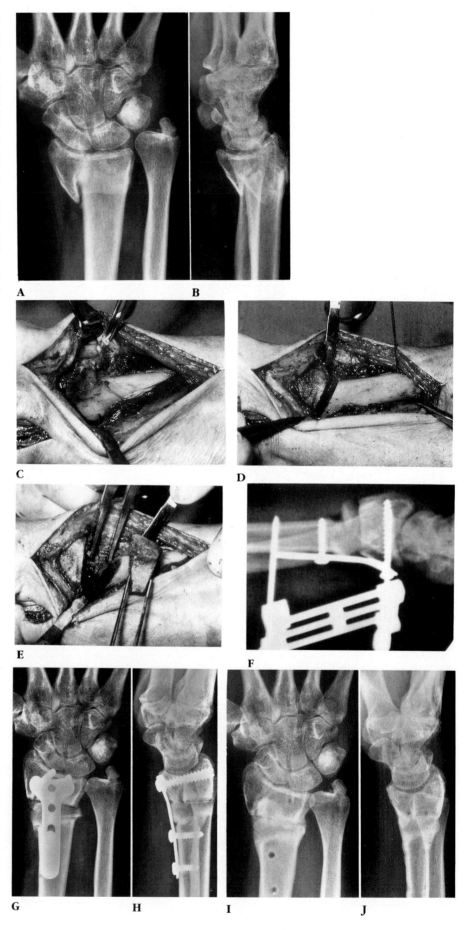

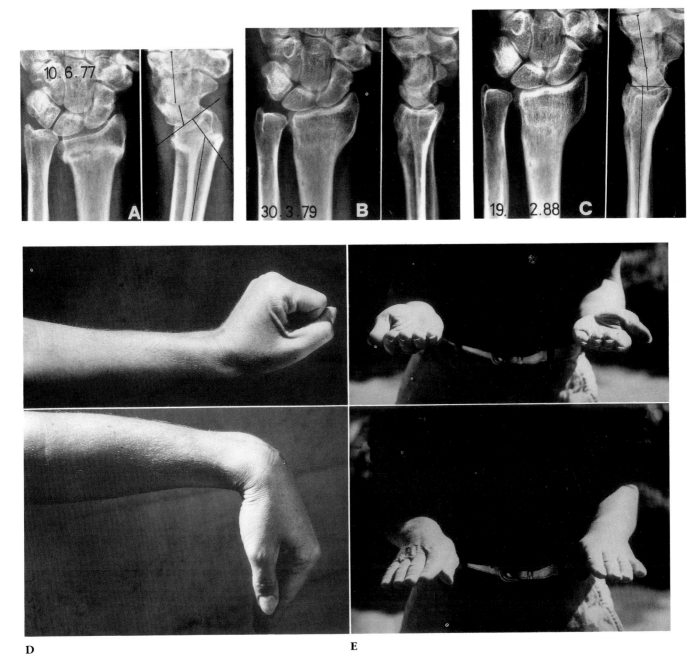

Figure 10.25. An 11-year follow-up after a distal radius osteotomy for a malunited distal radius fracture. A. Anteroposterior and lateral radiographs of the malunion seen preoperatively in 1977. B. Anteroposterior and lateral radiographs almost 2 years postosteotomy. C. Anteroposterior and lateral radiographs 11 years following the osteotomy. D. Wrist extension and flexion at 11-year follow-up. E. Full forearm rotation is noted at 11-year follow-up.

(Fig. 10.25A–E). Since that time, both authors' experience with over 120 osteotomies support the conclusion that careful patient selection, correct indications, and some refinements of the surgical technique can result in well over 80 percent good to excellent results. We have also learned to recognize the possibility of associated incongruity of the distal radioulnar joint and plan for the potential for a distal radioulnar joint procedure. In the experience of osteotomies by Fernandez (Table 10.5), an operation on the ulnar side of the wrist was required in 38 cases (Table 10.6) (see salvage procedures).

Table 10.4. Rating scale for evaluation of outcome of distal radius osteotomy.

Rating	Criteria
Excellent	No pain. Normal or near-normal motion Grip strength not less than 80 percent of normal No visible deformity
Good	No pain. Moderate limitation of motion Grip strength not less than 70 percent of normal No deformity
Fair	Moderate pain with activity Limitation of motion of 40 to 65 percent of normal Grip strength of 50 to 70 percent of normal Mild deformity
Poor	Failure of treatment due to pain; severe loss of motion; reduced grip strength less than 40 percent of normal; impairment of hand function

Table 10.5. Corrective osteotomies of the distal radius.

Malunion after	
Colles' fractures	37
Smith's fractures	20
Comminuted fractures	15
Reversed Barton's fractures	2
Children's fractures	6
Total	80

Table 10.6. Operations on the ulnar side of the wrist.

Darrach	8
Ulnar shortening	3
Partial ulnar head resection	19
Partial ulnar head resection and ulnar shortening	3
Sauvé-Kapandji	3
Epiphysiodesis—distal ulna	2
Total	38

Intraarticular Malunion: Radiocarpal Joint

The role of osteotomy of an intraarticular malunion of the radiocarpal joint following distal radius fracture is limited by both chronology and type of injury. The osteotomy should be done as early as possible following fracture, as the fracture plane can be readily identified upwards of 8 to 12 weeks post fracture (see Technique: "Nascent" Malunion, above). In addition, it is preferable to reserve such a procedure for those malunited fractures which have a relatively simple intraarticular component. Those include malunited radial

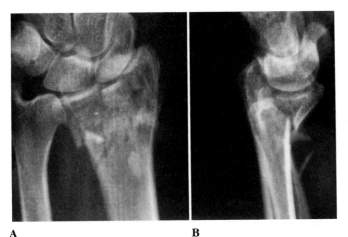

Figure 10.26. Intraarticular malunion in a volar shearing (Barton's) fracture in a 40-year-old woman seen 8 weeks postfracture. A,B. Anteroposterior and lateral radiographs 8 weeks post fracture. Healing callus is visible. C,D. Preoperative drawings of the malunion. The callus is represented by the black shadow. E,F. Two years postosteotomy. Mild articular congruity is apparent. The patient regained good wrist motion with only occasional discomfort.

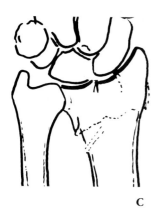

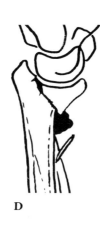

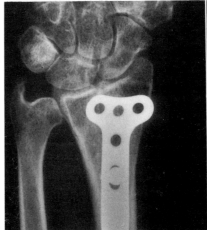

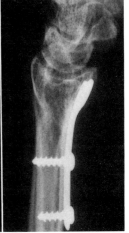

styloid fractures, volar or dorsal shearing (Barton's) fractures (Fig. 10.26A–F), and dorsal die-punch fractures (Fig. 10.27A–G).

In executing such osteotomies, caution must be taken to minimize the soft tissue dissection around the malunited articular fragment in order to offset the potential for avascular necrosis. Similarly, internal fixation must be gentle to avoid fragmentation of these tenuous articular fragments.

Postoperative Management Following Distal Radius Osteotomy

As a general rule, we prefer to immobilize the wrist in a volar plaster splint for 10 to 14 days to permit the surrounding soft tissue to heal. Once suture removal is accomplished, gentle active wrist motion is permitted in those cases in which stable internal fixation was accomplished in the presence of good bone quality. A thermoplast splint is advisable, which the patient can remove early on to perform such exercises.

In those cases in which Kirschner wire fixation is used, a below-elbow cast is used for about 4 weeks.

Strenuous activities are reserved until there is radiographic evidence of

Figure 10.27. A complex intra- and extra-articular malunion in a 65-year-old general surgeon (also see Figure 10.12A–I) at 3 months postinjury. A,B. The anteroposterior radiographs of the original fracture and malunion show the impacted dorsal die-punch malunion of the lunate facet as well as the dorsal angula tion and shortening of the distal metaphyseal fragment. C. Intraoperative view of the lunate facet osteotomized through the original fracture (*arrow*). The reduction was held with a cannulated 3.5-mm screw over a washer. D,E. Anteroposterior and lateral radiographs showing the reduction of both the intra- and extraarticular malunions. A modified Darrach resection was done. F,G. One year postoperatively, radiographs demonstrate maintenance of the articular restoration. The patient was extremely satisfied with the outcome. (Reprinted with permission. Jupiter JB, Ruder J: Computergenerated bone models in the planning of osteotomy of multidirectional distal radius malunions. *J Hand Surg* 17A: 406–415, 1992.)

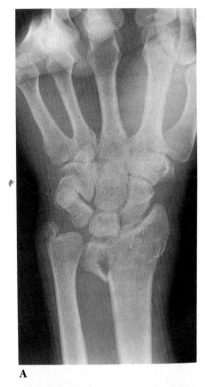

A

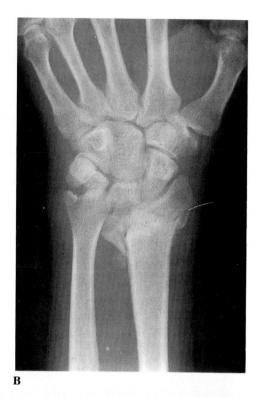

B

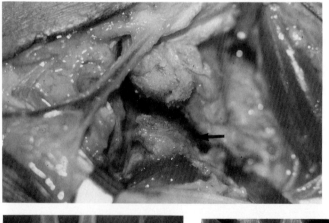

C

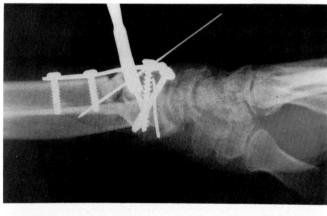

E

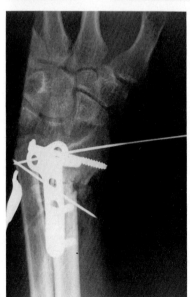

D

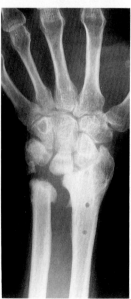

F

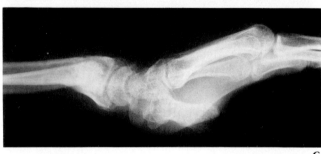

G

bony healing, which will not be present for a minimum of 8 to 12 weeks following the osteotomy.

We have found it necessary to remove most dorsally placed plates due to limitation of the overlying extensor tendons, whereas more commonly the volar plates can be left in place.

Salvage Procedures

In cases in which intraarticular malunion following extensive joint comminution has resulted in pain and associated disability, a salvage procedure such as arthrodesis or arthroplasty should be considered (Fig. 10.28A and B). The type of salvage procedure depends on a number of factors, including the functional requirements of the wrist, hand dominance, level of pain, patient age, and occupation.

Limited arthrodesis of the radiocarpal joint (radioscapholunate fusion) is a good alternative for localized degenerative changes secondary to incongruity of the radial joint surfaces. The outcome of this procedure is dependent the anatomic and functional integrity of the midcarpal joint. The requirements, therefore, should include a well-preserved midcarpal joint space as well as the absence of carpal collapse or a fixed midcarpal instability (Fig. 10.29A–D).

The joint is approached through a dorsal transverse capsulotomy centered between the third and fourth compartments. The posterior interosseous nerve is identified and its distal 3 to 4 cm are resected. Wrist flexion will facilitate exposure as well as removal of any remaining articular cartilage from the

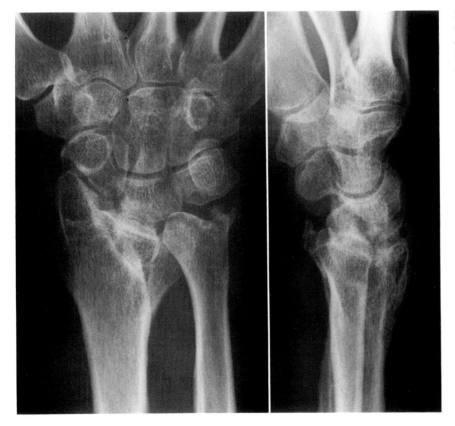

Figure 10.28. A severe intraarticular fracture of the distal radius resulted in a painful disability. Note the evidence of an associated intercarpal instability. Ultimately a wrist arthrodesis was performed.

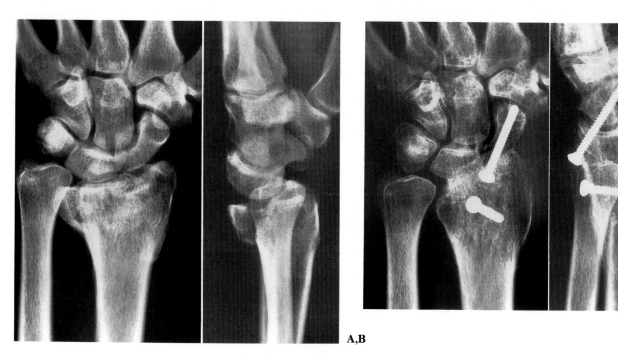

A,B

C,D

Figure 10.29. A 34-year-old roofer sustained a complex intraarticular fracture of the distal radius with resultant painful radiocarpal arthrosis. A,B. The anteroposterior and lateral radiographs show the localized radiocarpal posttraumatic changes and dorsal carpal subluxation. C,D. A radiocarpal arthrodesis was chosen as a salvage procedure. The radiographs were taken 3 years following the fusion. The patient lost 40 percent of normal wrist extension and flexion. (Reprinted with permission, Fernandez DF: Reconstructive procedures for malunion and traumatic arthritis. In: Melone C, ed. Distal radius fractures. *Orthop Clin North Am* 24: 341–336, 1993.)

scaphoid, lunate, and distal radius. Cancellous bone can be obtained from either the distal radius or the iliac crest and used to fill up the intercarpal space. Fixation of the arthrodesis may be achieved with Kirschner wires, screws, or a dorsal T plate with the distal screws centered in the scaphoid and lunate (Fig. 10.30A–D).

Should the patient decline a total or partial wrist arthrodesis, a motion preserving procedure can be considered. The proximal row carpectomy, although appealing, has a limited place because the lunate facet is often distorted by the fracture. If, however, the degenerative changes are localized on the radial side of the radiocarpal joint with both the lunate and capitate articular surface, intact a proximal row carpectomy can be considered.

Lastly, a total wrist arthroplasty may also have a place in the treatment of posttraumatic arthrosis after intraarticular fractures, although in our experience, this has only been reserved for those patients who require the use of their wrist for nonstrenuous activities of daily living (Fig. 10.31A–D).

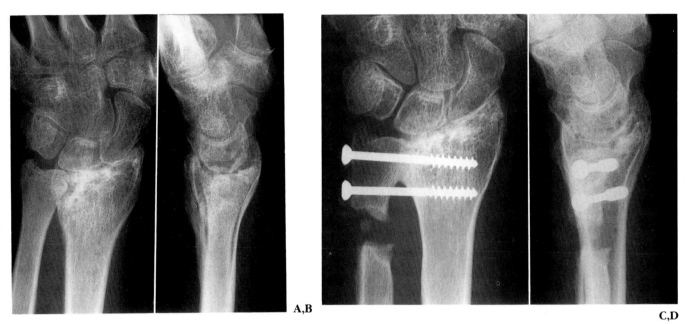

A,B

C,D

Figure 10.30. Posttraumatic radiocarpal and radioulnar arthritis following an intra-articular fracture of the distal radius. Forearm rotation was locked in 10 degrees of supination. A,B. The preoperative anteroposterior and lateral radiographs reveal extensive radiocarpal and radioulnar arthritis. C,D. Anteroposterior and lateral radiographs taken 3 years following radioscapholunate fusion and a Sauvé-Kapandji procedure for the distal radioulnar joint. (Reprinted with permission, Fernandez DF: Reconstructive procedures for malunion and traumatic arthritis. In: Melone C, ed. Distal radius fractures. *Orthop Clin North Am* 24: 341–336, 1993.)

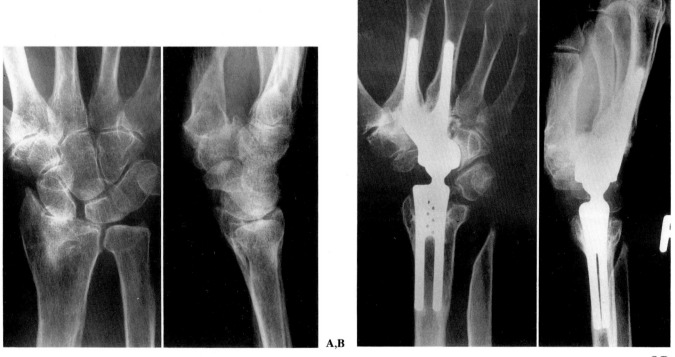

A,B

C,D

Figure 10.31. Posttraumatic arthrosis and chronic scapholunate dissociation following an intraarticular fracture of the distal radius in a 67-year-old retired postal clerk. A,B. The anteroposterior and lateral radiographs show radioscaphoid arthrosis, chronic scapholunate dissociation, and ulnar translation of the carpus. C,D. Radiographs 5 years following a noncemented titanium Meuli total wrist arthroplasty.

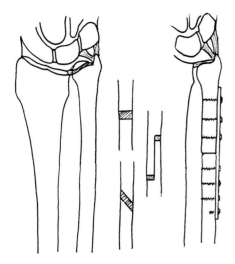

Figure 10.32. Schematic representation of three methods of shortening the ulnar for an ulnar plus variance. These include a transverse, oblique, and step-cut Z osteotomy. Plate fixation is preferred to stabilize the ulnar. (Reprinted with permission, Fernandez DF: Reconstructive procedures for malunion and traumatic arthritis. In: Melone C, ed. Distal radius fractures. *Orthop Clin North Am* 24: 341–336, 1993.)

Reconstructive Procedures for Distal Radioulnar Joint Incongruity

When the primary focus of the patient's complaints rests in the distal radioulnar joint and the angulation of the radioulnar joint surfaces are less than 10 degrees in both the sagittal and the frontal planes, a reconstructive procedure at the radioulnar joint alone is indicated without the need of a radial osteotomy.

For posttraumatic positive ulnar variance and associated ulnocarpal impingement and an acceptable relationship between the head of the ulnar and the sigmoid notch (best judged by a CT scan), a shortening osteotomy of the ulnar should be considered[35] (Fig. 10.32). Ulnar shortening can serve not only to reestablish congruency of the distal radioulnar joint, but also to decompress the ulnar compartment of the wrist and help stabilize the distal ulnar by tightening the triangular fibrocartilage. The method of shortening may vary from oblique to step-cut to transverse osteotomy, but whatever the type of bony cut, it is advisable to stabilize the ulnar with a compression plate (Fig. 10.33A–D).

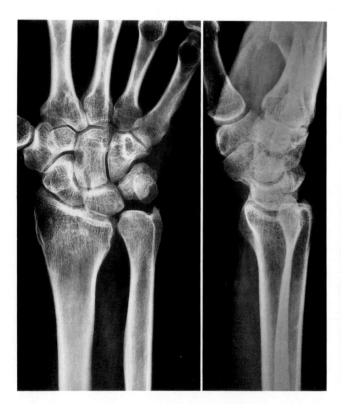

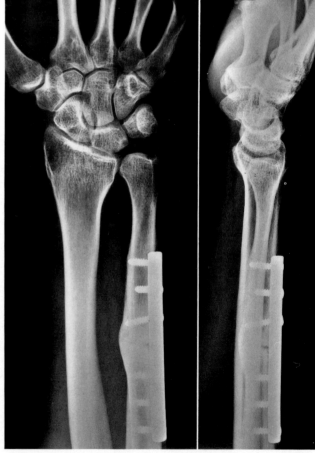

Figure 10.33. Ulnocarpal impingement and subluxation of the distal radioulnar joint following a distal radius fracture treated with an ulnar shortening osteotomy. A,B. Anteroposterior and lateral radiographs demonstrate the impingement associated with a positive ulnar variance. C,D. An ulnar shortening osteotomy restored a more normal distal radioulnar congruency and eliminated the ulnocarpal impingement. Stability of the distal radioulnar joint was also enhanced.

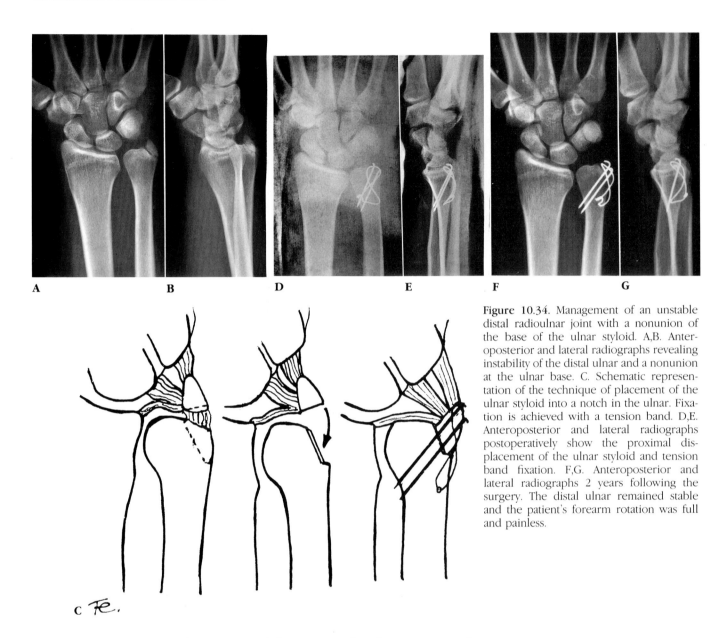

A　　　　　　　B　　　　　　　D　　　　　　　E　　　　　　　F　　　　　　　G

c

Figure 10.34. Management of an unstable distal radioulnar joint with a nonunion of the base of the ulnar styloid. A,B. Anteroposterior and lateral radiographs revealing instability of the distal ulnar and a nonunion at the ulnar base. C. Schematic representation of the technique of placement of the ulnar styloid into a notch in the ulnar. Fixation is achieved with a tension band. D,E. Anteroposterior and lateral radiographs postoperatively show the proximal displacement of the ulnar styloid and tension band fixation. F,G. Anteroposterior and lateral radiographs 2 years following the surgery. The distal ulnar remained stable and the patient's forearm rotation was full and painless.

When faced with radioulnar joint instability associated with a nonunion of the base of the ulnar styloid, resection of the sclerotic margins at the nonunion and displacement of the styloid proximally into a notch created in the lateral aspect of the ulnar can work effectively to stabilize the distal ulnar by tightening the triangular fibrocartilage complex. The styloid can be secured with either a tension band technique or a screw and tension wire (Fig. 10.34A–G).

In some circumstances, a positive ulnar variance, ulnocarpal impingement, and ulnar styloid nonunion may effectively be treated by a combination of an ulnar shortening osteotomy and tension band fixation of the ulnar styloid nonunion (Fig. 10.35A–H).

If the plain radiographs or CT scans suggest posttraumatic incongruity or degenerative changes of the radioulnar joint, consideration should now be extended toward alternative approaches, such as a resection arthroplasty or distal radioulnar joint arthrodesis. The advantage of attempting to preserve part of the ulnar head over complete resection is that the ulnocarpal ligaments and triangular fibrocartilage complex remain in continuity with the distal ulnar (Fig. 10.36).[2,51] Partial ulnar resection, however, will not affect ulnar variance.

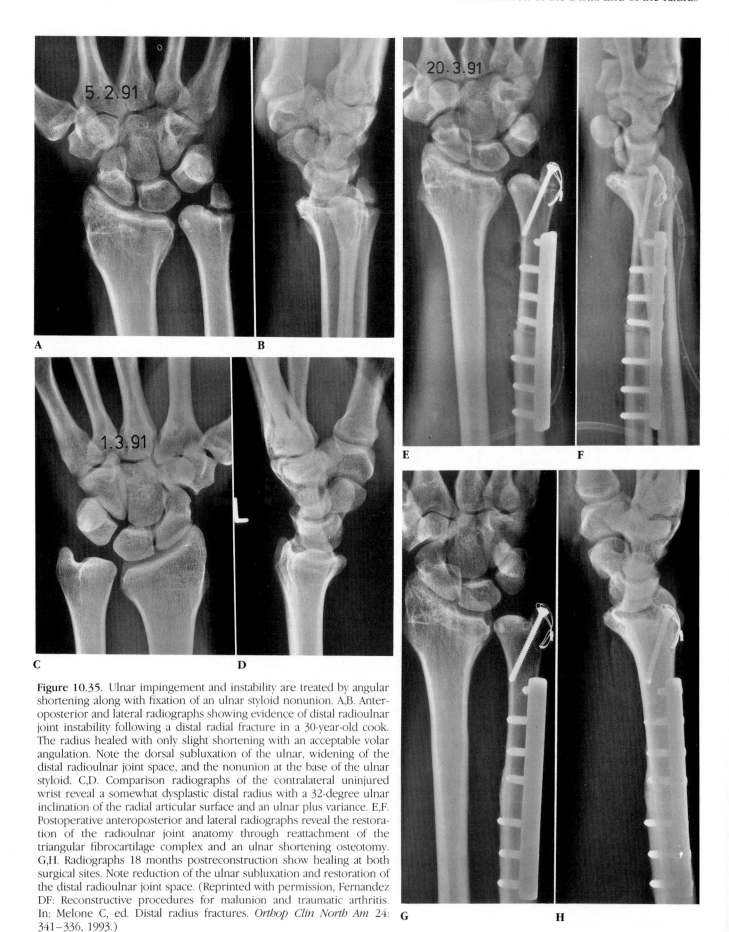

Figure 10.35. Ulnar impingement and instability are treated by angular shortening along with fixation of an ulnar styloid nonunion. A,B. Anteroposterior and lateral radiographs showing evidence of distal radioulnar joint instability following a distal radial fracture in a 30-year-old cook. The radius healed with only slight shortening with an acceptable volar angulation. Note the dorsal subluxation of the ulnar, widening of the distal radioulnar joint space, and the nonunion at the base of the ulnar styloid. C,D. Comparison radiographs of the contralateral uninjured wrist reveal a somewhat dysplastic distal radius with a 32-degree ulnar inclination of the radial articular surface and an ulnar plus variance. E,F. Postoperative anteroposterior and lateral radiographs reveal the restoration of the radioulnar joint anatomy through reattachment of the triangular fibrocartilage complex and an ulnar shortening osteotomy. G,H. Radiographs 18 months postreconstruction show healing at both surgical sites. Note reduction of the ulnar subluxation and restoration of the distal radioulnar joint space. (Reprinted with permission, Fernandez DF: Reconstructive procedures for malunion and traumatic arthritis. In: Melone C, ed. Distal radius fractures. *Orthop Clin North Am* 24: 341–336, 1993.)

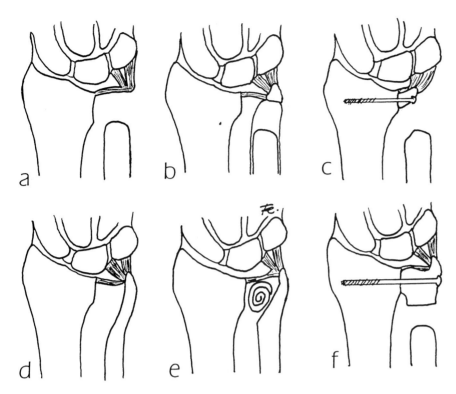

Figure 10.36. Schematic of the various operative procedures for the distorted distal radioulnar joint. (a) Darrach, (b) Darrach-Dignman, (c) Darrach-Zancolli, (d) Watson matched ulnar resection, (e) Bowers' hemiresection interposition arthroplasty, (f) Sauvé-Kapandji arthrodesis.

Therefore, an additional ulnar shortening will need to be done either at the styloid level or in the ulnar diaphysis (Fig. 10.37A–D).

Although loss of grip strength, loss of ulnar support of the carpus, and instability of the distal ulnar stump are recognized adverse sequelae associated with the Darrach procedure,[8] the most common cause of failure is excessive resection of the distal ulnar.[15]

Zancolli's modification of the Darrach procedure (Fig. 10.36C), in which the ulan styloid is fixed to the sigmoid notch, has the added advantages of retaining the ulnocarpal ligaments and enlarging the ulnar shelf of the lunate facet of the radius. Furthermore, tightening of the ulnocarpal ligament complex in a radial direction controls ulnar translation of the carpus. For stabilization of the distal stump of the ulnar, he recommends a careful closure of the sheath of the extensor carpi ulnaris tendon.[53]

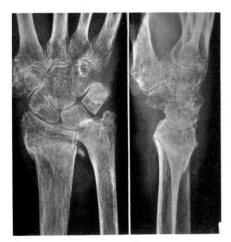

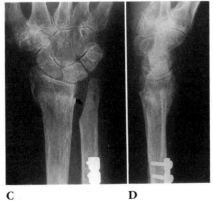

Figure 10.37. Ulnocarpal impingement and traumatic arthrosis of the distal radioulnar joint following a distal radius fracture in a 70-year-old active woman. A,B. Anteroposterior and lateral radiographs reveal a malunited distal radius along with ulnocarpal impingement and arthritic changes in the distal radioulnar joint. C,D. The malalignment was addressed by an ulnar shortening and Bowers hemiresection arthroplasty.

A   **B**

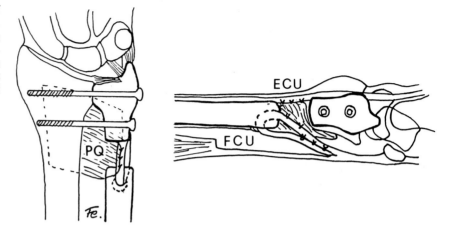

Figure 10.38. Schematic representation of our modified Sauve-Kapandji procedure. The ulnar head is secured with two lag screws. The proximal ulnar stump is stabilized with a strip of the flexor carpi ulnaris (FCU). The pronator quadratus (PQ) is sutured to the sheath of the extensor carpi ulnaris (ECU).

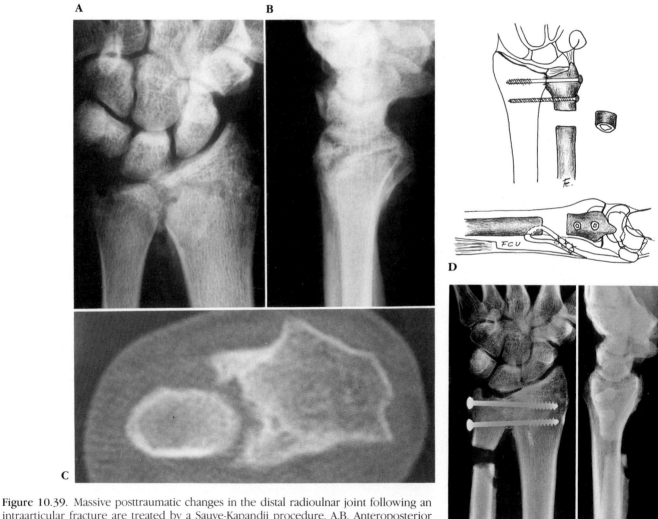

Figure 10.39. Massive posttraumatic changes in the distal radioulnar joint following an intraarticular fracture are treated by a Sauve-Kapandji procedure. A,B. Anteroposterior and lateral radiographs of the wrist showing the distal radioulnar joint disruption. C. The CT scan clearly shows the disruption of the distal radioulnar joint. D. Schematic of the procedure. E,F. Anteroposterior and lateral radiographs of the successful Sauve-Kapandji procedure.

Distal radioulnar joint arthrodesis combined with the creation of a proximal pseudarthrosis preserves both the ulnocarpal ligaments and the bony support of the carpus (Fig. 10.36F). We have found this operation extremely useful for the restoration of forearm rotation in patients with fixed distal radioulnar joint subluxation following articular fractures of the distal radius with extensive destruction of the radioulnar joint.

In the original technique described by Sauvé and Kapandji,[47] fusion of the ulnar head to the sigmoid notch is stabilized by a single screw. A 15- to 20-mm ulnar segment is resected just proximal to the ulnar neck. The periosteal sleeve is removed to prevent reossification, and the pronator quadratus is pulled dorsally through the pseudarthrosis gap and sutured to the sheath of the extensor carpi ulnaris tendon. To prevent painful instability of the proximal ulnar stump, we prefer to use a distally based tendon strip of the flexor carpi ulnaris as a palmar tenodesis (Figs. 10.38A and B, 10.39A–F).

Combined Radial Osteotomy and Distal Radioulnar Joint Procedure

The decision to perform an associated primary procedure on the ulnar side of the wrist during an osteotomy of the distal radius is dependent on a careful assessment of the status of the distal radioulnar joint. It is the authors' belief that partial resection of the ulnar head should be performed as a primary operation in combination with radial osteotomy when the patient's primary symptom is painful limitation of forearm rotation due to posttraumatic arthritis of the radioulnar joint (Fig. 10.40A and B). There may, in fact, be occasions when the correction of the ulnocarpal impingement may also require an ulnar shortening through the distal diaphysis (Fig. 10.41A–F).

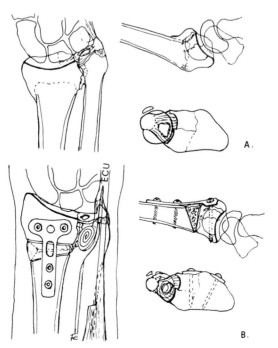

Figure 10.40. Schematic representation of a malunion of a four-part articular fracture with resultant ulnocarpal impingement, incongruity of the sigmoid notch, radial shortening, and increased dorsal tilt. A. Pictorial representation of the deformity. B. Pictorial representation of the radial osteotomy and Bowers arthroplasty. (Reprinted with permission, Fernandez DL: Radial osteotomy and Bowers arthroplasty for malunited fractures of the distal end of the radius. *J Bone Joint Surg* 70A: 1538–1551, 1988.)

Figure 10.41. Complex deformity following a dorsal bending (Colles') distal radius fracture. Associated ulnocarpal impingement and incongruity of the distal radioulnar joint resulted in a painful limitation of forearm rotation. The patient is a 60-year-old college professor. A,B. Preoperative anteroposterior and lateral radiographs of the complex deformities. Note the incongruity of the sigmoid notch. C,D. The preoperative plan shows the decrease in ulnar inclination of the distal radial articular surface to 12 degrees and a 7-mm radial shortening. The planned surgical tactic includes an ulnar shortening and Bowers hemiresection arthroplasty. E,F. Anteroposterior and lateral radiographs of the healed osteotomy showing the ulnar inclination restored to 25 degrees and radial length restored by the ulnar shortening. Full pain-free forearm rotation was recovered.

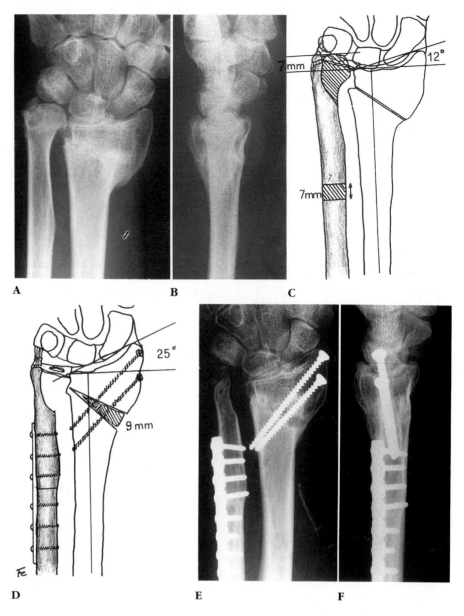

There have been occasions in which distal radioulnar joint instability and ulnocarpal impingement due to shortening, angulation, or malrotation of the distal end of the radius could be corrected by radial osteotomy alone, yet the patient continued to experience distal radioulnar joint symptoms postosteotomy. In these instances we have performed a hemiarthroplasty or Sauve-Kapandji procedure at a later date (Figs. 10.42A–D).[1]

One of us (Diego Fernandez) reported on 15 patients who had a combination of a radial osteotomy and hemiresection arthroplasty for a malunited fracture of the radius associated with symptoms predominantly in the radioulnar joint and limited forearm rotation.[12] The length of follow-up averaged 3 years after the osteotomy. Thirteen patients had no pain in the distal radioulnar joint, and two noted only mild pain with extremes of forearm

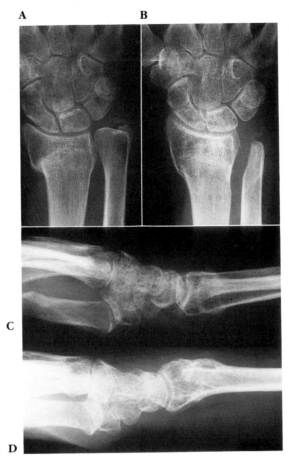

Figure 10.42. Malunited Colles' fracture with associated midcarpal instability, and painful forearm rotation. The osteotomy was combined with a hemiresection arthroplasty of the distal radioulnar joint. A,B. Preoperative radiograph of malunion with midcarpal instability (DISI) and sever limitation of forearm rotation. C,D. Radiographs 2 years after radial osteotomy and hemiresection arthroplasty. Full forearm rotation was achieved. (Reprinted with permission, CV Mosby, Inc. Fernandez DL: Malunion of the distal radius. *AAOS Instructional Course Lectures*, p. 100, 1993.)

rotation. Dorsal subluxation of the distal ulnar was not seen in any patient. An average increase in grip strength of 30 percent over the preoperative strength was seen in all patients, and each patient noted substantial improvement in overall function (Table 10.7). The outcomes were rated very good in four patients, good in eight, and fair in three.

Complex Deformity

A number of unique clinical situations may present with resultant deformity of the distal radius and distal radioulnar joint incongruity. These include complex fractures (Fig. 10.43A–H), fractures with bone loss, or complex deformity following distal radius fracture in the pediatric age group (Fig. 10.44A–M).

The surgical tactics in these particular situations must be individualized to accomplish the specific demands presented by the injury pattern. What is consistent, however, is the recognition that reconstruction of the distal radioulnar joint with restoration of functional forearm mobility is critical for overall hand and wrist function.

Table 10.7.1. Combined radial osteotomy and druj hemiarthroplasty.

Case	Sex, age (yrs)	Type of fracture	Radiographic measurements				Level of pain*		Findings before operation		Motion of the wrist‡ (degrees)				Grip strength‡ (kgf)
			Dorsal tilt (degrees)	Volar tilt (degrees)	Ulnar tilt (degrees)	Radioulnar index (mm)	Radiocarpal	Radioulnar	Radiog. degen. changes†		Dorsiflex.	Palmar Flex.	Pronat.	Supinat.	
									Radiocarpal	Radioulnar					
1	M, 48	Smith	–	34	20	6	–	++	None	Severe	30/70	85/75	85/80	15/85	25/45
2	M, 37	Colles' fractured ulna	–	30	10	5	+	++	None	Moderate	25/75	70/75	30/80	0/80	15/52
3	F, 20	Colles' intraarticular	25	–	18	4	+	+++	None	Mild	90/80	45/80	40/90	0/85	12/35
4	F, 48	Colles' intraarticular	15	–	22	6	++	+++	Mild	Severe	40/70	30/75	45/85	20/90	10/30
5	M, 51	Colles'	35	–	10	1	–	++	None	Mild	60/75	20/70	35/80	40/90	29/42
6	F, 45	Smith	–	27	25	9	–	++	None	Mild	40/80	90/75	80/85	10/90	9/22
7	M, 49	Colles' intraarticular	28	–	17	5	–	++	None	Mild	60/70	5/80	35/80	40/90	23/41
8	M, 57	Colles' intraarticular	5	–	12	7	+	+++	Mild	Moderate	45/75	43/70	20/85	0/80	18/43
9	F, 59	Colles' intraarticular	–	25	15	6	+	++	None	Moderate	20/65	45/70	65/80	0/85	7/25
10	F, 51	Colles'	30	–	13	6	–	+++	None	Mild	80/70	10/75	40/90	50/90	16/29
11	F, 74	Colles'	5	–	–10	9	+	++	None	Mild	60/70	50/65	5/85	45/85	8/19
12	F, 70	Colles' intraarticular	45	–	10	3	++	+++	Mild	Severe	70/70	15/75	35/60	20/70	12/27
13	F, 63	Colles' intraarticular	–	15	12	4	+	++	Mild	Moderate	15/70	40/75	40/75	25/85	9/20
14	M, 43	Colles' intraarticular	–	20	–	5	–	++	Mild	Mild	35/80	60/70	35/80	0/90	21/47
15	M, 69	Smith, fractured ulna	–	26	19	3	–	++	None	Moderate	45/65	60/70	60/85	30/85	15/37

* – = none, + = mild, ++ = moderate, and +++ = severe. See text for a full description of each level of pain.
† Severe = narrowing of the joint space, subchondral sclerosis, formation of osteophytes, subluxation, and incongruity of the joint; moderate = narrowing of the joint space, subchondral sclerosis, and incongruity of the joint; mild = minimum narrowing of the joint space; and none = none of these radiographic findings.
‡ Affected/normal.

Table 10.7.2 Combined radial osteotomy and druj hemiarthroplasty.

Time to union (wks)	Length of follow-up (mos)	Radiographic measurements				Results at latest follow-up				Motion of the wrist‡ (degrees)				Grip strength‡ (kgf)
		Dorsal tilt (degrees)	Volar tilt (degrees)	Ulnar tilt (degrees)	Radioulna index (mm)	Level of pain*		Radiog. degen. changes†		Dorsiflex.	Palmar Flex.	Pronat.	Supinat.	
						Radiocarpal	Radioulnar							
6	54	—	4	21	0	—	—	None		55/70	65/75	80/80	75/75	38/42
6.5	52	—	7	18	0	—	—	None		65/75	55/75	75/80	70/80	41/50
5	48	—	5	22	0	—	+	None		70/75	70/80	85/90	80/85	25/32
6.2	44	—	7	25	1	+	—	Mild		50/70	45/70	80/85	80/90	22/30
7	42	—	5	19	0	+	—	None		50/75	60/70	75/80	80/90	37/42
6	41	—	6	25	3	—	—	None		70/80	65/75	85/85	75/90	18/24
6.1	38	—	5	21	0	—	—	Mild		55/70	5/75	65/80	80/90	37/43
8	35	0	—	25	1	—	—	Mild		50/75	45/70	75/85	80/80	35/40
6.5	34	—	5	20	1	+	—	None		45/65	40/70	70/80	65/85	15/23
7.2	32	—	3	18	0	—	—	None		65/70	50/75	75/90	80/90	23/30
8.1	29	0	—	15	2	+	—	None		55/70	50/65	60/85	55/85	12/18
6.5	27	4	—	20	0	—	—	Mild		55/70	45/75	75/60	80/70	15/25
8	27	3	—	17	0	+	—	Moderate		40/70	35/75	80/75	80/85	13/21
7.1	25	0	—	15	1	—	—	Mild		60/80	50/75	60/80	65/90	30/45
8	24	—	5	20	0	—	+	None		50/65	45/70	75/85	60/85	24/35

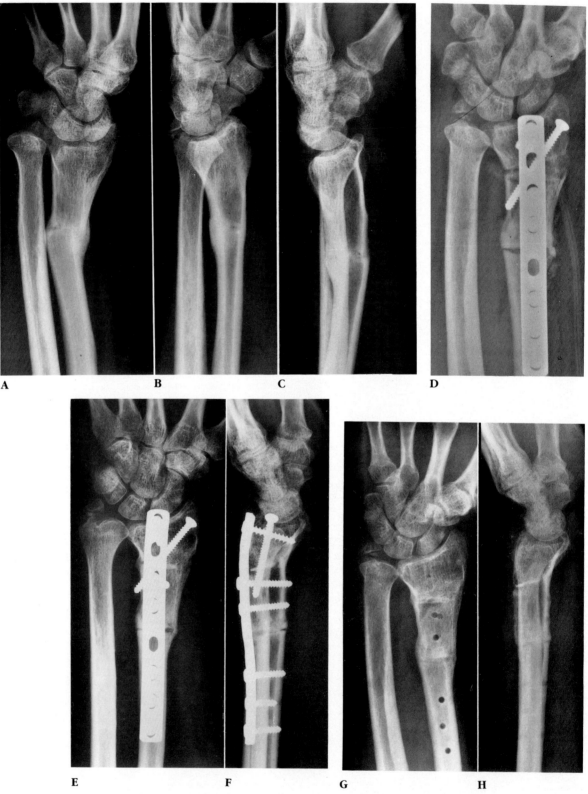

Figure 10.43. Complex malunion of both a distal radius and Galeazzi fracture treated with a double-level osteotomy. A-C. Anteroposterior, oblique, and lateral radiographs reveal the complex double-level deformity with alteration of the distal radioulnar joint. D. A double osteotomy was performed and secured with a 3.5-mm DC plate and oblique lag screw. E,F. Union progressed with both osteotomies and the distal radio-ulnar joint remained congruent. G,H. At 1 year follow-up, excellent function resulted.

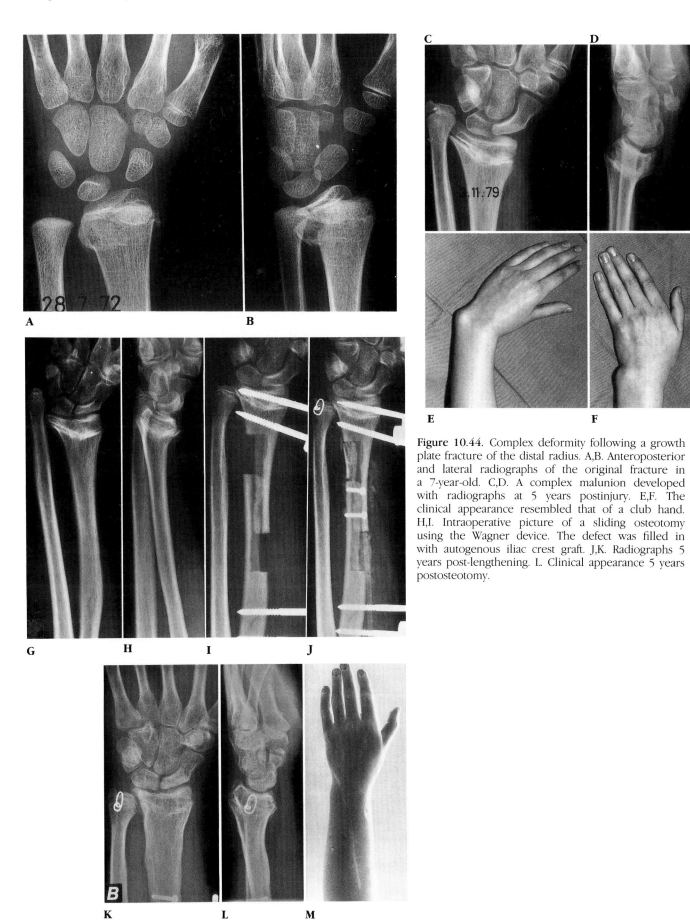

A **B** **C** **D** **E** **F** **G** **H** **I** **J** **K** **L** **M**

Figure 10.44. Complex deformity following a growth plate fracture of the distal radius. A,B. Anteroposterior and lateral radiographs of the original fracture in a 7-year-old. C,D. A complex malunion developed with radiographs at 5 years postinjury. E,F. The clinical appearance resembled that of a club hand. H,I. Intraoperative picture of a sliding osteotomy using the Wagner device. The defect was filled in with autogenous iliac crest graft. J,K. Radiographs 5 years post-lengthening. L. Clinical appearance 5 years postosteotomy.

References

1. Baciu C: L'opération de Sauvé-Kapandji du traitement des cals vicieux de l'éxtremité inférieure du radius. *Ann Chir* 31: 323–330, 1976.

2. Bowers WH: Distal radioulnar joint arthroplasty: The hemi-resection interposition technique. *J Hand Surg* 10A: 169–178, 1985.

3. Boyd HB, Stone MM: Resection of the distal end of the ulnar. *J Bone Joint Surg* 26: 313–321, 1944.

4. Bunnell S (ed): *Surgery of the Hand.* 2nd edition. Philadelphia: JB Lippincott 596: 681–682, 1948.

5. Campbell WC: Malunited Colles' fractures. *JAMA* 109: 1105–1108, 1937.

6. Castaing J: Les fractures récentes de l'extrémité inférieure du radius chez l'adulte. *Rev Chir Orthop,* 50: 581–696, 1964.

7. Cooney WP III, Dobyns JH, Linscheid RL: Complications of Colles' fractures. *J Bone Joint Surg [Am]* 62A: 613–619, 1980.

8. Darrach W: Partial excision of the lower shaft of the ulnar for deformity following Colles' fracture. *Ann Surg* 57: 764–765, 1913.

9. Desault M: Extrait d'un mémoire de M. Desault sur la luxation de l'extrémité inférieure du cubitus. *J Chir* 1: 78, 1791.

10. Durman DC: An operation for correction of deformities of the wrist following fracture. *J Bone Joint Surg* 17: 1014–1016, 1935.

11. Durman DC: Malunited Colles' fracture, abstract: Discussion of Dr. Campbell's article. *JAMA* 109: 1105–1108, 1937.

12. Fernandez DL: Radial osteotomy and Bowers arthroplasty for malunited fractures of the distal end of the radius. *J Bone Joint Surg* 70A: 1538–1551, 1988.

13. Fernandez DL: Correction of posttraumatic wrist deformity in adults by osteotomy, bone grafting, and internal fixation. *J Bone Joint Surg* 4A: 1164–1178, 1982.

14. Fernandez DL: Correction of posttraumatic wrist deformity in adults by osteotomy, bone grafting, and internal fixation. *J Bone Joint Surg* 64A: 1164–1178, 1982.

15. Fernandez DL: Osteotomias del antebrazo distal. Indicación, técnica y resultados. *Acta Orthop Latinoamerica* 11: 55–72, 1984.

16. Fernandez DL, Albrecht HU, Saxer U: Die Korrekturosteotomie am distalen Radius bei posttraumatischer Fehlstellung. *Arch Orthop Unfallchir* 90: 199–211, 1977.

17. Fernandez DL, Geissler WB: Korrektureingriffe bei Fehlstellung am distalen Radius. *Z Unfallchir Med Berufskr* 82: 34–44, 1989.

18. Forgon M, Mammel E: Unsere Korrekturosteotomie in Fehlstellung geheilter Frakturen der Speiche an der typischen Stelle. *Unfall Chir* 9: 318–324, 1983.

19. Fourrier P, Bardy A, Roche G, Cisterne JP, Chambon A: Approche d'une définition du cal vicieux du poignet. *Int Orthop (SICOT)* 4: 299–305, 1981.

20. Ghormley RK, Mroz RJ: Fractures of the wrist: A review of one hundred and seventy six cases. *Surg Gynecol Obstet* 55: 377–381, 1932.

21. Hobart MH, Kraft GL: Malunited Colles' fracture. *Am J Surg* 53: 55–60, 1941.

22. Jupiter JB, Ruder J, Roth DA: Computer-generated bone models in the planning of osteotomy of multidirectional distal radius malunions. *J Hand Surg* 17A: 406–415, 1992.

23. Kaukone JP, Karaharju EO, Porras M: Functional recovery after fractures of the distal forearm: Analysis of radiographic and other factors affecting the outcome. *Ann Chir Gyn* 77: 27–31, 1988.

24. Kazuki K, Masakata K, Shimazu A: Pressure distribution in the radiocarpal joint measured with a densitometer designed for pressure sensitive film. *J Hand Surg* 16A: 401–408, 1991.

25. King GJ, McMurtry RY, Rubenstein JD, et al: Computerized tomography of the distal radioulnar joint. A correlation with ligamentous pathology in a cadaveric model. *J Hand Surg* 11A: 711–717, 1986.

26. Knirk JL, Jupiter JB: Intraarticular fractures of the distal end of the radius in young adults. *J Bone Joint Surg [Am]* 68A: 647–659, 1986.

27. Lichtman DM, Schneider JR, Swafford AR, et al: Ulnar midcarpal instability: Clinical and laboratory analysis. *J Hand Surg* 6: 515–523, 1981.

28. Linscheid RL, Dobyns JH, Beabout JW, et al: Traumatic instability of the wrist. Diagnosis, classification, and pathomechanics. *J Bone Joint Surg [Am]* 54A: 1612–1632, 1972.

29. Marsh JL, Vannier MW: Surface imaging from computerized tomographic scans. *Surgery* 94: 159–165, 1983.

30. Martini AK: Die sekundäre Arthrose des Handgelenkes bei der in Fehlstellung verheilten und nicht korrigierten distalen Radiusfrakturen. *Aktuel Traumatol* 16: 143–148, 1986.
31. McQueen M, Caspers J: Colles' fracture: Does the anatomic result affect the final function? *J Bone Joint Surg [Br]* 70B: 649–651, 1988.
32. Meine J: Die Früh- und Spätkomplikationen der Radiusfraktur loco classico. *Z Unfallchir Vers Med Berufsk* 82: 25–32, 1989.
33. Merle d'Aubigné R, Joussement L: A propos du traitement des cals vicieux de l'extrémité inférieure du radius. *Mem Acad Chir* 71: 153–157, 1945.
34. Merle d'Aubigné R, Tubiana R: Séquelles de traumatismes du poignet. In: *Traumatismes Anciens: Généralités Membre Supérieur*. Paris: Masson, 1958, pp. 361–376.
35. Milch H: Cuff resection of the ulnar for malunited Colles' fracture. *J Bone Joint Surg* 23: 311–313, 1941.
36. Moore EM: Three cases illustrating luxation of the ulnar in connection with Colles' fracture. *Med Rec NY* 17: 305–308, 1880.
37. Mino DE, Palmer AK, Levinsohn M: The role of radiography and computerized tomography in the diagnosis of subluxation and dislocation of the distal radioulnar joint. *J Hand Surg* 8A: 23–31, 1983.
38. Palmer AK, Werner FW: Biomechanics of the distal radioulnar joint. *Clin Orthop* 187: 26–35, 1984.
39. Palmer AK, Glisson RR, Werner FW: Ulnar variance determination. *J Hand Surg* 7: 376–379, 1982.
40. Poque DJ, Viegas SF, Patterson RM, et al: Effects of distal radius fracture on wrist joint mechanics. *J Hand Surg* 15A: 721–727, 1990.
41. Posner MA, Ambrose L: Malunited Colles' fracture. Correction with a biplanar closing wedge osteotomy. *J Hand Surg* 16A: 1017–1026, 1991.
42. Rodriguez-Megthiaz AM, Chamay A: Traitement des cals vicieux extra-articulaires du radius distal par ostéotomie d'ouverture avec interposition d'une greffe. *Med Hyg* 46: 2757–2765, 1988.
43. Sakai K, Doi K, Ihara K, et al: Carpal alignment after fractures of the distal radius, abstract. Presented at the International Symposium on the Wrist, Nagoya, Japan, 1991. p. 117.
44. Shaw JA, Bruno A, Paul EM: Ulnar styloid fixation in the treatment of post-traumatic instability of the radioulnar joint. A biomechanical study with clinical correlation. *J Hand Surg* 15A: 712–720, 1990.
45. Short WH, Palmer AK, Werner FW, et al: A biomechanical study of distal radius fractures. *J Hand Surg* 12A: 529–534, 1987.
46. Speed JS, Knight RA: Treatment of malunited Colles' fractures. *J Bone Joint Surg* 27: 361–367, 1945.
47. Sauvé L, Kapandji M: Une nouvelle technique de traitement chirurgical des luxations recidivantes isolées de l'éxtrémité cubitale inférieure. *J Chir* 47: 589–594, 1936.
48. Taleisnik J, Watson HK: Midcarpal instability caused by malunited fractures of the distal radius. *J Hand Surg* 9A: 350–357, 1984.
49. Vannier MW, Totty WG, Stevens WG, et al: Musculoskeletal application of three-dimensional surface reconstructions. *Orthop Clin North Am* 16: 543–555, 1985.
50. Villar RN, Marsh D, Rushton N: Three years after Colles' fracture. A prospective review. *J Bone Joint Surg [Am]* 69B: 635–638, 1987.
51. Watson HK, Ryu J, Burgess RC: Matched distal ulnar resection. *J Hand Surg* 11A: 812–817, 1986.
52. Weeks PM, Vannier MW, Stevens WG, et al: Three-dimensional imaging of the wrist. *J Hand Surg* 10A: 32–39, 1985.
53. Zancolli EA: personal communication.

Chapter Eleven

Early Complications

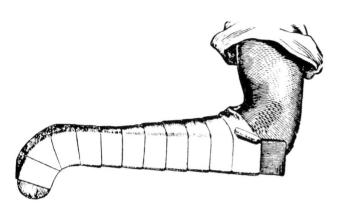

The first application of the bandages ought to be only moderately tight, and as the inflammation and swelling develop in these structures with rapidity, they should be attentively watched and loosened as they become painful. It must be constantly borne in mind that, to prevent and control inflammation, in this fracture, is the most difficult and by far the most important object to be accomplished, while to retain the fragments in place once reduced, is comparatively easy and unimportant.

F.H. Hamilton, M.D. 1860[67]

Introduction

Complications associated with fractures of the distal end of the radius are, unfortunately, all too common. Whether related to the injury itself or to the method of treatment, the sequelae of early complications can result in a profound and lasting disability.

In addition to the fact that the distal radius fracture is a common injury, unique anatomic features of this region of the upper limb contribute to the frequency of associated soft tissue problems. The overlying tendons, nerves, vascular channels, and integument are closely oriented to the underlying radius. Furthermore, these structures are confined by specific anatomic boundaries to well-defined, albeit crowded, zones that are prone to injury, both direct and indirect, from swelling or local compression.[81,90,99]

The complications surrounding soft tissue elements associated with the management of fractures of the distal end of the radius are evident in the earliest descriptions of Colles as well his European contemporaries.[33] The complications of constricting bandages were at times tragic, leading to loss of limb and even life. This is well depicted in the description of the origin of specimen No. 1038 in the Warren Anatomical Museum of Harvard Medical School:

Comminuted fracture of the lower end of the radius, just above and into the joint, and a second fracture, 2½ inches above the joint. From a man who received a very violent blow from a piece of machinery, December 24. On the 26th, he entered the hospital with gangrene of the limb, consequence of the exceeding tightness of the bandage that had been applied, and on the 29th day he died.

Prepared by Mr. R.H. Derby
One of the House Pupils, 1867
Dr. H.J. Bigelow[79]

With the development of plaster of Paris bandaging, the late nineteenth century saw increasing enthusiasm for longer periods of immobilization in ever more cumbersome plaster casts. As noted by Frederick Amendola, M.D., in 1938:[5]

A fracture about the wrist meant the encasement of the whole arm from the fingertips to the shoulder in a cast which sometimes immobilized the patient as well as the wrist.

On removal of the cast some months later, it was the general rule to find a rigid hand, a withered arm, and a deformity of the fracture which had not been reduced in the first place.

It is not surprising, therefore, to appreciate why the concepts of shortening the duration of immobilization combined with early joint manipulation and massage promoted by Lucas de Champonnière[102] attracted so many converts. The results of limited immobilization and aggressive massage and therapy, however, soon lost favor as treating surgeons came to recognize that unsupported fractures led to a persistence of pain, limited digital mobility, displacement of the fracture, and late deformity.

This chapter will focus on a number of early complications related to fractures of the distal end of the radius. Although it is not always readily apparent whether these complications are due to the injury itself on the methods of treatment, this chapter will address problems related to the overlying skin, tendons, nerves, and articulations.

Complications of Applied Techniques

Unfortunately, many principles of treatment of Colles' fractures are insufficiently known or their applications are not enforced. Consequently, one constantly sees patients who originally sought care for a disabled wrist and later seek care for a disabled hand.

W.H. Cassebaum, M.D., 1950[28]

Colles warned his colleagues against the dangers of ill-applied casts or splints, and unfortunately that admonition holds true today. The incorrect timing or method of application of a circumferential cast can lead to any number of problems, not the least of which involve distortion or damage to the underlying skin or the production of distal edema with resultant small joint contraction, peritendinous fibrosis, or intrinsic muscle contraction. These, in turn, will limit the mobility of the hand, leading to a stiff hand, which has long been identified as one of the most deleterious and yet common problems associated with the use of circumferential cast immobilization in the management of fractures of the distal end of the radius.[5,28,35,37,51,55,62,65,87,99,103,128,129]

Positioning of the hand and wrist in the extremes of palmar flexion and ulnar deviation (the Cotton-Loder position) has been condemned largely for its association with median nerve dysfunction.[1,28,106,165,176] This wrist position, it should be pointed out, was promoted in large part to help maintain the reduction of unstable fractures associated with loss of the integrity of the distal radioulnar joint. Its promoters stressed that this position should be held for no longer than 7 to 10 days, after which the wrist must be restored to a neutral position.[144,166] Its early advocates cautioned that the duration of immobilization in this position should be limited and that daily massage of the hand and active mobility exercises under supervision should be instituted immediately upon application of the casting. In spite of these precautions, problems still were commonplace. This is well documented in the following case from the fracture records of the Massachusetts General Hospital in 1924 (Fig. 11.1).

Even when a cast has been applied with the hand and wrist in what has become a more accepted position of immobilization, consisting of modest flexion and ulnar deviation, distal edema can substantially inhibit the ability of the patient to obtain full digital mobility. If this position is combined with traction in an external fixator with the pins placed above the center of rotation of the wrist joint, further inhibition will result as a consequence of tightening of the extrinsic extensor tendons. This will lead to the recognizable claw position of the digits.[2,83]

Case 78. 50, boilermaker (bench job). Inj. Nov. 13, 1924: fell (20 inches); adm. same date. X-RAY: comminuted Colles' fracture left radius, distal fragments displaced posteriorly and rotated upward.
Other Injuries: none.
Treatment: ether: immediate closed reduction attempted; antero-posterior splints. Position improved but not perfect. 6 days a.i.: ether: closed reduction; arm in extension in plaster cylinder from axilla to mid palm, hand in palmar flexion and extreme pronation. X-RAY: good position. 12 days a.i.: original plaster removed; antero-posterior molded plaster splints to forearm, wrist in comfortable palmar flexion and normal pronation. Discharged Dec. 2, 1924 (19 days a.i.); posterior splint discarded. 30 days a.i.: plaster cock-up splint; fingers very stiff; physiotherapy advised. 7 mos. a.i.: returned to work. 8 mos. a.i.: complained of anesthesia of finger.
Complication: none.
End-result: 1 yr. a.i.: incomplete extension of fingers at proximal interphalangeal joints, finger tips could not be approximated to palm; grip strong; limitation in rotation at wrists; limited but good extension at wrist. Patient satisfied. $A_3F_3E_4$

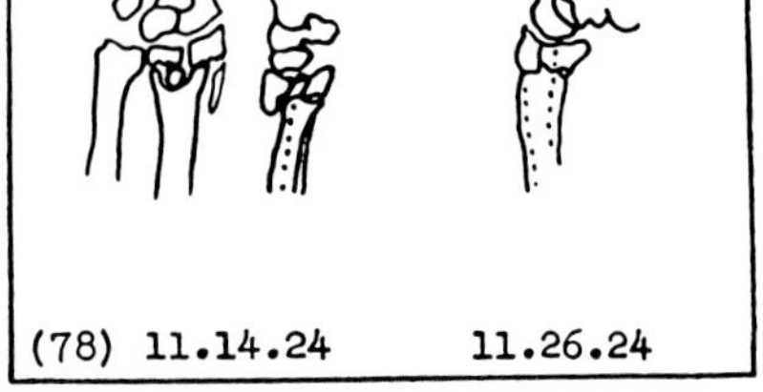

(78) 11.14.24   11.26.24

Figure 11.1. Case 78 from the Fracture Registry of Massachusetts General Hospital, 1924.

Figure 11.2. An improperly applied cast or splint is a common cause of swelling of the hand and digits. A. The cast extends beyond the distal palmar flexion crease. Note the distal swelling. B. Despite 6 months of hand therapy, the patient remained with residual loss of flexion due to intrinsic tightness, capsular contracture, and peritendinous fibrosis.

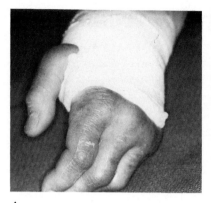

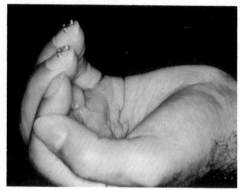

A

B

The unfortunate combination of postcast edema and a dysfunctional hand position can be further complicated by a cast extending beyond the metacarpophalangeal joints. A common occurrence, this too has a potential for inducing the development of the stiff claw hand recognizable by the extension contractures of the metacarpophalangeal joints, flexion contractures of the proximal interphalangeal joints, and a loss of wrist extension (Fig. 11.2).[99]

Edema will also have an adverse effect on the interosseous muscles within the hand. Intrinsic tightness accentuates the patient's difficulty in achieving full digital mobility both while in the cast and after removal of the cast.[154,156]

It is apparent, therefore, that measures should be taken early on in the treatment program to avoid or minimize the development of edema and maintain digital mobility. This was recognized as early as 1896 by Braatz[23] and soon after by Böhler in 1919,[20] with the latter having developed a program for active functional range of motion as well as coordinated exercises for patients during the time that they were treated for fractures of the distal end of the radius. This has been well accepted today with the addition of modalities such as Coban wrap* or an Isotoner glove.** These devices, combined with range of motion exercises accentuating metacarpophalangeal joint flexion under the supervision of a hand therapist, can offset many of the problems associated with edema.[34,99,122]

The adverse consequences of edema may overshadow the initial problem represented by the fracture and ultimately prove far more disabling than any skeletal deformity. This was clearly pointed out by Ford and Key:[51]

It is far better to lose position of a reduced Colles' fracture in order to spread a cast as a means of preventing interference with circulation if, by doing so, one can maintain full digital function.

Patients with marked residual stiffness of the fingers because swelling in the cast was unrelieved would have been better off in the final analysis if they had accepted the position of deformity and had simply maintained finger motion with or without splinting of the fracture.

The problems associated with an improperly padded or applied cast also involve the underlying skin. Pressure points, such as those over the radial styloid and the distal ulnar, should be well padded, and care should be taken to avoid creation of sharp edges at the proximal or distal limits of a cast. Even the degree of pressure that occurs under a cast has been investigated.[108,123]

---

*®3M Corporation, St. Paul, MN
**®Aris Isotoner Glove, New York, NY

Investigators have noticed that the highest pressures occurred immediately after application of a plaster of Paris cast, with a second rise an pressure an average of 13 hours after cast application. Yet the pressures were not sustained, and there was no correlation found between the development of edema of the hand and digits and pressures recorded under the plaster cast, which suggested to the investigators that edema was due more to dependency and the tracking of fluid than to persistent or increasing elevation or pressure under the cast. Yet with the advent of fiberglass cast materials, some investigators have suggested that considerably higher pressures will be generated under a fiberglass cast than with similar casts made of plaster of Paris.[90]

Although cast immobilization of fractures of the distal end of the radius has been well accepted historically and even in contemporary practice, many problems that have been attributed to the fracture may well be related to the applied techniques of immobilization. This is illustrated quite clearly in a case from a study by Siegel and Weiden:[151]

Case Report 2

P.D. a 29-year-old repairman fell off a ladder and sustained a patellar fracture and a closed comminuted fracture of the distal radius with probable extension into the joint...No evidence of nerve injury was found by the admitting house officer.

The patient underwent patellectomy, and a closed reduction of the wrist fracture under general anesthesia. A long arm cast with the wrist in moderate volar flexion was applied. Four days after reduction, the cast was bi-valved because of edema. During a change of plaster 3½ weeks after injury, fracture blisters and a small area of non-viable skin were seen on the volar surface of the wrist. The swelling of the hand and wrist persisted. By four weeks a complete median and ulnar nerve palsy distal to the wrist was present and confirmed by electrical testing. A carpal tunnel release was performed 12 weeks after injury. The patient signed out of the hospital after the operation and was lost to follow-up.

Problems associated with the application of pins and operative techniques cannot be minimized and are defined for the reader in preceding chapters.

Nerve Injury

A laborer, A.E.T. 45, of robust health, was admitted during 1853, having fallen from the roof of a house...The hand was cold and numb...The forearm throughout was tense and emphysematous. Mr. Stanley amputated immediately below the elbow. The muscles, tendons and cellular tissue were found bruised and torn about the broken bones, the median nerve was lacerated.

GW Callender, M.D. 1865[26]

The incidence of nerve-related complications in association with a fracture of the distal end of the radius is unclear. Whereas numerous reports in the past have suggested a relatively limited incidence,[14,28,54,55,112,152] others have implicated this to be far more commonplace.[11,22,35,106,159,161]

It is not unusual for patients with fractures of the distal end of the radius to experience paresthesias in the median nerve distribution at the time of injury, although in most cases these symptoms resolve in a relatively short time. Sponsel and Palm, in describing eight cases of acute and chronic median nerve injury following Colles' fractures, noted five patients with deficits identified from the time of injury which they felt were due to trauma of the median nerve, while three had the onset of symptoms 24 hours postinjury, which were thought to be associated with immobilization in the position of flexion.[157]

Nerve injuries may occur at the time of fracture, after fracture manipulation, or following application of circular casts or external fixation devices. Later nerve dysfunction (tardy) may be related to exuberant callus or chronic carpal tunnel compression.[150] With fractures of the distal radius, most often swelling or direct contusion will produce symptoms of nerve dysfunction with the median nerve most commonly involved.[91,96,109,110,113,120,138] The ulnar nerve is much less involved,[168,177] and least of all of the radial nerve.[98,99] Seddon's classification[145] (focal demyelination with axonal degeneration) is by far the most common problem seen in association with the most extreme injury. Neurotmesis (severe axonal disorganization or division), is rarely seen, with the exception of those unusual cases associated with extensive soft tissue injury or devascularizing trauma. In rare circumstances, direct nerve injury, either partial or complete, has been reported, with less extreme injuries in some instances attributed to entrapment of the nerve at the fracture site.[42,60,91,105,160,164,173]

Acute nerve dysfunction, especially that of the median nerve, has been associated with immobilization of the wrist in positions of extreme flexion.[1,57] Abbott and Saunders in 1933 used injection studies of the forearm flexor musculature to demonstrate that acute flexion and ulnar deviation, as found with the Cotton-Loder position, would prevent the contrast from passing distal to the proximal extent of the transverse carpal ligament. With elimination of flexion, the contrast was observed to flow freely into the palm. Robbins,[135] in an anatomic study, observed that with palmar flexion of the wrist, the anterior part of the lunate projected palmarward. Robbins felt that the hemorrhage and edema following a fracture of the distal end of the radius, in combination with this observed lunate rotation with the wrist flexed, would decrease the volume of the carpal tunnel and lead to compression of the median nerve. Using intercarpal canal interstitial fluid pressure measurements, Gelberman and co-workers[57] evaluated 22 patients with 23 fractures at the distal end of the radius. Although the mean values of pressure measurements were 18 mm of mercury in the neutral position, this increased to a mean of 47 mm of mercury in 40 degrees of wrist flexion and 35 mm of mercury in 20 degrees of wrist extension. It is noteworthy that 4 of these 22 patients had symptoms of acute median nerve compression, with 3 of these 4 having carpal tunnel pressure measurements in excess of 50 mm Hg in the 40-degree flexed position.

What then are the recommended treatment considerations when one is faced with a patient who presents with altered median or ulnar nerve function in conjunction with an acute fracture of the distal end of the radius? In the first place, one should attempt to reduce the fracture, as an accurate reduction in some instances can eliminate bony encroachment on the carpal canal.[54,56,90,99,109,176] The sensory function should be controlled by some objective means by using either von Frey pressure measurements, vibratory sensibility testing, or two-point discrimination. It is noteworthy that two-point discrimination represents the least reliable of these three methods in reflecting early changes in nerve function in response to trauma.[58] If no improvement is noted over the succeeding 4 to 6 hours, particularly if there is dense sensory loss and/or motor weakness, one should consider either testing intercarpal canal interstitial pressure or proceeding directly to operative decompression.[56]

Should the nerve dysfunction occur or worsen after the patient has been immobilized in a cast, the cast should be removed and the wrist placed in a neutral position. A soft bulky dressing will help support the wrist and allow for observation of distal sensory and motor function.[16] Likewise, if no improvement is noted over the next 6 hours, one can consider decompression of the

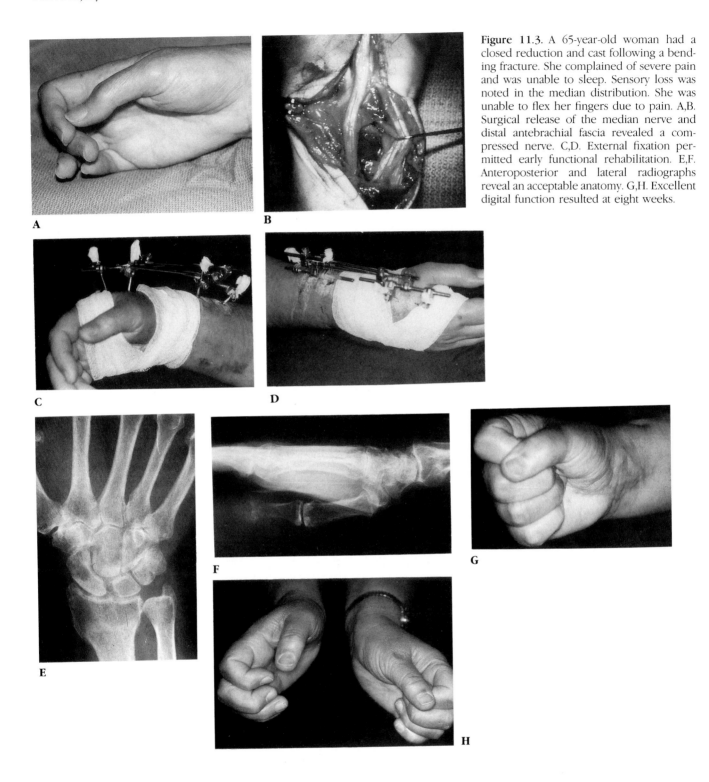

Figure 11.3. A 65-year-old woman had a closed reduction and cast following a bending fracture. She complained of severe pain and was unable to sleep. Sensory loss was noted in the median distribution. She was unable to flex her fingers due to pain. A,B. Surgical release of the median nerve and distal antebrachial fascia revealed a compressed nerve. C,D. External fixation permitted early functional rehabilitation. E,F. Anteroposterior and lateral radiographs reveal an acceptable anatomy. G,H. Excellent digital function resulted at eight weeks.

median nerve or, alternatively, monitoring the intercarpal canal interstitial pressure measurements to determine if they are elevated. If this proves to be the case, then operative release should be done.

In the event that operative release is decided upon, the procedure should include release of not only the carpal tunnel and canal of Guyon, but also the distal forearm antebrachial fascia. In conjunction with this procedure, it would be our preference to immobilize the fracture with percutaneous pins in conjunction with external fixation (Fig. 11.3).

One further situation which is likely related to acute nerve compression or injury is that in which the patient is noted to have pain far in excess of what would be expected with his or her fracture and early treatment. In these instances, the potential for the development of sympathetic-maintained pain syndrome (reflex sympathetic dystrophy) is considerable, and the patient should have the cast or splint loosened or removed and observed closely. Consideration should be given as well to the measurement of the intercarpal canal interstitial pressure. If the latter is elevated or if the pain symptoms persist in association with sensory or motor dysfunction, operative release of the median nerve may well abort the development of a sympathetic-maintained pain syndrome.

Acute ulnar nerve lesions appear more likely to be seen with higher-energy injuries associated with wide displacement of the fracture fragments, especially with co-existent distal ulnafracture.[36,49,90,113,138,147,151,165,168,177] The incidence of ulnar nerve involvement is considerably less than that of median nerve involvement, in part due to the variability of the neural anatomy in relationship not only to the end of the radius but also to their anatomic "tunnels" as they enter the proximal palm. The ulnar nerve will be less prone to compression by associated edema in the canal of Guyon, which is more distal than the proximal limit of the transverse carpal ligament. By the same token, the approach to ulnar nerve dysfunction should be much the same as with the median nerve.[35]

The radial nerve is vulnerable to compression neuropathy from a constricting cast and to direct trauma from the placement of pins percutaneously for fracture fixation or as part of an external fixation device.[35,99,141,161] Recognition of the anatomic relationship between the branches of the radial sensory nerve and the various loci for pin placement will help avoid local injury. In addition, the use of either an oscillating attachment to a drill or a drill guide when placing pins through limited incisions will also minimize the potential for direct nerve injury.

A late "tardy" median neuropathy may occur months or even years after the radius fracture has healed. In addition to chronic perineural fibrosis from the original injury or the original swelling, late median nerve dysfunction may be seen in association with a malunited fracture or with exuberant callus along the palmar aspect of the distal radius.[22,90,165] The approach to this problem, however, is little different from that with other compression neuropathies.[6,27,35,36,149,175]

Tendons

In fact, if treated by a quack, whose ignorance leads him to treat the injury as a sprain with an ointment, poultice, or with "faith", often a better result is obtained in such ordinary cases than by the learned medial neophyte, who after having made a most erudite diagnosis, immobilizes the joint for too long a period in the zeal to keep the fragments together; there will be no deformity, but adhesions will be formed, and the wrist will remain immobile.

Carl Beck, M.D. 1898[17]

The anatomic confinements of both the flexor and the extensor tendons at or about the level of the end of the radius make them vulnerable to either trauma, peritendinous swelling, or compression from encircling casts. Although the most dramatic complication involving a tendon is that of a secondary rupture, the more common problems, in fact, involve the development of peritendinous adhesions. These represent part of the "stiff hand syndrome" that results from edema and leads to residual loss of function. The optimal approach to this is prevention with early mobilization and methods taken to reduce edema. If the patient is seen at a later period after fracture healing, a vigorous program of exercise under the supervision of a trained therapist can overcome many of the problems associated with peritendinous adhesions. On occasion, however, late tenolysis will be necessary, but this is more likely to be required in more severe cases of stiffness.

Tendon injuries include those of tendon entrapment at the fracture site, tenosynovitis such as de Quervain's stenosing tenosynovitis, and tendon ruptures, most notably involving the extensor pollicis longus tendon.

Entrapment of tendons involving either the flexor or extensor tendons is exceedingly uncommon yet should be thought of if a mechanical block appears to be present preventing complete reduction of a fracture.[49,76,78,85,117,118,120,148,163] Residual fracture malalignment and individual tendon dysfunction can be a difficult sequela if an entrapped tendon is not recognized. Early recognition should lead to considerations for operative intervention.

Entrapment of the extensor carpi ulnaris tendon has been identified as a particular problem with fractures of the distal radius with distal radioulnar joint involvement. Radiographic demonstration of widening of the distal radioulnar joint as well as the inability to reduce the radial fracture should suggest the possibility of this lesion. Surgical exploration should then be considered in addition to operative fixation of the radius fracture. Extirpation of the extensor carpi ulnaris, repair of the distal radioulnar joint capsule, and relocation of the extensor carpi ulnaris with a sling made of the extensor retinaculum is generally required (Fig. 11.4).[78,121]

Tenosynovitis noted soon after fracture treatment most often affects the tendons within the first dorsal extensor retinacular compartment.[28,176] The etiology of this could involve localized swelling, compression from a cast, irritation from a percutaneous pin, or localized fracture hematoma. Whatever the cause, it is generally approached very much in the way one might approach a patient with isolated de Quervain's stenosing tenosynovitis. This would include the use of a long opponens splint combined with local instillation of a corticosteroid and administration of oral nonsteroidal antiinflammatory drugs. Surgical release would be recommended in those cases that do not respond to conservative treatment.

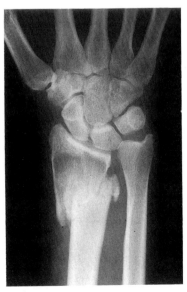

A

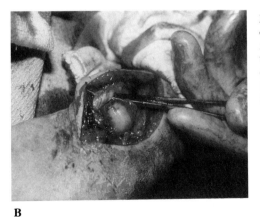

B

Figure 11.4. A 30-year-old woman with a complex fracture of the radius with a disrupted distal radioulnar joint. A. At exploration the extensor carpi ulnaris was found displaced below the ulnar head, blocking reduction. B. The tendon was relocated and a new retinacular sheath constructed.

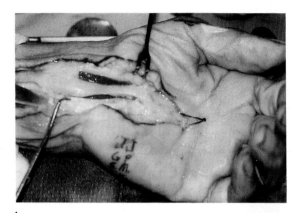

A   **B**

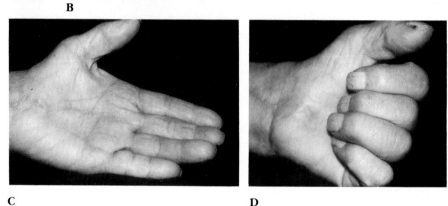

Figure 11.5. A 64-year-old man presented with an inability to flex the interphalangeal joint of his thumb as well as distal interphalangeal joint of his index 4 months following a fracture of the distal radius. A. At surgery an attrition rupture was found involving the flexor pollicis longus and flexor digitorum profundus to the index. The median nerve was also severely compressed. B. The sublimis tendon to the ring finger was transferred to the profundus of the index. The thumb interphalangeal joint was fused and the palmaris longus tendon was transferred to the abductor pollicis brevis. C,D. Excellent flexion and thumb abduction were gained.

C   **D**

Rupture of both flexor and extensor tendons has been reported in association with a fracture of the distal end of the radius. Attritional ruptures can result from abrasion of a tendon over a bony exostosis or malunited fragment.[140]

On the flexor side, isolated rupture of the flexor pollicis longus tendon,[8,35,136,173] the flexor profundus tendon to the index finger[35,139,155,174] as well as multiple ruptures[24,41,173] have all been reported. These for the most part have been identified as secondary to attritional rupture over a bony prominence. In most cases, a tendon graft or tendon transfer will be required, as the extent of damage and local ischemia to the injured tendon would preclude repair (Fig. 11.5A–D).

The tendon most often identified with rupture in association with a fracture of the distal end of the radius is the extensor pollicis longus tendon.[28,29,30,35,43,48,53,54,70,71,72,80,90,99,107,111,165,167,170,176] Yet even so, tendon rupture is extremely unusual. Helal noted an incidence of spontaneous rupture of the extensor pollicis longus following all distal radius fractures of <0.2 percent. Although reports have suggested various time intervals from the fracture to the clinical presentation of the rupture, what is unique regarding the extensor pollicis longus rupture is that most occur within 2 to 3 months of fracture[31,35,48,71,107] and most have been reported in association with non-displaced or minimally displaced fractures.[7,10,19,35,48,54,72,101,162,167,172] According to most reports, the tendon ruptured at the level of Lister's tubercle under the third extensor retinacular compartment.

The first case of extensor pollicis longus rupture has been attributed to Duplay in 1876.[47] Kleinschmidt identified 27 cases in a report in 1929.[86] Other cases were reported by McMaster (1932),[111] Moore (1936),[116] Kwedan and

Mitchell (1940),[92] Smith (1946),[153] and Trevor (1950),[167] who added 9 additional cases and totalled approximately 90 cases reported to that time. Of interest is the fact that age does not appear to be a factor, with some patients reported as young as 16[31,72] and two as old as 78.[72]

The etiology of the extensor pollicis longus rupture has been the subject of some debate. While some have suggested the rupture to be due to attrition over a prominent bony spike,[13,86] the fact that most have occurred in the setting of nondisplaced fractures has led many to feel otherwise. Several studies have been done to look at the blood supply to the extensor pollicis longus tendon at the level of Lister's tubercle.[3,48,71,72] These studies have suggested that the extensor pollicis longus receives a dual blood supply from a proximal and distal perfusion from the anterior interosseous artery and a dorsal carpal branch of the radial artery distally as well as through a well-vascularized tenosynovium. There appears to be a zone at or about the beginning of the extensor retinaculum of approximately 5 to 10 mm which is not well perfused, and the tendon is apparently nourished by diffusion from the overlying tenosynovium. Many have suggested that the etiology of the rupture is a combination of a mechanical cause of direct trauma to the tendon at the time of fracture which is accentuated by secondary ischemic changes as localized pressure within the intact retinacular compartment compromises the extrinsic synovial sheath nutrition of the underlying tendon.[39,71,72,80,90]

When faced with a patient complaining of increasing pain with movements of the thumb in the setting of a nondisplaced fracture of the distal end of the radius, a high index of suspicion should alert the treating physician to the possibility of an impending rupture of the extensor pollicis longus tendon. The authors would prefer to remove a circular cast if present and apply a long opponens splint immobilizing the thumb. If symptoms persist, then a corticosteroid injection or, preferably, opening the third extensor compartment may prevent a complete rupture from occurring.[25]

When a complete rupture has in fact occurred, most have recommended either transfer of the extensor indicus proprius tendon[71,72,134,142,162,167] or a free tendon graft.[40,66,107] The advocates of the free tendon graft have felt that patients would regain function more quickly than with the extensor indicus proprius transfer, as the original muscle belly is used and the flexor pollicis longus would get back its original antagonist.

Finally, it should be noted that there have been occasional reports of rupture of the extensor pollicis longus due to prominent screw heads from a dorsally applied plate[104,171] or to the tip of the screw from a palmarly applied plate.[32]

Reflex Sympathetic Dystrophy

A satisfactory result following Colles' fracture means a complete restoration within a reasonable time of muscle power and motion in the hand, wrist, forearm and elbow and in the upper arm and shoulder as well.

Frederick Amendola, M.D. 1938

Although the descriptive terminology has varied over the past century, dystrophy or, as it is currently termed, sympathetic-maintained pain, has been well described as an early complication associated with fractures of the distal end of the radius. Given the fact that a number of terms have been used to identify this entity, including posttraumatic reflex sympathetic dystrophy, post-traumatic sympathetic dystrophy, shoulder-hand syndrome, osteoneurodystrophy, Sudeck's atrophy, and causalgic syndrome, it is quite hard to glean from the literature what might be an accurate incidence of this problem.[4,15,44,77,124,126,127,143,161]

In 1877 von Lesser[169] noted trophic changes in the hands following otherwise unremarkable distal radius fractures, and in 1915 Le Breton described 10 cases of what would appear to the reader to be consistent with dystrophic changes.[95] These early descriptions were soon followed by those of Hansen in 1926,[68] Kotrnetz and Geiringen in 1937,[89] and Rosen[137] in 1947, who noted no fewer than 10 out of 280 fractures to be troubled by symptoms suggestive of dystrophy.

Several subsequent investigations attempted to identify the incidence of dystrophy with distal radius fractures. Bacorn and Kurtzke in 1953[14] identified a 0.1 percent incidence of "acute causalgia" and a 0.1 percent incidence of "Sudek's atrophy"; Lidström in 1959 using the term "post-traumatic causalgia" found an incidence of 10.3 percent (53 out of 515 fractures).[97] Of note is the fact that in follow-up of these patients, Lidström identified an unsatisfactory result in 67 percent. Raschle in 1965 noted a 6.5 percent incidence, while Rehn in the same year noted an 8.5 percent incidence.[132,133] Frykman in 1967,[54] using the term "shoulder-hand syndrome," identified 9 cases out of 430 fractures, giving an incidence of 2.1 percent.

Atkins and colleagues in two studies using the criteria of pain and tenderness, vasomotor and pseudomotor instability, swelling and dystrophy, and impairment of joint mobility, identified 13 of 109 patients who had all four groups of symptoms 9 weeks postfracture, with 11 others having three of these groups of symptoms.[11,12] These investigators felt that this could reflect a milder form of sympathetic-maintained pain following fractures, which is transient in nature. Field reviewed a series of patients 10 years after fracture finding 26 percent having some residual symptoms.[50] Vasomotor symptoms were found in 64 percent of these, with small joint stiffness in 14 percent.

A number of etiologies have been offered to explain the development of sympathetic-maintained pain with fracture at the distal end of the radius. These include sympathetic overactivity, traumatic fracture reduction, frequent cast changes, psychological factors, or malposition of the fracture fragments.[9,18,21,37,38,46,47,52,54,94,114,115,119,125,130]

Likewise, any number of treatments have been attempted for this problem, including sympathetic blockade, intravenous guanethidine, corticosteroids,vasodilators, hydroxy radical scavengers, and vigorous physical therapy.[46,52,59,63,73,94,100,119,131,143]

Although many theories have been proposed to explain the pathophysiologic changes responsible for sympathetic-maintained pain, there exists a group of patients who exhibit a true causalgic picture in whom an acute or chronic injury to a nerve focus has been identified.[63,82,158] It is the authors' belief that there is a strong likelihood that many of the patients who exhibit these signs and symptoms and have signs consistent with vasomotor and pseudomotor instability in conjunction with a fracture of the distal radius have in common a compressed median nerve. Treatment should consist of controlling the sympathetic-maintained pain with sympathetic blockade, evaluation of neural function with electrodiagnostic testing, and, if indicated, measurement of intercarpal canal interstitial pressures followed by surgical release of the nerve if the findings confirm this to be under compression. If the patient is seen 2 to 3 months postinjury, we have also utilized local muscle flaps to cover the nerve at the time of surgical release in order to provide a protective covering and enhance the local environment surrounding the nerve (Fig. 11.6A–C).

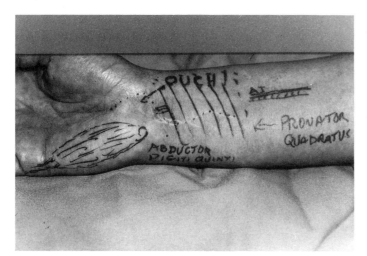

A

Figure 11.6. A 50-year-old woman presented with a profound causalgic picture 3 months following a distal radius fracture and an attempt at carpal tunnel release. A. Upon exploration the median nerve was severely scarred. B. A microscopic-assisted neurolysis identified normal fascicular orientation. C. An abductor digiti quinti muscle flap was elevated and rotated to cover the nerve in the proximal palm. D,E. At 2 years follow-up, nearly full motion is maintained. No symptoms of sympathetic-maintained pain have recurred.

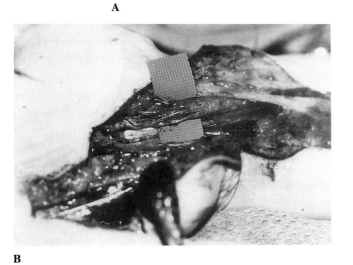

B

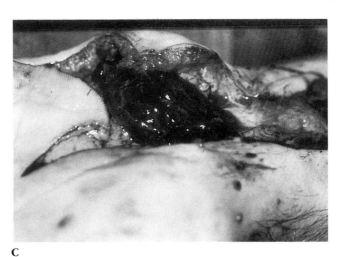

C

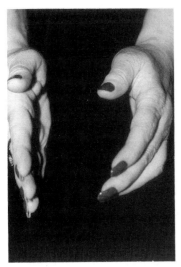

D

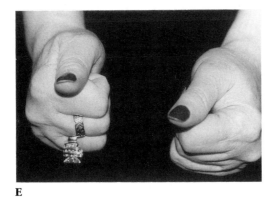

E

Dupuytren's Contracture

The exact role of trauma in relationship to the development of Dupuytren's contracture remains controversial. Hueston has suggested that a single episode of injury can lead to the development of this process, particularly in those who have a preexisting propensity or evidence of the disorder.[74,75] There are a number of reports in the literature, probably starting with the first report by

Figure 11.7. Nonunion of a complex fracture of the end of the radius associated with a scaphoid fracture. A,B. The anteroposterior and lateral radiographs reveal the nonunion. C,D. Treatment consisted of an intercalated iliac crest graft and small plate and smooth Kirschner wires. E,F. The nonunion was healed by 3 months following surgery.

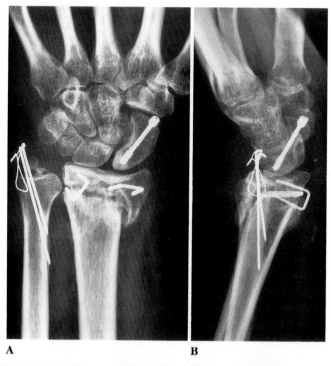

A   B

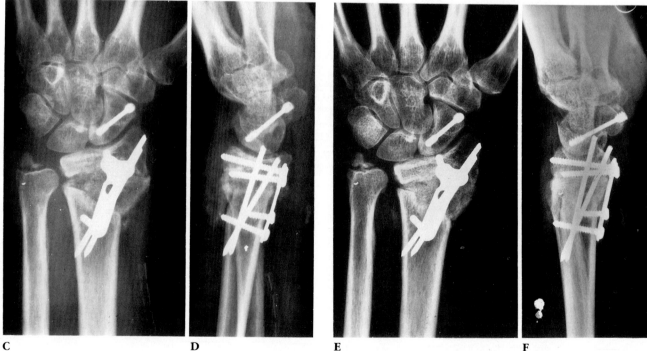

C   D   E   F

Table 11.1. A summary of the incidence of Dupuytren following Distal Radicus Fractures.

Author	Number (Incidence)	Number of patients
Kohlmeyer, 1935	6 (5.4%)	110 ♂
	4 (0.75%)	530 ♀
Bacorn and Kurtzke, 1953	4 (0.2%)	2,132
Castaing, 1964	2 (0.45%)	440
Smaill, 1965	2 (4.9%)	41
Stuart et al, 1985	22 (9.3%)	235
De Bruijn, 1987	5 (2.5%)	196

Goyrand in 1835.[61,88] Since then, a number of reports, with an incidence varying from 0 to 11 percent, have been put forth in the literature. Kelly and colleagues summarized the incidence of this condition in a table drawing on a number of prior articles (Table 11.1).[84]

Nonunion

Although uncommon, delayed union and nonunion can occur when the bone substance in the immediate subchondral bone is deficient from comminution or osteoporosis or there has been extended overdistraction usually associated with external fixation.[64,69,93,99,146]

In the presence of a nonunion, the authors have found that autogenous bone graft with internal fixation can gain successful union (Fig. 11.7A–F). In some instances, however, if the radiocarpal articulation has been disrupted, a wrist arthrodesis should be considered.

References

1. Abbott LC, Saunders JB: Injuries of the median nerve in fractures of the lower end of the radius. *Surg Gynecol Obstet* 57: 507–516, 1933.
2. Agee JM: External fixation. Technical advances based upon multiplanar ligamentotaxis. *Orthop Clin North Am* 24: 265–274, 1993.
3. Akiyoshi T: A study of microangiography on the extensor pollicis longus tendon. *J Kyoto Prefectural Univ Med* 95: 177–188, 1986 (In Japanese with English summary).
4. Amadio PC, Mackinnon SE, Merritt WH: Reflex sympathetic dystrophy syndrome: Consensus report of an ad hoc committee of the American Association for Hand Surgery on the definition of reflex sympathetic dystrophy syndrome. *Plast Reconstr Surg* 87: 371–375, 1991.
5. Amendola FH: The after-treatment of Colles' fracture. *JAMA* 112: 1803–1806, 1938.
6. Aro H, Koirunen J, Katevuo K, Nieminen S, Aho AJ: Late compression neuropathies after Colles' fractures. *Clin Orthop Rel Res* 233: 217–225, 1988.
7. Aronson H: Ett bidrag till kännedom om den s.k. efterrupturen sv tummens länga efter handlestrauma. *Nord Med* 2: 1985 and 1939.
8. Aschall G: Flexor pollicis longus rupture after fracture of the distal radius. *Injury* 22: 153–155, 1991.
9. Ascherl R, Blümel G: Zum Krankheitsbild der Südeck's Dystrophe. *Fortschr Med* 99: 712–720, 1980.
10. Ashurst APC: Rupture of tendon of extensor pollicis longus following a Colles' fracture. *Ann Surg* 78: 398–400, 1923.
11. Atkins RM, Duckworth T, Kanis JA: Features of aligodystrophy after Colles' fracture. *J Bone Joint Surg* 72B: 105–110, 1990.
12. Atkins RM, Duckworth T, Kanis JA: Aligodystrophy following Colles' fracture. *J Hand Surg* 14B: 161–164, 1989.
13. Axhausen G: Die Spätruptur der Sehne des Extensor Pollicis Longus bei der typischen Radiusfraktur. *Beiträge Klin Chir* 133: 78–88, 1925.

14. Bacorn RW, Kurtzke JF: Colles' fracture: A study of 2,000 cases from the New York State Workers' Compensation Board. *J Bone Joint Surg [Am]* 35A: 643, 1953.

15. Baitsch R, Heller HR: Speichenbruch an der typischen Stelle und Südecksches Syndrom. *Muench Med Wschr* 101: 665–701, 1959.

16. Bauman TD, Gelberman RH, Murbarak SJ, et al: The acute carpal tunnel syndrome. *Clin Orthop* 156: 151–156, 1981.

17. Beck C: Colles' fracture and the roentgen rays. *Med News* February: 230–232, 1898.

18. Bennett GJ: The role of the sympathetic nervous system in painful peripheral neuropathy. *Pain* 45: 221–223, 1991.

19. Björkroth J: Bidrag till Kännedom om den posttraumatiska spontan-rupturen av tummens länga sena. *Nord Med* 12: 3022, 1941.

20. Böhler L: Die funktionelle Behandlung der "typischen" Radiusbrueche auf anatomischer und physiologischer Grundlage. *Muenchen Med U* 66: 1185, 1919.

21. Bonica JJ: Causalgia and other reflex sympathetic dystrophies. In: Bonica JJ ed. *Advances in Pain Research and Therapy*, pp. 141–166. New York: Raven Press, 1979.

22. Bourrel P, Ferro RM: Nerve complications in closed fractures of the lower end of the radius. *Ann Chir Maine* 1: 119–126, 1982.

23. Braatz E: Zur Behandlung der typischen Radiusbrüche. *Verhandl Deutsch Gesellsch Chir* 25: 300, 1896.

24. Broder H: Rupture of flexor tendons associated with a malunited Colles' fracture. *J Bone Joint Surg* 36A: 404–405, 1954.

25. Bunata RE: Impending rupture of the extensor pollicis longus tendon after a minimally displaced Colles' fracture. *J Bone Joint Surg* 65A: 401–402, 1983.

26. Callender GW: Fractures injuring joints—Fractures interfering with the movements at the wrist and with those of pronation and supination. *Saint Bartholomews Hospital Reports* 281–298, 1865.

27. Cannon BW, Love JG: Tardy median palsy; median neuritis; median thenar neuritis amenable to surgery. *Surgery* 20: 210–216, 1946.

28. Cassebaum WH: Colles' fractures. A study of end results. *JAMA* 143: 963–965, 1950.

29. Castaing J: Les fractures récentes de l'extremité inférieure du radius chez l'adulte. *Rev Chir Orthop* 50: 581–696, 1964.

30. Chemell S, Light TR, Blair SJ: Rupture of the extensor pollicis longus tendon. *Orthopedics* 6: 565–570, 1973.

31. Christophe K: Rupture of the extensor pollicis longus tendon following Colles' fracture. *J Bone Joint Surg* 35A: 1003–1005, 1953.

32. Chung JW, Quinlan W: Rupture of extensor pollicis longus following fixation of a distal radius fracture. *Injury* 20: 375–376, 1989.

33. Colles A: On the fracture of the carpal extremity of the radius. *Edinburgh Med Surg J* 10: 182–186, 1814.

34. Collins DC: Management and rehabilitation of distal radius fractures. *Orthop Clin North Am* 24: 365–378, 1993.

35. Cooney WP III, Dobyns JH, Linscheid RL: Complications of Colles' fractures. *J Bone Joint Surg [Am]* 62A: 613–618, 1980.

36. Cotton FJ: Wrist fractures. Disabilities following restorative operations. *Trans Am Surg Assoc* 11: 289, 1922.

37. de Bruijn HP: Functional treatment of Colles' fractures. *Acta Orthop Scand* Suppl. 223: 1–95, 1987.

38. De Brunner AM: Distale Radiusfrakturen. *Schweiz Med Wochenschr* 25: 820–822, 1967.

39. Denman EE: Rupture of the extensor pollicis longus, a crush injury. *Hand* 11: 295–298, 1979.

40. Denmark van RE, Cotton GW: Translocation tenorraphy and the extensor pollicis longus after spontaneous rupture in Colles' fracture. *Clin Orthop* 31: 106–109, 1963.

41. Diamond JP, Newman JH: Multiple flexor tendon ruptures following Colles' fracture: A case report. *J Trauma* 29: 1295–1297, 1989.

42. Dickson FD: Peripheral nerve injuries associated with fractures of the long bones. *South Med J* 19: 37–42, 1926.

43. Djørup F: Fractura extremitas inferioris radii. *Nord Med* 67: 685–690, 1962.

44. Doupe J, Cullen CR, Chance GQ: Post-traumatic pain and the causalgic syndromes. *J Neurol Neurosurg Psychiatry* 7: 33–48, 1944.

45. Droury D, Dirheimer Y, Pattin S: Algodystrophy: Diagnosis and therapy of a frequent disease of the locomotor appartus. Berlin: Springer-Verlag, 1981.

46. Dunningham TH: The treatment of Sudeck's atrophy in the upper limb by sympathetic blockade. *Injury* 12: 139–144, 1980.

47. Duplay S: Rupture sous-cutanée du tendon du long extenseur du pouce de la main droite au niveau de la tabatière anatomique. Flexion permanente du pouce. Rétablissement de la faculté d'éxtension par une opération (suture de l'extremité du tendon rompu avec le premier radial externe). *Bull Mem Soc Chir Paris* 2: 788–791, 1876.
48. Engkvist O, Lundborg G: Rupture of the extensor pollicis longus tendon after fracture of the lower end of the radius. A clinical and microangiographic study. *Hand* 11: 76–86, 1979.
49. Fernandez DL: Irreducible radiocarpal fracture-dislocation and radioulnar dissocia- tion with entrapment of the ulnar nerve, artery, and flexor profundus II–V. *J Hand Surg* 6A: 456–461, 1986.
50. Field J, Warwick D, Bannister GC: Features of algodystrophy ten years after Colles' fracture. *J Hand Surg* 17B: 318–320, 1992.
51. Ford LT, Key JA: Present day management of Colles' fracture. *J Iowa State Med Soc* 324–327, 1955.
52. Freund E, Hüttner HJ, Schröder H: Morbus Südeck als Komplikation des Radiusfraktur. *Mschr Unfallheilk* 73: 569–574, 1970.
53. Fritsche K: Konservative oder operative Therapie der typischen Radiusfraktur. *Zentralblatt Chir* 103: 435–438, 1978.
54. Frykman GK: Fracture of the distal radius including sequelae—Shoulder hand finger syndrome. Disturbance in the distal radioulnar joint and impairment of nerve function. A clinical and experimental study. *Acta Orthop Scand* Suppl. 108: 1–155, 1967.
55. Gartland JJ, Werley CW: Evaluation of healed Colles' fractures. *J Bone Joint Surg [Am]* 33A: 895–907, 1951.
56. Gelberman RH: Acute carpal tunnel syndrome. In: Gelberman RH ed. *Operative Nerve Repair and Reconstruction*. Philadelphia: JB Lippincott, 1991, pp. 940– 948.
57. Gelberman RH, Szabo RM, Mortensen WW: Carpal tunnel pressures and wrist position in patients with Colles' fractures. *J Trauma* 24: 747–749, 1984.
58. Gelberman RH, Szabo RM, Williamson RV, et al: Sensibility testing in peripheral nerve compression syndromes—a human experimental study. *J Bone Joint Surg* 65A: 632–638, 1983.
59. Girgis FL, Wynn Parry CB: Management of causalgia after peripheral nerve injury. *Int Disabil Studies* 11: 15–20, 1989.
60. Goldie BS, Powell JM: Bony transfixation of the median nerve following Colles' fracture: A case report. *Clin Orthop* 273: 275–277, 1991.
61. Goyrand G: De la rétraction permanente des doigts. *Gaz Med Paris* 253: 481–486, 1835.
62. Green JT, Gay FH: Colles' fracture, residual disability. *Am J Surg* 21: 636–642, 1956.
63. Grundberg AB, Reagan DS: Compression syndromes in reflex sympathetic dystrophy. *J Hand Surg* 16A: 731–736, 1991.
64. Hamada G: Extraarticular graft for nonunion in Colles' fracture. *J Bone Joint Surg* 26: 833–835, 1944.
65. Hamburg HJ, Watson J, Toole A: The use of differential skin-temperature measure- ments in the evaluation of post-traumatic edema control. *Med Biol Eng* 13: 202–208, 1975.
66. Hamlin C, Littler JW: Restoration of the extensor pollicis longus tendon by an intercalated graft. *J Bone Joint Surg* 59A: 412–414, 1977.
67. Hamilton FH: *A Practical Treatise on Fractures and Dislocations*. Philadelphia: Blanchard & Lea, 1860.
68. Hansen PN: Discussion: *Dansk Kirurgiske Selskabs Forhandlinger* 27: 44, 1926.
69. Harper WM, Jones JM: Nonunion of Colles' fracture: Report of two cases. *J Hand Surg* 15B: 121–123, 1990.
70. Heineke D: Spontanruptur der Sehne des langen Daumenstreckers. *Münch Med Wschr* 40: 560, 1913.
71. Helal B, Chen SC, Iwegbu G: Rupture of the extensor pollicis longus tendon in undisplaced Colles' type of fracture. *Hand* 14: 41–47, 1982.
72. Hirasawa Y, Katsumi Y, Akiyoshi T: Clinical and microangiographic studies on rupture of the extensor pollicis longus tendon after distal radius fracture. *J Hand Surg* 15B: 51–57, 1990.
73. Hobelman CF Jr, Dellon AL: Use of prolonged sympathetic blockade as an adjunct to surgery in the patients with sympathetic-maintained pain. *Microsurgery* 10: 151–153, 1989.

74. Hueston JT: Dupuytren's contracture and specific injury. *Med J Aust* 1084–1085, 1968.

75. Hueston JT: The incidence of Dupuytren's contracture. *Med J Aust* 2: 999–1002, 1960.

76. Hunt DD: Dislocation of the extensor pollicis longus tendon in Smith's fracture of the radius: A case report. *J Bone Joint Surg* 51A: 991–994, 1969.

77. International Association for the Study of Pain; Subcommittee on Taxonomy. Reflex sympathetic dystrophy (I-5). *Pain* Suppl 3: 529–530, 1986.

78. Itoh Y, Horiuchi Y, Takahashim H, et al: Extensor tendon involvement in Smith's and Galeazzi fracture. *J Hand Surg* 12A: 535–540, 1987.

79. Jackson JBS: *A Descriptive Catalogue of the Warren Anatomical Museum*. Boston: A. Williams and Co., 1870, pp. 175–176.

80. Jenkins NH, Mackie IG: Late rupture of the extensor pollicis longus tendon: The case against attrition. *J Hand Surg* 13B: 448–449, 1988.

81. Jupiter JB: Current Concepts review: Fractures of the distal end of the radius. *J Bone Joint Surg* 73A: 461–469, 1991.

82. Jupiter JB, Seiler JG, Zienowicz R: Sympathetic-maintained pain (causalgia) associated with a demonstrable peripheral nerve lesion. Operative treatment. *J Bone Joint Surg* 76A: 1376–1384, 1994.

83. Kaempffe FA, Wheeler DR, Peimer CA: Severe fractures of the distal radius: Effects of amount and duration of external fixator dislocation on outcome. *J Hand Surg* 18A: 33–41, 1993.

84. Kelly SA, Burke FD, Elliot D: Injury to the distal radius as a trigger to the onset of Dupuytren's disease. *J Hand Surg* 17B: 225–229, 1992.

85. Kilgore ESJ, Graham WP: *The Hand. Surgical and Nonsurgical Management*. Philadelphia: Lea & Febiger, 1977.

86. Kleinschmitt K: Versuche zur Erklärung der Spätruptur der langen Daumenstrecksehne nach Radius-fraktur. *Beitr Klin Chir* 146: 530–535, 1929.

87. Knapp ME: Treatment of some complications of Colles' fracture. *JAMA* 148: 825–827, 1952.

88. Kohlmayer H: Zur Frage der traumatischen Entstehung der Dupuytrenschen Fingerkontraktur. *Zentralblatt Chir* 33: 1928–1931, 1935.

89. Kotrnetz H, Geiringen F: Speichbrüche des erwachsenen an typischer Stelle. *Arch Orthop Unfall Chir* 37: 504–514, 1937.

90. Kozin SH, Wood MB: Early soft tissue complications after distal radius fractures. *AAOS Instructional Course Lectures* Chapter 6: 89–98, 1993.

91. Kumar A: Median and ulnar nerve injury secondary to a comminuted Colles' fracture. *J Trauma* 30: 118–119, 1990.

92. Kwedan AT, Mitchell CL: Late rupture of extensor pollicis longus tendon following Colles' fracture. *J Bone Joint Surg* 22: 429–435, 1940.

93. Lachman JW: *In* Report of meeting of the Orthopedic Association of the English-speaking World. *J Bone Joint Surg* 40B: 596, 1958.

94. Lankford LL, Thompson JE: Reflex sympathetic dystrophy, upper and lower extremity. Diagnosis and management. In: *AAOS Instructional Course Lectures* Volume 26. St. Louis: CV Mosby, 1977.

95. Le Breton P: Arthritis of the joints of the hand following Colles' fracture. *Surg Gynec Obstet* 20: 450–456, 1915.

96. Lewis MH: Median nerve decompression after Colles' fracture. *J Bone Joint Surg [Am]* 60B: 195–196, 1978.

97. Lidström A: Fractures of the distal end of the radius. A clinical and statistical study of end results. *Acta Orthop Scand* 30 (Suppl 41): 1–118, 1959.

98. Linscheid RL: Injuries to the radial nerve at wrist. *Arch Surg* 91: 942–946, 1965.

99. Linscheid RL, Dobyns JH: Complications of fractures and dislocations of the wrist. In: *Complications in Orthopaedic Surgery*. 3rd ed. Charles Epps Jr. ed. Philadelphia: JB Lippincott, 1994, pp. 321–338.

100. Linson M, Leffert RD, Todd D: The treatment of upper extremity reflex sympathetic dystrophy with prolonged continuous stellate ganglion blockade. *J Hand Surg* 8: 153–159, 1983.

101. Lipschutz B: Late subcutaneous rupture of the tendon of the extensor pollicis longus muscle. *Arch Surg* 31: 816–820, 1935.

102. Lucas-Champonnière J: Traitement des fractures du radius et du péroné par le massage. Traitement des fractures pararticulaires simples et compliquées de plaie sans immobilisation, mobilisation et massage. *Bull Mem Soc Chir Paris* 12: 560, 1886.

103. Lucas GL, Sachtjen KM: An analysis of hand function in patients with Colles' fracture, treated by Rush rod fixation. *Clin Orthop* 155: 172–179, 1981.

104. Lugger IJ, Pechlaner S: Tendon rupture as a complication after osteosynthesis of the distal radius. *Unfallchirurgie* 10: 266–299, 1984.
105. Lusthaus S, Matan Y, Finsterbush A, et al: Traumatic section of the median nerve: An unusual complication of Colles' fracture. *Injury* 24: 339–340, 1993.
106. Lynch AC, Lipscomb PR: The carpal tunnel syndrome and Colles' fractures. *JAMA* 185: 363–366, 1963.
107. Mannerfelt L, Oetker R, Ostlund B: Rupture of the extensor pollicis longus tendon after Colles' fracture and by rheumatoid arthritis. *J Hand Surg* 153: 49–50, 1990.
108. Marson BM, Keenan MAE: Skin surface pressures under leg casts. Presented at American Academy of Orthopaedic Surgeons meeting, Washington DC, February 20–25, 1992.
109. McCarroll HR Jr: Nerve injuries associated with wrist trauma. *Orthop Clin North Am* 15: 279–287, 1984.
110. McClain EJ, Wissinger HA: The acute carpal tunnel syndrome: Nine case reports. *J Trauma* 16: 75–78, 1976.
111. McMaster PE: Late ruptures of the extensor and flexor pollicis longus tendons following Colles' fractures. *J Bone Joint Surg* 14: 93–101, 1932.
112. Meadoff N: Median nerve associated with in the region of the wrist. *Calif Med* 70: 252–256, 1949.
113. Melone CP Jr: Articular fractures of the distal radius. *Orthop Clin North Am* 15: 217–236, 1984.
114. Melzack R, Wall P: Pain mechanisms: A new theory. *Science* 150: 971–979, 1965.
115. Mitchell SW, Morehouse GR, Keen WW: *Gunshot Wounds and Other Injuries to the Nerves*. Philadelphia: J.B. Lippincott, 1864.
116. Moore T: Spontaneous rupture of the extensor pollicis longus tendon associated with Colles' fracture. *Br J Surg* 23: 721–726, 1936.
117. Morrissey RT, Nalebuff EA: Distal radial fractures with tendon entrapment. A case report. *Clin Orthop* 124: 205–208, 1977.
118. Murakami Y, Todani K: Traumatic entrapment of the extensor pollicis longus tendon in Smith's fracture of the radius—case report. *J Hand Surg* 6: 238–240, 1981.
119. Nigst H: Zur Prophylaxe der posttraumatischen Osteoporose und des Sudeckschen Syndroms. *Landartz* 43: 167–169, 1967.
120. Paley D, McMurtry RY: Median nerve compression by volarly displaced fragments of the distal radius. *Clin Orthop* 215: 139–147, 1987.
121. Paley D, McMurtry RY, Murray JF: Dorsal dislocations of the ulnar styloid and extensor carpi ulnaris tendon into the distal radioulnar joint: The empty sulcus sign. *J Hand Surg* 12A: 1029–1032, 1987.
122. Pasila M, Karaharju EO, Lepisto P: Role of physical therapy in recovery of function after Colles' fracture. *Arch Phys Med Rehabil* 55: 130–134, 1974.
123. Patrick JH, Levack B: A study of pressures beneath forearm plasters. *Injury* 13: 37–41, 1981.
124. Plewes LW: Sudeck's atrophy in the hand. *J Bone Joint Surg* 38B: 195–203, 1956.
125. Pollack HJ, von Neumann R, Pollack E: M. Sudeck und Psyché. *Beitr Orthop Traumatol* 27: 463–468, 1980.
126. Pool C: Colles' fracture. A prospective study of treatment. *J Bone Joint Surg [Br]* 55B: 540, 1973.
127. Poplawski ZJ, Wiley AM, Murray JF: Post-traumatic dystrophy of the extremities. *J Bone Joint Surg* 65A: 642–655, 1983.
128. Porter M, Stockley I: Fractures of the distal radius. Intermediate and end results in relation to radiograph parameters. *Clin Orthop Rel Res* 220: 241–251, 1987.
129. Pritchard DJ, Linscheid RL, Svien HJ: Intraarticular median nerve entrapment with dislocation of the elbow. *Clin Orthop Rel Res* 90: 100–103, 1973.
130. Procacci P, Maresca M: Reflex sympathetic dystrophies and aligodystrophies: Historical and pathogenic considerations. *Pain* 31: 137–146, 1987.
131. Raj PP, Calodney A, Janisse T, Cannella J: Reflex sympathetic dystrophy. In: Browner BD, Jupiter JB, Levine AM, Trafton PG, eds. *Skeletal Trauma*. Philadelphia: WB Saunders, 1991, pp. 471–499.
132. Raschle R: Unsere Erfahrungen in der Behandlung der Radiusfrakturen. *Z Unfallmed Berufskr* 58: 113–122, 1965.
133. Rehn J: Behandlungsergebnisse typischen Radiusfrakturen. *Chirurgie* 36: 206–214, 1965.
134. Riddell DM: Spontaneous rupture of the extensor pollicis longus. The results of tendon transfer. *J Bone Joint Surg* 45B: 506–510, 1963.
135. Robbins H: Anatomical study of the median nerve in the carpal tunnel and etiologies of carpal tunnel syndrome. *J Bone Joint Surg* 45A: 953–960, 1963.

136. Roberts JO, Regan PJ, Roberts AH, et al: Rupture of the flexor pollicis longus as a complication of Colles' fracture. A case report. *J Hand Surg* 15B: 370–372, 1990.

137. Rosen E: Fractura extremitatis distalis radii. *Ugesk Laeger* 109: 603, 1947.

138. Rychak JS, Kalenak A: Injury to the median and ulnar nerves secondary to fracture of the radius: A case report. *J Bone Joint Surg [Am]* 59A: 414–415, 1977.

139. Rymaszewski LA, Walker AP: Rupture of the flexor digitorum profundus to the index finger after a distal radial fracture. *J Hand Surg* 12B: 115–116, 1987.

140. Sadr B: Sequential rupture of extensor tendons after a Colles' fracture. *J Hand Surg* 9A: 144–145, 1984.

141. Sanders RA, Keppel FL, Waldrop JI: External fixation of distal radius fractures. Results and complications. *J Hand Surg* 16(A): 385–391, 1985.

142. Schneider LH, Rosenstein RG: Restoration of extensor pollicis longus function by tendon transfer. *Plast Reconstr Surg* 71: 533–537, 1983.

143. Schutzer SF, Gossling HR: Current concepts review. The treatment of reflex sympathetic dystrophy syndrome. *J Bone Joint Surg [Am]* 66A: 625–629, 1984.

144. Scudder CL: *Treatment of Fractures*. Philadelphia: WB Saunders, 1938.

145. Seddon HJ: *Surgical Disorders of the Peripheral Nerves*. 2nd ed. Edinburgh and London: Churchill Livingstone, 1975, p. 119.

146. Seiler JG III, Nayagam S, Gelberman RH, Jupiter J, Manning M: Nonunion after open fractures of the distal radius. *J Southern Orthop Assoc* 2: 112–115, 1993.

147. Shea JD, McClain EJ: Ulnar nerve compression syndromes at and below the wrist. *J Bone Joint Surg* 51A: 18–21, 1969.

148. Shively JL, Lesnick DS: Distal radius fracture with tendon entrapment. *Orthopedics* 5: 1330–1332, 1982.

149. Short DW: Tardy median nerve palsy following injury. *Glasgow Med J* 32: 315–320, 1951.

150. Siegal DB, Gelberman RH: Peripheral nerve injuries associated with fractures and dislocations. In: Gelberman RH, ed. *Operative Nerve Repair and Reconstruction*. Philadelphia: JB Lippincott, 1991, pp. 619–620.

151. Siegel RS, Weiden I: Combined median and ulnar nerve lesions complicating fractures of the distal radius and ulnar. *J Trauma* 8: 1114–1118, 1968.

152. Smaill GB: Long-term followup of Colles' fracture. *J Bone Joint Surg [Br]* 47B: 80–85, 1965.

153. Smith FM: Late rupture of extensor pollicis longus tendon following Colles' fracture. *J Bone Joint Surg [Am]* 28A: 49–59, 1946.

154. Smith RJ: Intrinsic contracture. In: Green DP, ed. *Operative Hand Surgery*, 2nd ed. New York: Churchill Livingstone, 1988, pp. 609–631.

155. Southmayd WW, Millender LH, Nalebuff EA: Rupture of the flexor tendons of the index finger after Colles' fracture. *J Bone Joint Surg* 57A: 562–563, 1975.

156. Spinner M, Aiache A, Silver L, et al: Impending ischemic contracture of the hand. Early diagnosis and management. *Plast Reconstr Surg* 50: 341–349, 1972.

157. Sponsel KH, Palm ET: Carpal tunnel syndrome following Colles' fracture. *Surg Gynecol Obstet* 121: 1252–1256, 1965.

158. Stein AH: The relationship of median nerve compression to Sudeck's syndrome. *Surg Gynecol Obstet* 115: 713–720, 1962.

159. Stark WA: Neural involvement in fractures of the distal radius. *Orthopedics* 10: 333–335, 1987.

160. Sterling AP, Habermann ET: Acute post-traumatic median nerve compression associated with a Salter II fracture-dislocation of the wrist. *Bull Hosp Joint Dis* 34: 167–171, 1973.

161. Stewart HD, Innes AR, Burke PD: The hand complications of Colles' fractures. *J Hand Surg* 10B: 103–106, 1965.

162. Strandell G: Post-traumatic rupture of the extensor pollicis longus tendon—pathogenesis and treatment. Survey based on 207 cases, including 14 personal cases. *Acta Chir Scand* 109: 81–96, 1955.

163. Stuart MJ, Beckenbaugh RD: Flexor digitorum profundus entrapment after closed treatment of a displaced Colles' fracture. *J Hand Surg* 12A: 413–415, 1987.

164. Sumner JM, Khuri SM: Entrapment of the median nerve and flexor pollicis longus tendon in an epiphyseal fracture-dislocation of the distal radioulnar joint: A case report. *J Hand Surg* 9A: 711–714, 1984.

165. Taleisnik J: Complications of fracture-dislocations and ligamentous injuries of the wrist. In: *Complications in Hand Surgery*, Boswick JA, ed. Philadelphia: WB Saunders, 1986, pp. 154–196.

166. Taylor GW: Fractures of the lower end of the radius. In: *The Management of Fractures and Dislocations*, Wilson P, ed. Philadelphia: WB Saunders, 1929, pp. 67–106.

167. Trevor D: Rupture of the extensor pollicis longus tendon after Colles' fracture. *J Bone Joint Surg [Br]* 32B: 370–375, 1950.

168. Vance RM, Gelberman RH: Acute ulnar neuropathy with fractures at the wrist. *J Bone Joint Surg* 60A: 962–965, 1978.

169. von Lesser L: Zur Behandlung fehlerhaft geheilter Brüche der karpalen Radiusepiphyse. *Zbl Chir* 14: 265, 1887.

170. Weinberg ED: Late spontaneous rupture of the extensor pollicis longus tendon following Colles' fracture. *JAMA* 142: 979–983, 1950.

171. Weiss H, Schmit-Neuerburg KP: Indikation, Technik und Ergebnisse von Sechsig Plattenosteosynthesen am distalen Radius. *Hefte Unfallheilkunde* 148: 716–720, 1980.

172. Witter H: Ruptur der Sehne des Musculus extensor pollicis longus als Komplikation der Radiusfraktur. *Beitr Klin Chir* 201: 448–452, 1960.

173. Wong FYH, Pho RWH: Median nerve compression with tendon ruptures, after Colles' fracture. *J Hand Surg* 9B: 139–141, 1984.

174. Younger CP, de Fiore JC: Rupture of the flexor tendons to the fingers after a Colles' fracture. *J Bone Joint Surg* 59A: 828–829, 1977.

175. Zachary RB: Thenar palsy due to compression of the median nerve in the carpal tunnel. *Surg Gynecol Obstetr* 81: 213–217, 1945.

176. Zemel, NP: The prevention and treatment of complication of fractures of the distal radius and ulnar. *Hand Clin* 3: 1–8, 1987.

177. Zoëga H: Fracture of the lower end of the radius with ulnar nerve palsy. *J Bone Joint Surg* 48B: 514–516, 1966.

Index

References to figures are marked with *f*; references to tables are marked with *t*.

ISBN 0-387-94239-4